CALIFORNIA STATE UNIVERSITY, SACRAMENTO

This book is due on the last date stamped below
Failure to return books on the date due will resul
of overdue fees.

Integrated Behavioral Healthcare

Positioning Mental Health Practice
with Medical/Surgical Practice

Integrated Behavioral Healthcare
Positioning Mental Health Practice
with Medical/Surgical Practice

Nicholas Cummings, Ph.D., Sc.D.,
William O'Donohue, Ph.D.
Steven C. Hayes, Ph.D.
Victoria Follette, Ph.D.
University of Nevada, Reno

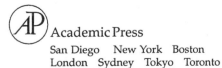
Academic Press
San Diego   New York   Boston
London   Sydney   Tokyo   Toronto

Academic Press
A Harcourt Science and Technology Company
525 B Street, Suite 1900, San Diego, California 92101-4495, USA
http://www.academicpress.com

Academic Press
Harcourt Place, 32 Jamestown Road, London NW1 7BY, UK
http://www.academicpress.com

Library of Congress Catalog Card Number: 2001088744

International Standard Book Number: 0-12-198761-2

PRINTED IN THE UNITED STATES OF AMERICA
01 02 03 04 05 06 07 SB 9 8 7 6 5 4 3 2 1

Foreword

Healthcare is now practiced in a radically different financial and delivery system than it was two decades ago. Behavioral healthcare has been trasnformed from a cottage craft into an industry. Once industrialization occurs it is never reversed. Thus, we will not go back to the solo practice funded by indemnity insurance no matter how much this is pined for by individual practitioners or their guild organizations. Organized behavioral healthcare has defined and will continue to define who is treated for what kinds of problems, how, by whom, and for what reimbursement. Moreover, the situation is still not stable: after recent mergers many of the large behavioral healthcare companies are facing serious financial difficulties.

Mental health professionals have been greatly impacted by these developments and yet there is little understanding of exactly what has happened, what has caused these events, what are the resultant strengths and weaknesses, what the behavioral healthcare professional should do in response to these, and what the future will look like. This book is edited by four mental health care professionals, including the "father" of behavioral managed care, Nicholas Cummings, and attempts to provide some answers to these key questions.

This book is an outgrowth of a conference held in Reno, Nevada in January, 1999. We would like to thanks the presenters as well as Vice President for Research Ken Hunter and Dean Robert Mead for their support of that conference. We would also like to thank Erin Northouse for her assistance in all phases of this project.

Contents

Preface

For most of the 20th Century there has been a conceptual as well as a practical division between those professionals that help people with physical/medical problems and those that help people with mental/behavioral problems. In this dualism, traceable philosophically to Descartes, individuals with clear physical problems like a broken bone go to a medical doctor such as their family practitioner or orthopedic surgeon, and individuals with depression or marital problems go to a mental health professional such as a psychologist or social worker.

This would be a felicitous state of affairs if all medical problems were solely due to physical causes and all medical problems were solely treated by physical therapies. It would also be a happy state of affairs if all mental problems were caused by nonphysiological, psychosocial causes and entirely treated by nonphysiological "talk" psychotherapy. However, this is not the case. Broken bones are caused by behavioral problems (e.g., marital abuse, alcoholism, poor diet). Medical problems are treated by behavioral changes (diet, exercise, and other lifestyle changes). And most medical treatments require and can be defeated by behavioral compliance problems with the prescribed regimen (pill taking, showing up for the scheduled procedure, etc.). Moreover, mental health problems can be caused and treated by physiological factors (neuron-chemical imbalances, endocrine problems, and psychotropic drugs). Thus, fragmenting the treatment of the mental and physical problems to two distinct realms makes little conceptual or practical sense.

This is further compounded by the fact that mental health has traditionally been surrounded by problems of stigma. A mental health diagnosis seems like the "booby prize" to many patients and thus is to be avoided. This attitude can cause avoidance and therefore poor penetration rates and continued health problems. A seamless integrated team dealing with the whole patient can avoid much of this stigma and therefore result in more appropriate and complete treatment.

The book describes the promise of integrating behavioral and medical care in the primary care setting-a move that recently has been gaining momentum. It also describes the many complex problems associated with this movement. At times there is a focus on a particular problem; at other times these problems are only briefly mentioned. Below, we will describe some of these major problems as these set an important research and practical problem solving agenda. We do this very much in the spirit of Gertrude Stein's deathbed words. When she was asked what is the answer? she responded by saying, "Damn the answer; What is the question?"

MAJOR PROBLEMS AND QUESTIONS

What kind of skill sets in what kind of team produces what kinds of effects in what kinds of patients with what kinds of problems?

How does one define the target problems-by DSM diagnosis? By treatment focus (e.g., treatment adherence, stress management), by both etc.?

What interventions produce more appropriate future medical usage? Is this more appropriate medical usage less so that the increased costs of the behavioral interventions are offset and even leveraged?

How does one obtain "buy in" for integrated care from all the relevant stakeholders?

How should the professionals be trained to work together and to have the requisite clinical and managerial skills?

What sort of clinical and operational protocols should be developed and used? To what extent, for example, are practice guidelines useful?

How is care to be coordinated? What is the role of case management and how is this do be done well?

How are stepped care models developed and to what extent are these useful?

To what extent are interventions community based v. clinic based?

To what extent is a public health/population management perspective useful?

What is the government's role? To what extent should it
provide regulation or payment?

What should the ideal health benefit look like?

What are the issues surrounding different kinds of delivery systems such as staff models, networks models,
fee for service models v. capitated models?

What do mental health parity laws mean in an integrated
care environment?

How does this system ideally interface with an Employee
Assistance Program?

What are the roles of processes such as utilization review,
pre-certification, and credentialing?

What is the role of integrated care in specialty medical
practice such as oncology?

What are the implications of integrated care for the carve
in or carve out contract?

What sort of accountability and quality assurance process should occur?

What is the role of the various guild organizations such
as the American Psychological Association or the
American Medical Association?

What are the implications for solo practice and hospitals?

How does the issue of the art v. science of practice impact
on this movement?

What sort of management information system is ideal?

What are the implications for long-term psychotherapy
and proponents of the diverse "schools" of psychotherapy?

What sort of outcome research and program evaluation
projects are priorities and how can these be done in
relatively cost-effective and unobtrusive ways?

How does one develop and implement sound financial
models for integrated care so that these systems are
seen as good business practices?

How does one appropriately screen, assess, and triage in
an integrated practice? What assessment devices
need to be developed and what are the psychometric
properties of existing strategies?

To what extent does an integrated care model improve
    penetration rates?

To what extent does it decrease stigma?

To what extent should treatment be individual therapy
    and to what extent should it be conducted in groups?

To what extent do these professionals need to have man-
    agement, business, and entrepreneurial skills?

To what extent should tele-medicine and web-based
    technologies be involved?

What are the roles of different disciplines in this effort
    (e.g., the nutritionist)?

To what extent can the cost-savings of integrated care
    reverse the very controversial problems of the cost-
    containment strategies used by some existing man-
    aged care companies in denying services?

What is the appropriate relationship between psychotro-
    pic drugs vs. psychotherapy?

To what extent can integrated care help resolve the seri-
    ous and perineal issue of treatment compliance?

How can psychotherapy be adapted to the 'world of
    primary care' in which interventions are generally
    much more brief, focused, and "on the fly"?

What will be the attitude of employers-one of the largest
    payers for medical services-regarding integrated care?
    Can one show higher employee functioning and
    lower absenteeism, for example?

How should special populations defined in various ways
    (e.g., geriatrics or African-Americans) be addressed?

How can integrate care teams more effectively rule out
    psychological problems so that actual medical prob-
    lems can be more effectively identified and treated?

What are the best marketing strategies for this type of
    delivery system?

How is this approach to resolve issues of research dis-
    semination and knowledge utilization?

Is health care, including integrated care, a commodity or
    are there substantive and particularly quality dis-
    tinctions?

What is the role of outside accrediting agencies such as
    NCQA?

What is the relevant actuarial knowledge that needs to be obtained, and how is this best gathered?

What is the role of bench marking and report cards?

How are "housekeeping tasks" such as claims processing best accomplished?

What are the best grievance procedures?

How does one decrease unwanted treatment variability?

How are providers justly compensated and how are they properly incentived? What are the advantages of equity models? How is the problem of decreased provider income to be addressed?

What is the role of the masters-level psychotherapist v. doctoral level professional?

What changes in the formal training of professionals are called for?

How does one monitor adherence and competence to protocols? What are the best supervision, case conferencing, and continuing education programs?

Should there be specialty certification or degrees relevant to integrated care?

What is the role of alternative medicine in integrated care?

What are the role of prevention and wellness programs and other programs targeting generally lifestyle issues?

How does one structure the physical setting so co-location is optimized?

How does one handle the handoff or the consult between a PCP and a behavioral health specialist?

How does one handle emergencies?

How is record keeping handled?

What is the role of natural helpers in the patient's environment such as ministers and friends?

How does one educate and manage office staff?

How does one enhance provider satisfaction?

How is the problem of relapse addressed?

How does one handle patient choice and patient rights?

What disease management programs are critical and what are the specifics of these?

These are some of the major conceptual and practical problems surrounding health care in general but also involved in integrated care. These are often both fascinating intellectually and nettlesome practically. However, these must be addressed in order to painfully produce more optimal healthcare. We think the chapters in this book represent steps in this direction.

Finally, we note that this structure of this book is a bit unusual. We have main chapters followed by commentaries. These commentaries are meant to address some of the most important issues in the chapters as well as to reflect on some of the more controversial issues contained in the chapters. We hope that this format allows the reader to see the important dialogue around all these important issues.

1

CHAPTER

A History of Behavioral Healthcare: A Perspective From a Lifetime of Involvement

Nicholas A. Cummings, Ph.D., Sc.D.
University of Nevada, Reno,
and
The Nicholas and Dorothy Cummings Foundation

The History of Capitation
American Healthcare in the 1930's
The Birth of the Blues
The Federal HMO Enabling Act
The Jackson Hole Group
Behavioral Healthcare
Diagnosis Related Groups (DRGs)
The Birth of the Carve-out
The Biodyne Model
A Vision Rejected
Consolidation, Competition, and Chaos
What Went Right and What Went Wrong?
The Future of Managed Behavioral Healthcare
References

1

Integrated Behavioral Healthcare: Positioning Mental Health Practice with Medical/Surgical Practice

The history of managed healthcare, and particularly managed behavioral care, has never been succinctly delineated, leaving professional psychologists entering the field without clear knowledge of how healthcare evolved from a cottage industry into complete industrialization in a matter of a few decades. This account is from the first-hand experience of the author, whose more than half a century as a psychologist was lived as a key player in the events described.

THE HISTORY OF CAPITATION

A method of prospective reimbursement which is based on a set amount of payment per member (i.e., enrollee) per month (known in the industry as *pmpm*) is not new. A woman physician whose name is lost in history, and is the only event this author is recounting that precedes his birth, formed a one-physician delivery system in a rural area of Oklahoma circa 1920. Her practice flourished in spite of more often being paid in farm produce rather than cash, and the farming families benefited by having a doctor when this was a rarity in the rural communities of the era. Capitation did not appear again in any significant form until the 1930s when the Ross-Loos Group was formed in Los Angeles, and "Dr. Callan and Staff" offered a prepaid plan in the San Francisco Bay Area. Both of these plans solicited subscribers from the general public, as employer sponsored health insurance offered as a fringe benefit was still almost a decade away. This fact, coupled with the propensity of medical care in the 1930s which made access easy, rendered prepaid healthcare not very compelling, or even financially attractive. The latter will be discussed below, but suffice it to say that the Callan plan suffered an early demise, while the better financed and aggressively marketed Ross-Loos Group survives to this day.

Even the successful Ross-Loos program remained small during the 1930s, but capitation was finally launched on a large scale on the Mojave Desert of California. A man who was to become one of America's most celebrated industrialists, Henry J. Kaiser, bid on the construction of the aqueduct carrying the Hoover Dam (then still Boulder Dam) water to Los Angeles. Not only was his bid surprisingly lower than the next lowest, he completed the project for significantly less money than his own anticipated cost. Few realize, however, that his endeavor would have failed without the participation of a young physician from Los Angeles who had tried private practice and did not like it. Even though it was during the Great Depression with high unemployment, construction workers were reluctant to bring their families to the desert where they were isolated from any medical care whatsoever for many hours across dirt roads. Kaiser was about to fail because he could not hire workers when Dr. Sidney Garfield approached him with an offer he could not refuse. For five cents, a worker hour Garfield would build and staff the outpatient and inpatient facilities that would guarantee treatment for both his employees and their families.

That day in the early 1930s capitated healthcare, embodying both the management of care and the acceptance of risk, was born in a big way and for all time. While the facilities were being built Garfield launched a prevention program, spending a significant part of the capitation dollars to educate the workers and their families on the avoidance of the hazards of the desert: rattlesnake and tarantula spider bites, scorpion stings, heat stroke and heat exhaustion. He strongly believed this would pay off in reduced treatment costs in the future. He was right, of course, but by implementing this aspect he defined the concept that capitation, which allows the spending of the money as the providers see fit, includes prevention. It was not long before his ideas expanded to include wellness, an integral part of the most successful capitated programs today.

After the aqueduct was completed, Kaiser transported what was still called Sidney Garfield and Associates to Northern California to provide capitated healthcare to his huge new shipyard operations. World War II had been raging in Europe since 1939, and by 1941 when the United States was thrown into the conflict following the attack on Pearl Harbor, Hitler had conquered most of Europe. Great Britain was vulnerable as only isolated islands dependent on the outside for supplies would be. Kaiser's California shipyards (Vallejo and Richmond) startled the world by building "victory ships" in five days from keel to launch. These ships, which Kaiser built faster than the German U-boats could sink, transported all of the supplies, food and munitions, that saved England. Again, Kaiser could not have done this without Dr. Garfield who provided all of the medical care that enticed millions of workers to migrate from Arkansas, Oklahoma, Texas, and other parts of the South and Midwest to California to fill the important jobs in the shipyards. The genius of Henry Kaiser trained farmers to be ship fitters; Sidney Garfield took care of their health through capitated medicine.

Following the end of World War II, Kaiser invited Garfield to offer capitated healthcare to the general public, and in 1946, the Kaiser Permanente Health System was founded. Kaiser borrowed the name from the Permanente Cement Company, a small bankrupt plant in Fontana that he had acquired. Not only did this astute purchase have the nostalgia that it helped him succeed with the aqueduct, he liked the sound of the Spanish word for permanence. With its beginnings in Oakland across the Bay from San Francisco, the Kaiser Permanente Health System grew rapidly and, as we shall see below, became the national model for what was later known as the Health Maintenance Organization (HMO). It was two decades, however, before the success of the Kaiser Permanente model spurred the government and the private healthcare system to adopt capitation as a significant payment vehicle on a national scale.

AMERICAN HEALTHCARE IN THE 1930s:
A REMARKABLE ROBIN HOOD MODEL

Let us return to the 1930s, known as the Great Depression, characterized by hunger, high unemployment, and economic stagnation. Surprisingly, medical care was readily accessible, a seeming contradiction that forestalled the development of prepaid health plans. How was this possible?

During the 1920s, medicine finally cleaned up its act and became a profession to be emulated. Medical practices acts were adopted in all states, medical schools were graded A and B with the eventual shutting down of all B grade schools, and medical apprenticeships, which were the principle way in which one learned to be a doctor in the 1910s and 1920s, were eliminated. It was only a matter of time before those who had been "grand-fathered" into the new state licensing laws would retire or pass on. In 1954, I met the last practicing "physician" in the State of Illinois who had been grandfathered because, as a veterinarian before medical licensure, he had occasionally treated the farm family members along with their livestock. For those involved in healthcare today, it is startling to learn medicine only relatively recently became a true profession.

The new breed of physician was altruistic, dedicated, and proud of the calling. The Hippocratic oath was taken seriously, and in spite of a shortage, physicians saw everyone who wanted to see them, even if this meant a 16-hour workday. A request for a house call was never denied. It was further unthinkable to press a bill for payment, and no physician would ever consider using a collection agency. Patients were seen and house calls were made even when a patient had not paid the accumulated bill for three or four years. Physicians knew people were strapped financially, and they saw themselves truly as caregivers without regard to compensation. The physician of the time was over-worked and never wealthy. They looked old by age fifty, and usually died from over-work by their late fifties. It was not unusual for a patient whose economic status improved with the passing of the Great Depression to send the doctor payment many years later. More likely, it went to the surviving spouse.

What of the patient who was financially well fixed? The answer was simple: the physician doubled or even quadrupled the bill, depending on the patient's status. My father, who was well off but not wealthy, told me about this, and explained it was up to him and others like him to pay for those who could not. Greed on both sides was remarkably absent.

Consider this remarkable availability, regardless of ability to pay, whereas prepaid health insurance would cost the kind of money that families during the Great Depression simply did not have. The system was not perfect, especially in rural areas that required considerable travel to the nearest physician. Furthermore, some persons were too ashamed to see the physician if they owed money, and the physicians tended to burnout from over-work at a relatively early age. However, it was a non-system in which the doctor-patient relationship was decidedly one of mutual respect. This author was immersed in this tradition. I was in the independent practice of psychology in San Francisco for 44 years and never sent a bill beyond the third mailing. Non-payment indicated to me that either the patient was unable to pay, or unwilling because I had not helped him or her. If it were the latter, I felt I did not deserve payment. Whatever the reason, I respected the patient's right to make the decision. The thought of a collection agency is still anathema to me. In today's competitive reimbursement climate, all of this seems quaint.

When did this remarkable, easily accessed system go awry? It was in the mid-1960s when Titles 18 and 19 of the Social Security Act and known as Medicare and Medicaid, were enacted into law. This put the government bureaucrat in every physician's office, burying the practitioner in a mountain of paperwork. Physicians rebelled, and they tried to compensate for the time lost in red tape by over-billing the government. The bureaucratic response was increased surveillance through more paperwork. The cat and mouse game between providers and third party payers began, and would increase exponentially. Physicians were typically disgruntled, an emotion which seemed to justify previously unthinkable behavior. Cynicism crept in and soon was rampant; it was okay to manipulate the payer, as long as it was not done to the patient. The triangulation among doctor, patient, and third party payer seemed to put a new distance between the physician and the Hippocratic Oath. Lamentably, greed was back into healthcare.

THE BIRTH OF THE BLUES

For decades prior to Medicare and Medicaid, no one thought of a hospital as making a profit or even breaking even. Most were non-profit and owned by religious and other charitable organizations, or were community sponsored.

At least twice a year each hospital held a fundraising drive to make up the financial shortfall. No one who needed hospitalization was turned away, regardless of ability to pay. The now ever-present insurance card demanded at the reception desk of every hospital was non-existent.

To create a much needed revenue stream the hospitals organized into an organization named Blue Cross. For those who could afford the monthly premium, small by today's standards, any needed hospitalization was prepaid. Care became inpatient-based, as the entire plan was hospital-oriented. A common joke of the era was that if you needed to have a hangnail removed, you would have to first be admitted to the hospital.

In defense, the physicians organized into a parallel organization named Blue Shield, which prepaid physicians' services and was, in contrast to Blue Cross, essentially outpatient care. The Blues plans were locally based, and the more populous states might have several Blues plans. For example, until the current era Ohio had eight. As they were autonomous and potentially competitive among themselves, they belonged to a loosely organized national organization based in Chicago, the National Association of Blue Cross and Blue Shield Plans, which managed to keep jurisdictional and other disputes to a minimum. In my experience, however, most of the decisions were made on the golf course by the presidents of these companies at the semi-annual resort-area meetings of the Blues plans.

There was such a perceived need for prepaid health during the Great Depression that the states cooperated in exempting the Blues from requirements imposed on the insurance industry. Special laws were enacted creating *medical services corporations*, applying only to Blues type plans, and making it possible for them to get by with a much lesser dollar reserve than was required of full-fledge insurance companies. They were also shielded from laws prohibiting the corporate practice of medicine, which restricted physicians from forming partnerships with anyone but other physicians. These laws were originally enacted to prevent the exploitation of medicine by non-medical interests, but later were used to discourage progress into medical-business alliances.

In recent years, Blue Cross and Blue Shield have tended to merge, but with glaring exceptions as notably found in California. Furthermore, financially troubled Blues plans in such states as West Virginia and Nevada have been bought out by other Blues plans, and Blues plans have been known to encroach on each other's territory. Formed as the bastions of fee-for-service healthcare, many have launched HMOs with frequently disastrous results.

THE FEDERAL HMO ENABLING ACT

The stellar success of the Kaiser Permanente Health System prompted the federal government to conceptualize the HMO as the solution to the spiraling health costs that followed the enactment of Medicare in Medicaid. Kaiser Permanente had grown to eight million covered lives on the West Coast and had pioneered such innovations as health education and wellness programs, and as early as 1963 had developed a large-scale automatic multiphasic health screening with 29 laboratory and other tests, including an electronic mental health/substance abuse screening. The patient went through the procedure in less than an hour, at the end of which she or he saw a physician who already had the multiphasic results in hand. This was remarkable in the era far preceding the current electronic data systems and the PC, and earned for Morris F. Collen, M.D., the co-founder with Garfield of the post-war Kaiser Permanente System, and Lester Breslow, M.D., his consultant, the appellation "fathers of computerized medicine." This kind of progress was noted by the health planners in government - who were grappling with how to bring down health costs - and in 1975, Congress passed the HMO Enabling Act, which gave start-up money to encourage the formation of new HMOs.

It was during this era that the name HMO was coined. Sidney Garfield, who referred to most health insurance plans as "sickness" plans because the provider made money only when the patient was sick, delivered his now famous speech, "An Organization to Maintain Health." He pointed out that health plans should be rewarded not just for treating the sick, but also for keeping people healthy. Capitation was the vehicle for this, because indemnity (fee-for-service) insurance did not pay for prevention. Paul Ellwood, M.D. picked up on Garfield's description of the prevention-oriented capitated entity and called it a Health Maintenance Organization, or HMO. This term was immediately seized upon by the federal government, which incorporated the name in the new legislation. Dan Patterson, a physician, was appointed to head the first "HMO shop" in Washington, and this author was privileged to be a consultant. In this capacity, he made sure that the regulations allowed for a single-purpose HMO, having anticipated the advent of the managed behavioral healthcare organization (MBHO).

Before the federal government espoused the HMO concept, the road had been rocky for Kaiser Permanente, which would not have survived without the militant support of the labor unions in California. The American Medical Association regarded this new system as "socialized medicine," and the Permanente physicians were barred from membership in the county medical societies. Harry Bridges, the head of the International Longshoremen's and Warehousemen's Union, who had the power to shut down shipping on both coasts in five minutes, was on the board and threw his enormous weight toward what he perceived to be a consumer-oriented system. During the time I knew and worked with Harry Bridges the government several times attempted to deport him to his native Australia for allegedly having lied on his naturalization application for U.S. citizenship. This bombastic man was acquitted on all counts, and in spite of his legal problems, he always found time to be a staunch supporter of this unique health system. He once told me that I need not worry about longshoremen missing behavioral health appointments, saying, "Any member of our union who misses a medical appointment is fined two days pay."

To capture the flavor of those difficult times it would help to recall the story of how Permanente physicians were finally admitted to membership in the county medical societies. During that era a physician who was not a member of these AMA affiliates would find it almost impossible to practice. Essentials ranging from the availability of malpractice insurance to community acceptance were all dependent upon being a member in good standing of the county medical society. Henry J. Kaiser and Garfield were traveling to Chicago by train, which was the customary mode in the mid-1950s. It was then that Kaiser first learned of the discrimination against Garfield's medical staff. In addition, when he further learned that the person to see was Morris Fishbein, the seemingly perpetual medical director of the AMA, he immediately asked to see him. Dr. Fishbein, not knowing there was a difficulty, was delighted to usher the celebrated industrialist into his offices. He reportedly was stunned when Kaiser announced that he was giving him sixty days to make eligible for membership the Permanente physicians, or face a lawsuit in federal court. However, it was done, and the Permanente physicians, once outcasts, became important by their large numbers in the county medical societies. At that time in the San Francisco Bay Area alone, there were over 2,000 Kaiser Permanente doctors.

By the time the HMO Enabling Act became law, Henry J. Kaiser had died. His son, Edgar Kaiser, decided we should give away the HMO technology. Many of us were assigned fledgling HMOs to mentor. In spite of this, seven of every eight new HMOs failed financially once the federal start up money was gone. I was fortunate to work with the Group Health Cooperative of Puget Sound (Seattle) and the Harvard Community Health Plan (Boston), both winners that survive to this day. Interestingly, the Group Health Cooperative of Puget Sound in 1998 merged with the Kaiser Plan.

By the 1980s, there were scores of HMOs throughout the United States, but the concept continued to be most successful in California and Minnesota. The market-penetration was sufficient in those states so the population was accepting of the *staff model*, a format that maximizes both clinical and financial efficiency. In most other states, patients who were expected to receive care in a staff model complained they were being managed. Being seen in the practitioner's office, as is the usual procedure in a network model, gave the illusion the patient was in "private care," resulting in greater acceptance. Capitated HMOs patterned after the network model could never keep up with Kaiser Permanente, which had the added advantage of *physician equity*. This was a model created by Garfield that made the doctors practitioner-owners. The founder of the system liked to say, "Doctors work hardest when they're working for themselves."

UNIVERSAL HEALTHCARE

The several years preceding the HMO Enabling Act saw a strong move in the Congress for government-sponsored universal healthcare. It was headed by Senator Edward (Ted) Kennedy, who was at that time chairing the Subcommittee on Health of the U.S. Senate Finance Committee. I testified before that Committee, and was invited subsequently by Senator Kennedy to act as a consultant. Convinced that universal healthcare was close to becoming a reality, I agreed to serve. It was during that time that the pendulum swung toward initiatives in the private sector, and Senator Kennedy lost the chair of the Subcommittee on Health to Senator Herman Talmadge. This was the decision of Senator Russell Long who chaired the over-arching U.S. Senate Finance Committee. It is worthy to note, because of the current era in which Republicans are viewed as the opposition party to expanding government-sponsored healthcare, that all the players at the time who "swung over" were Democrats.

Much of the conceptualization that interrupted the drive toward federally sponsored universal healthcare came from a group of influential health economists who were meeting regularly to address the spiraling costs which were created by the government getting into healthcare.

THE JACKSON HOLE GROUP

Other than the fact that the Federal Reserve Board likes to have retreat meetings in Jackson Hole, Wyoming, it is a beautiful spot that was adopted as a meeting place by a group of self-appointed health economists. It was led by Paul Ellwood, M.D. of Minnesota and included such diverse persons as Alain Enthoven (Stanford), Stuart Altman (Brandeis), Eli Ginsburg (Columbia), and

Uwe Rinehart (Princeton). Enthoven had been a consultant to the Kaiser Permanente System for many years, and much later, I was privileged to have him on the American Biodyne Board of Directors.

These health economists took note that the government had caused this inflation by fueling a non-competitive health economy, first by the Hill-Burton Act in 1959 which fostered what turned out to be the over-building of hospitals, and shortly thereafter by Medicare and Medicaid. They conceived of a system they termed *managed competition*, which was incorporated into the HMO Enabling Act, and in 1993 became the centerpiece of the Rodham-Clinton task force on healthcare. Several members of the Jackson Hole Group dissociated themselves from this task force when they no longer could recognize their original concept of managed competition. Under the Clinton Administration, it had become engulfed in proposals that would have plunged healthcare further into government control and regulatory red tape. As we all know, the Rodham-Clinton proposals met overwhelming opposition, and suffered their immediate defeat through the task force's self-created Achilles heal: it had violated all the sunshine laws by meeting in secrecy and had even failed to publish its list of members, reputed to number over 500. When the courts finally forced the disclosure, it was found that the overwhelming majority of task force members were not the nation's experts as had been trumpeted, but government employees instead.

Much of the thinking of the Jackson Hole Group found implementation in managed healthcare, with one of the problems, as we shall see below, becoming run-away or uncontrolled competition, resulting in the sacrifice of quality.

BEHAVIORAL HEALTHCARE

In the 1950s no health plan paid for psychotherapy. The thinking of the era was that psychotherapy was not subject to actuarial cost controls, as it was couched in psycho-babble and dispensed by long-term therapists who were unaccountable and staunchly believed that more is better. During that era when an actuary was asked how long psychotherapy should be, the response invariably was another question, "How long is a piece of string?" Psychotherapy was usually a named exclusion from the list of benefits in prepaid healthcare.

I was privileged to write the first comprehensive prepaid psychotherapy benefit at Kaiser Permanente as an experiment in the late 1950s. This was preceded by the discovery there that a startling 60% of patient visits to a physician were by persons somatizing stress, or whose physical condition was significantly exacerbated by emotional factors. Garfield and Collen were convinced of the importance of behavioral interventions, and made possible the experiment. Several years later, in following up on whether our interventions had made a difference, we were surprised to find that our brief therapy had yielded a 65% reduction in medical utilization, without a relapse into somatization. This *medical cost offset* became the principle reason why health plans began including psychotherapy as a benefit, and has been extensively chronicled elsewhere (Cummings, 1997). Those of us conducting the seminal research warned that medical cost offset could not be parachuted into a traditional system with positive results. This was borne out in our Hawaii Medicaid Project in the early 1980s, which became the proving ground for managed behavioral healthcare in that same decade. We also continued to experiment with the effectiveness of briefer models of psychotherapy, making the results the basis of managed behavioral healthcare. Our model we eventually named *brief, intermittent psychotherapy throughout the life cycle*. This extrapolated into behavioral care what we see in all other forms of healthcare: the patient sees the practitioner as needed during stressors in one's life cycle. Heretofore, the dominant mental health model was one in which the patient was seen continuously and indefinitely, ostensibly to prevent any further emotional conflict for all time. In our own managed care research, as well as the work of others, this hypothetical state was not only impractical, but unattainable nonsense.

DIAGNOSIS RELATED GROUPS (DRGs)

In the early 1980s the Congress of the United States inadvertently ushered in managed healthcare, and subsequently catapulted behavioral healthcare into managed care, none of which was its stated intent. Grappling unsuccessfully for months with run-away hospital costs in Medicare and Medicaid, literally at midnight of the last day of the budget process, it passed legislation that created Diagnosis Related Groups (DRGs). Under this system, almost 400 medical diagnoses were assigned maximum days of hospitalization for each. If the hospital exceeded the number of days for that particular condition, it lost money. On the other hand, if the hospital came under the requisite days, it made a profit. Almost immediately, medical/surgical beds were emptied. Hospitals, previously comfortable at a reimbursement rate of cost plus 15%, began going bankrupt. There was a national glut of hospital beds, with many hospitals showing less than 50% occupancy. Proprietary companies began buying the hospitals by the hundreds, applied sound business principles, and thrived on what later was called managed care. In other words, the care of each DRG was managed to fall within the prescribed number of days.

Cummings (1986) called this the beginnings of the industrialization of healthcare, and foresaw the impending industrialization of behavioral healthcare. This was to come about because no one in Washington could figure out how to do DRGs for mental health and substance abuse. Alert hospital administrators took advantage of this and converted these empty beds to psychiatry, substance abuse, and especially adolescent psychiatry. These new programs were huckstered on TV, and since insurance was paying, they were an immediate financial success. Families and employers could get rid of the alcoholic in their midst for 28 days or more, and parents could take a 60 to 90 day vacation from difficult or rebellious adolescent children. Where DRGs reduced the inflationary spiral in medicine and surgery from 12% annually to 8%, behavioral healthcare rocketed from 2% to 16% in two years. Now psychiatry was driving the inflationary rate for all healthcare for the first time in history.

The federal government, desperate for a solution, turned to the private sector and encouraged the participation of a new, emerging for-profit behavioral healthcare industry by tacitly ignoring the outmoded laws prohibiting the corporate practice of medicine. What soon was to be known as the behavioral managed care industry, or "carve-out," was born. These early and subsequent events have been extensively chronicled (Cummings, 2000).

THE BIRTH OF THE CARVE-OUT

By the early 1980s there were several companies that contracted with health plans to manage behavioral healthcare. Health plans, confronted with run-away costs in mental health and chemical dependency, were essentially left two choices: sign up with a company that guaranteed to bring down costs through utilization review, provider profiling, and pre-certification for hospitalization, or drop the behavioral care entirely. The trend, unfortunately, was toward the latter, and if it continued unabated, the hard-fought behavioral care benefit might well vanish. The health plans that were willing to experiment with early-managed behavioral care as just described spawned successful companies. Kenneth Kessler founded American PsychManagement, while Alex Rodriguez headed Preferred Health and Bud Larson founded the Metropolitan Clinics of Counseling (MCC). The first two leaders were psychiatrists, while Larson was a social worker. Suddenly a number of successful Employee Assistance Programs (EAPs), notably U.S. Behavioral Health (Saul

Feldman) and Human Affairs International, (Otto Jones), decided to convert their companies.

THE BIODYNE MODEL

During this time I was conducting the Hawaii Project, research sponsored by the Health Care Financing Administration (HCFA, the watch-dog of Medicare and Medicaid). We created a brand new staff model behavioral care system to serve the experimental group in Honolulu with 36,000 Medicaid recipients and 90,000 federal employees, one-third of which were randomly assigned to the existing system which served as the control group. Hawaii was chosen because it had the most liberal Medicaid psychotherapy benefit: 52 sessions per year renewable every year, with any licensed practitioner of the patient's choice. Thus, there was an experimental comparison between the effectiveness of the private practitioner in fee-for-service and a system of prospective reimbursement. The results were decidedly in favor of managed care over the traditional laissez-faire model.

Our program in Hawaii was so successful that we converted with government approval the non-profit Biodyne Institute into the first propri-etary managed behavioral care *delivery* system. Called American Biodyne, it was a clinically driven staff model in which each center of six professionals (plus support staff) were responsible for the mental health and substance abuse treatment, both outpatient and hospitalization, of 30,000 covered lives. If we should obtain 10,000 more enrollees in that locale, rather than adding these to the 30,000 and creating a larger center, we would split the population into two centers serving 20,000 lives each. The determination to keep each center the optimal, manageable size reflected our dedication to the clinical model, which in this case is antithetical to the business model that cannot tolerate redundancy even when it is clinically preferable.

American Biodyne developed 68 research-based psychotherapy proto-cols that were surprisingly effective and efficient. It reduced psychiatric hospitalization by 95% through the training and empowerment of psycholo-gists who were compelled to examine each patient presenting for hospitaliza-tion before admission, all night long. The approach was simple: outpatient treatment began in the emergency room in the middle of the night. If the patient responded, inpatient treatment was unnecessary and the patient was seen in immediate, daily (and often twice-daily) intensive psychotherapy. American Biodyne grew from zero to 14.5 million enrollees in a few years, far surpassing its competitors, even those that preceded it. Soon the Biodyne Model became the one to emulate. Eventually we had to modify our delivery system in response to the marketplace that preferred a network. We created the first *staff-network model*, a remarkably functional system that maintained the best of both approaches, but preserved the pre-eminence of the staff to manage and motivate the network. But the real advantage of American Biodyne was our insistence that 15% of all clinicians' time is devoted to quality assurance through clinical case conferencing, supervision, and research. This is an ideal that never existed before or after. But it worked. In the seven years I served as CEO of American Biodyne we never had a single malpractice suit. Contrast that record with an industry that today is surfeited with such lawsuits.

American Biodyne was confronted with a choice: either train businesspersons to think like clinicians (impossible), or train clinicians to also be proficient in business (improbable). We chose the latter, and all of our line managers were clinicians. In this way, clinical integrity was maintained because in a tough situation the final decision fell on the clinical, not the business side. We found creative ways to give business and financial training to our clinician-managers who, no matter how high their rank, had to spend no less than two-days per week in hands-on clinical work. This also included me as the CEO. I strongly believed that if I ever lost contact with the work in the trenches I would be ineffective as the company's leader. We further developed a post-doctoral masters degree in managed behavioral healthcare administration (MBHA, rather than MBA). This was conceived as a more effective way of training our psychologists in business. We offered to fund the program and to guarantee the student body, but no likely university we approached would face the opposition from its own anti-managed care psychology department.

American Biodyne grew rapidly because it was economically viable. I was able to say to a health plan that we could expand the benefit while reducing the cost to 80%, and that we could cap those costs for three years. All the while, we would take the risk. The response was immediate, and our greatest problem was limiting growth to 200% per year. To exceed that growth rate would jeopardize quality.

A VISION REJECTED

In founding American Biodyne it was my intent to give away the technology to the profession of psychology. I used the occasion of my acceptance address in 1985 for an APA award to announce a model that could be psychology's response to the imminent industrialization of behavioral healthcare. In 1986 the *American Psychologist* published an essentially do-it-yourself kit (Cummings, 1986) in which I indicated American Biodyne would be held to half a million enrollees and serve as a model which could be visited by psychologists who would learn how to go out and found a similar company. I stated there was easily room for 50 such half-million enrollee companies, all owned and run by psychologists. In this way, clinicians would own managed behavioral care, not Wall Street. For two years, I kept the company at the promised limit, watching as psychology ignored it while business interests were copying it. I then took my foot off the brake, and the subsequent explosive growth demonstrated that the Biodyne Model was the right concept at the right time.

The APA's response was disappointing, and eventually tragic. For several years, the leadership declared managed care was a passing fad. When it became apparent it was here to stay, the APA essentially declared war, refused opportunities for constructive engagement, and rendered itself essentially irrelevant to the decision-making process in American healthcare. Disappointed, I sold American Biodyne to McdCo/Merck, which spun it off as Merit, which eventually became part of Magellan. My worst fears were realized. Managed care became business-driven. Clinicians had thrown away an opportunity.

CONSOLIDATION, COMPETITION, AND CHAOS

As is the case in any industrialization, managed behavioral care has gone through a period of consolidation. It was inevitable that healthcare would succumb to the merger-mania that swept American business on its way to becoming global, but healthcare is not comparable to banking and electronics because in contrast it deals with life and death issues among our patients. Soon over 100 companies merged to the point where one company now owns 40% of the market, and nearly two-thirds is own by three companies. Clinical integrity was trampled as business considerations became paramount.

As would expected in any early industrialization with tremendous growth, the market became saturated and competition went out of control. "Bottom-feeding," or bidding on a project that is at the outset below the financial level that could support quality, and "low-balling," purposely bidding below cost with no intention of providing the contracted services, have become common. The hope is that capturing inordinate market share by any means, no matter how dubious, will result in an advantage over competitors, resulting in market primacy.

All of this has led to the chaos expected in any industrialization, and the three Cs of consolidation, competition, and chaos were included among our initial predictions.

WHAT WENT RIGHT AND WHAT WENT WRONG?

The outstanding accomplishment of managed behavioral care, and one that is seldom acknowledged by disgruntled practitioners, is that it saved the mental health benefit. In their complaint that their practices have been curtailed they fail to note they would have no practices at all had the trend of eliminating psychotherapy from insurance continued.

Managed behavioral health reduced drastically the shameful psychiatric over-hospitalization for profit that had become a national disgrace. It expanded outpatient care, and dramatically increased the continuum of care so that care became more appropriate. This included partial hospitalization, psychiatric rehabilitation, day treatment programs, consumer-run peer support, residential treatment, and crisis programs. This was at the expense of the psychiatric hospitals and the privately practicing psychotherapists who previously accounted for most of the behavioral healthcare dollar.

For the first time in history, accountability was introduced into behavioral health. Managed care has ushered in an era of data-based treatment, and has set the stage for the emergence of treatment guidelines and eventually standardized treatment protocols.

What went wrong, of course, is that the carve-out industry lost its clinical focus and began to manage costs, not care. Once practitioners forfeited their initial leadership, it was inevitable that business interests would take over. As the schism between managed behavioral care and the practitioners grew, the industry found itself at war with its own labor force. This, again, seems inevitable in the process of industrialization. By looking at the militancy of the labor movement during the industrialization of manufacturing at the beginning of the 21st Century, as well as the industrialization of the service sector in the middle of the century, the current antagonism between the healthcare industry and its providers is understandable. It is unfortunate that each wave of industrialization must repeat the mistakes of its predecessors, but few persons involved in healthcare today possess sufficient knowledge of economics to benefit from such a perspective.

Both the industry and its providers have been shortsighted, but the real culprits in the current chaos are the purchasers. Employers, who were being rendered non-competitive globally because healthcare inflation was pricing American goods and services out of the world market, are ecstatic. They and the federal government are delighted that managed care companies are taking the brunt of patient anger while no one is pointing the finger at them. Yet it is the big purchasers of healthcare, of which the federal government is the largest in the world that created a disastrous pricing-pressure. They have ratcheted down capitation rates to the point care is compromised. The fat in the system disappeared long ago, the muscle has been cut away, and the cost-cutting knife is well into the bone. Members of Congress smile agreeably as practitioners demand healthcare reform; smug in the fact the industry has gotten the blame while they have balanced the budgets of Medicare and Medicaid on the backs of the providers and their patients.

THE FUTURE OF MANAGED BEHAVIORAL HEALTHCARE

The purchasers have achieved their goal: the healthcare inflationary spiral has been held to 4% for the past several years. Costs are poised to increase again, but this time the purchasers have enough data to demand value (quality plus cost). Accountability is forever part of the system, and no one will be able to hide behind psychobabble or false concern with confidentiality, both intended to avoid scrutiny.

There will be increased micro-management of the industry by government, and this will add to costs. No industry can grow from almost nothing to 75% of the insured market in one decade without incurring regulation. The amount of regulation will be determined by how successful the industry is in regulating itself. Providers will continue to confuse patient concerns with practitioner concerns in an effort to regain control, but once industrialization has occurred, it continues to evolve; it never goes back to the previous cottage industry. In fact, the more managed care cleans up its act, the more acceptable it will be to the consumer.

It is time for the carve-out to carve-in. Behavioral care must be an integrated part of primary care. In accepting the formula for the establishment of the carve-out, the industry has ignored the admonition that this was intended for an interim of about ten years; i.e., the time needed to save the mental health and substance abuse treatment benefit from extinction. Once accomplished, it would be time for behavioral health to become indistinguishable with primary care, rendering moot for all time the question of parity between physical and mental health. However, the carve-out industry, now boasting 175 million covered lives, is loath to change. The fact that integration is best for patient care is a weak argument. In all of history, no entrenched group has stepped aside merely because it was asked to do so. It remains for someone to configure the economic viability of integration, thus making it attractive and possible. There is no longer fat in the carve-out system, but the waste in physical health because of stress and emotional problems is enormous. A 10% reduction in medical/surgical costs resulting from integrated behavioral care interventions would exceed today's entire mental health budget (Cummings, 2000).

REFERENCES

Cummings, N. A. (1986). The dismantling of our health system: Strategies for the survival of psychological practice. *American Psychologist, 41*, 426-431.

Cummings, N. A. (1997). Behavioral health in primary care: Dollars and Sense. In N. A. Cummings, J. L. Cummings, & J.N. Johnson, (Eds.), *Behavioral health in primary care: A Guide for clinical integration.* Madison, CT: Psychosocial Press.

Cummings, N. A. (1999). Managing a managed care organization. In W. O'Donohue, & J. E. Fisher, (Eds.), *Management and administrative skills for the mental health professional.* New York, NY: Academic Press.

Cummings, N. A. (2000). A psychologist's proactive guide to mental health care: New roles and opportunities. In A. Kent & M. Hersen (Eds.), *A psychologist's guide to managed mental health care.* Mahwah, NJ: Lawrence Erlbaum.

A New Vision of Healthcare for America

Nicholas A. Cummings, Ph.D., Sc.D.
University of Nevada, Reno,
and
The Nicholas and Dorothy Cummings Foundation

Integrated Behavioral Healthcare: Positioning Mental Health Practice with Medical/Surgical Practice

Once again behavioral healthcare is about to experience dramatic changes that will rival those of the mid-1980s. The behavioral health professions failed then to recognize the impending industrialization of healthcare and thus found themselves left out of the subsequent decision making process. Although the next leap forward will be evolutionary rather then revolutionary as was the period we are experiencing, the mental health professions will have the first real opportunity in several years to participate in the future of behavioral healthcare. In the previous decade the professional guilds ignored the trend toward industrialization, and remained oblivious to the disturbing fact the insurors were rapidly dropping mental health as a benefit. Within a short time the hard-fought psychotherapy benefits of health insurance would have disappeared were it not for the early managed behavioral care companies (American Biodyne, American Psych Management, MCC, and Preferred Health) had not demonstrated to the industry they could roll back costs and cap them for three years, all the while expanding the mental health benefit. The immediate losers were the psychiatric hospitals and the solo practitioners of long-term psychotherapy, for it was by reducing these overly utilized services that stability was quickly acquired. The beneficiaries were those who pay the costs and the patients who now had a new continuum of care. Managed behavioral care has resulted in an expansion of services as well as a substitution of services, with increases in psychiatric rehabilitation, day treatment, consumer-run peer support, residential treatment and crisis programs in lieu of psychiatric hospitalization and private practice psychotherapy, both of which declined and have never recovered (Cummings, 1999; Ross, 1998).

FINALLY THE TREND IS OUR FRIEND

The previous decade may well be known as the point in history which demonstrated that the introduction of business principles into the heretofore undisciplined healthcare system could not only tether costs, but expand the range of services available to the patient. Especially was this true in behavioral care where previously those who pay the bills were intimidated by a psycho-babble given credibility only because of the general lack of data. It also demonstrated that industrialization can proceed in spite of the fierce opposition of the practitioners. After fifteen years the so-called "carve-out" industry, named because the companies delivering behavioral healthcare were separate from those delivering the general healthcare, has outlived its usefulness. It has saved the mental health benefit, and it is time to "carve-in" with primary care where behavioral care belongs. This integration of primary and behavioral health, which involves behavioral health specialists being on site in the medical setting, is gaining momentum among primary care physicians even though mental health practitioners show continued reluctance to leave the tradition of their private offices. Again, the next evolutionary step in healthcare will occur with or without the concurrence of the professional guilds. There are far too many practitioners who are once again ready to break ranks with their respective societies, and seize the unprecedented opportunity that will accompany the new era of practitioner-dominated behavioral healthcare. These practitioners have learned to predict and control costs, and are prepared to participate in the future of integrated healthcare.

The new era will be dependent on data, which gives scientifically trained professional psychologist an unprecedented advantage. Future behavioral care will be evidence-based, and the mantra was enunciated by Yank Coble, addressing the industry on behalf of the American Medical association: "In God we trust. All others must have data" (as quoted in Time, November 24, 1998, p. 69). Before proceeding to what the new integrated healthcare delivery system may look like, it may be important to review the medical cost offset research which has attracted the attention of the healthcare industry, and especially the employers and other third party payors, and is contributing to the trend toward the integration of behavioral health with primary care.

MEDICAL COST OFFSET: THE VALUE ADDED

At the Kaiser Permanente Health System, the nation's prototype of the modern Health Maintenance Organization (HMO), in the early 1960s it was discovered that 60% of all physician visits were by patients who were somaticizing stress, or whose stress was exacerbating physical illness. It was further discovered that brief psychotherapeutic interventions had a surprising impact in that they reduced this over-utilization by addressing the patient's stress (Cummings, Kahn and Sparkman, 1962; Follette & Cummings, 1967; Cummings & Follette, 1968). Somaticization was defined differently than the Somatization Disorder found in DSM IV, and was seen simply as the translation of emotional problems into physical symptoms, or the exacerbation of a disease by emotional factors or stress. This somatization inevitably results in over-utilization of healthcare, overloading the system. The typical effect discovered by Cummings & Follette is portrayed in Figure 1, which demonstrates a steady reduction in the five years following behavioral healthcare intervention. There is a leveling-off at 62.5% reduction in the fifth year, which represents average utilization for a "healthy" population, and where on an eight-year follow-up (Cummings & Follette, 1976) it remained with no further somatization.

It is important to note that medical cost offset is not just about money. It is about appropriate treatment. Addressing the patient's emotional distress has the value-added of reducing healthcare costs even after paying for the effective psychotherapy.

More importantly, it spares the patient years of having to suffer painful physical symptoms in that the treatment of choice (psychotherapy rather than medical treatment) has been provided. But this body of research has not been without its methodological difficulties, many of which have been overcome during its three decades.

The medical cost offset literature can be divided into three generations. The first generation (1965 -1979) saw the discovery that 60% of physician visits were by somaticizers. The National Institute of Mental Health sponsored a number of replications, and published a summary of these (Jones & Vischi, 1979) which revealed a medical cost offset of 30 to 65%. That same year NIMH convened the Bethesda Consensus Conference in an effort to ascertain why some studies yielded impressive savings in medical/ surgical costs, while others did not produce enough offset to pay for the behavioral care interventions. All of the investigators in medical cost offset were invited to a three day session during which the studies to that date, 28 in all, were evaluated. A consensus emerged (Jones & Vischi, 1980) which included the following: (1) Medical cost offset is feasible only in organized settings where there exists a commitment, capability, and incentive, and where somaticizers can be identified, appropriately treated, and traced through sophisticated informatics. (2) The more traditional the behavioral interventions, the less the medical cost offset. The cost offset increases to the degree in which primary care and behavioral care are coordinated, collaborative, or integrated. (3) Medical cost offset increases to the degree that somatization is addressed through focused interventions, targeted to specific populations.

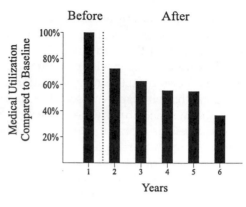

Figure 1

Reduction in medical utilization from the year before behavioral care intervention and through the succeeding five years following these interventions to an eventual reduction of 62.5% from the first year. Data are from Follette & Cummings, 1967

The Bethesda Consensus Conference enumerated a number of method-ological issues and recommended that a way be found to conduct randomized (prospective) studies rather than retrospective studies. The difficulty had been the contractual relationship with insured patients that prevented research in which those in the control group would be denied the treatment accorded to those in the experimental group. In an insured environment the denial of a contracted treatment to some patients, even for research purposes, is both illegal and unethical. The conclusions of the Bethesda Conference were not widely disseminated in that just two months later the government scientists who convened it were swept out of office when the Carter administration lost the election.

The second generation (1980-1990) saw the emergence of national orga-nized settings when the managed behavioral care industry came of age and captured most of the insured market. Unfortunately, with the carve-out arrangement, it was not possible to conduct medical cost offset between two companies that did not share informatics. Nonetheless, during this decade the role of stress, which was not adequately understood in the 1960s, was clarified in both somatization and unhealthy life styles (Ford, 1983, 1986; Pellitier, 1993; Sobel, 1995. The Health Care Financing Administration (HCFA), in conjunction with the State of Hawaii, sponsored the Hawaii Medicaid Project as the first comprehensive prospective study. Since this was a seven-year investigation, the results did not emerge until the following generation.

In the third generation (1990-1999) a number of organized settings attained the capability of conducting medical cost offset research, and man-aged behavioral care made a commitment to ongoing outcomes research. Not only were the new studies of a prospective (randomized) design, but they were of such a nature that they could be used in program planning and implemen-tation (Cummings, 1994). The Hawaii Medicaid Project became the prototype of this new generation of studies, which surprisingly confirmed the medical cost offset findings of previous, but retrospective research. It compared the impact of targeted, focused interventions, with the liberal 52-session annual Hawaii Medicaid psychotherapy benefit that could be obtained through any licensed privately practicing psychiatrist or psychologist of the patient's choice, and finally with those who received no treatment. Therefore, there were two experimental groups and one control group, all randomized. There were 36,000 beneficiaries in the Medicaid groups, to which were added in each of the conditions the 91,000 federal employees in Honolulu. The subjects were further identified between those who had no physical disease and those who had a chronic physical condition (asthma, diabetes, emphysema, hyperten-sion, ischemic heart disease, and rheumatoid arthritis, which together ac-count for 40% of the medical dollars in the ages 21 to 60 population) The results of the Hawaii Project are found in Figures 2 and 3, which reveal that targeted, focused interventions impressively reduced medical over-utilization, while the privately practicing psychotherapists increased costs. The difference is the greatest in the chronic disease groups (Figure 3). Targeted, focused interventions saved an average of $350 per year per patient, while the traditional setting raised medical costs by an average of $750 per year. In both the chronic and non-chronic groups the no treatment situation was preferable to traditional psychotherapy. The latter result was so baffling that psychotherapists were interviewed how they handled somatization. Surprisingly, instead of recognizing that their patient was somaticizing, the psychotherapists regarded the matter as an assertiveness issue and encouraged the patient to return to the physician demanding more and more tests to "prove" that the symptoms were, indeed, reflecting a yet undiagnosed physical disease. Consequently, unnecessary costs continued to mount.

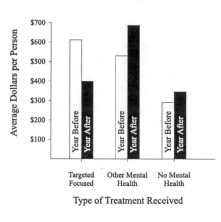

Figure 2

Average medical utilization in constant dollars for the Hawaii Project Non-Chronic Group for the year before (white columns) and the year after (black columns) receiving targeted and focused treatment, other mental health treatment in the private practice community, or no treatment. Data are from Cummings, 1993.

In a testimony before the United States Senate in which Cummings presented the Hawaii Project's preliminary findings, Senator Daniel K. Inouye of Hawaii who conducted the hearing, observed, "The most powerful argument for mental health benefits is the evidence that they reduce inappropriate medical utilization *(Congressional Record,* June 24, 1985, pp. S-8656 to S-8658). The lessons learned in the Hawaii Project, where an entire innovative behavioral care delivery system had to be created for the study, is that not only are organized settings imperative, but medical cost offset research can not be parachuted into a traditional setting. The importance of focused, targeted interventions in an integrated system is being elicited in a growing body of subsequent research (Cummings, Cummings & Johnson, 1997; Kent & Gordon, 1997; Strosahl, 1997).

WHY IS SOMATIZATION SO EXPENSIVE?

It is not uncommon for a somaticizer, finally having exasperated the physician who then makes a referral for psychotherapy, to abandon that physician and begin the investigation all over again with another doctor. Figure 4 illustrates the incidence of the fourteen most common complaints confronting the primary care physician, and reveals that only 5% of these symptoms on average are based on physical, rather than psychological conditions. These most common complaints are chest pain, fatigue, dizziness, headache, edema, back pain, dyspnea, insomnia, abdominal pain, numbness, impotence, weight loss, cough, and constipation. Figure 5 addresses the first five of these and reveals that in 1,000 primary care patients a surprising amount of money is required for evaluation of those manifesting stress, while a very small amount of money is adequate for the diagnosis of those with actual physical disease. For example, where $21,760 is spent to establish the somatization of chest pain, only $1,360 will diagnose the presence of an actual, existing organic cause (Kroenke & Mangelsdorf, 1989).

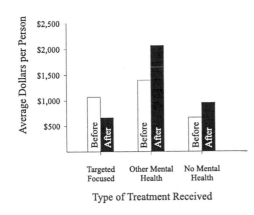

Figure 3

Average Medical Utilization in constant dollars for the Hawaii Project Chronically III Group for the year before (white columns) and the year after (black columns) receiving targeted and focused treatment, other mental health treatment in the private practice community, or no treatment. Data are from Cummings, 1997.

It is not so much that somaticizers are intractable, as it is the system which discourages their seeking appropriate psychotherapy. In an era of the "physician glut," the fee-for-service primary care physicians are reluctant to refer high utilizing patients for psychological treatment because this results in loss of income to themselves. In a capitated system primary care physicians hesitate to refer to psychologists because the cost must come out of their risk pool, resulting in less profit. But even in an enlightened system where physicians recognize the need and refer appropriately, only 10% of these referrals ever follow through and actually visit a psychotherapist. However, by having the psychologist on site in the primary care setting, the number of patients who accept the referral and enter treatment jumps to 80% (Slay & McLeod, In Press).

Supply Side Versus the Demand Side in Integrated Healthcare

Cost containment characteristically attempts to reduce costs by limiting the supply of unnecessary healthcare services. For example, in instances where short-term psychotherapy can be effective, long-term therapy is not reimbursed. Or where partial hospitalization is sufficient, full hospitalization is not authorized. The managed behavioral healthcare industry has now wrung all the fat out of the mental health/chemical dependency treatment system. There remains, however, a great deal of waste in the medical/surgical

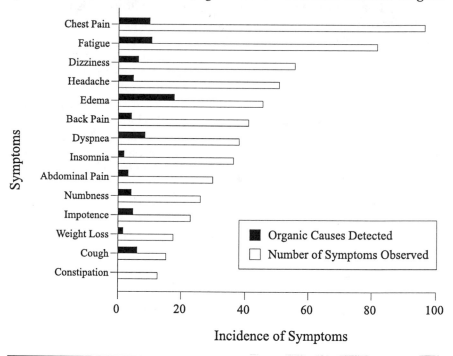

Figure 4

The incidence of 14 common symptoms (lighter shading) in 1,000 internal medicine outpatients, compared with those in which an organic disorder was detected (darker shading). Data are from Kroenke & Mangelsdorf, 1989

system where costs continue to rise from (1) expensive technology and (2) inappropriate care. Addressing the demand side of the economic equation (i.e., reducing demand) through the use of population-based group programs may constitute true prevention.

Cummings & Cummings (1997) reported a comparison of supply side versus demand side economics in two outpatient behavioral care centers in the same system. Center A (experimental) implemented several psychoeducational programs and every patient who presented during two successive periods of six months, and who fell into any of five categories, was assigned to the corresponding psychoeducational program. These programs with their designated patients were as follows: (1) adult children of alcoholics; (2) agoraphobia and multiple phobias; (3) borderline personality; (4) independent living for chronic schizophrenia; (5) perfectionistic personality life style. In Center B (control), every patient falling into any of the above five categories was routinely assigned to individual psychotherapy for two successive periods of six months each. All of the study patients for both centers were followed for a period of two years after their six months in treatment. Although there was not a randomized assignment of patients to control and experimental conditions because this would be tantamount to denying available services in Center A, the two groups from the two centers were comparable in all demographic characteristics (age, gender, socioeconomic level, education, ethnicity). Further, this arrangement permitted direct comparison between individual psychotherapy and population-based psychoeducational programs which was not possible within the randomized assignment of patients in the Hawaii Project.

As noted, there were two different periods of patient selection of six months duration each in both centers. All patients had a two-year follow-up after the initial six months. The total time of the experiment was three years, but only two-and-a-half years

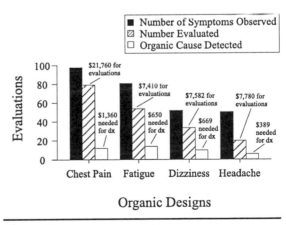

Figure 5

Evaluations and the cost per organic diagnosis for five symptoms in 1,000 internal medicine outpatients in 1988 dollars. Data are from Kroenke and Mangelsdorf, 1989.

A Comparison in the Use of Various Behavioral Health Services between an Experimental Group Assigned to a Psychoeducational Model, and the Control Group Assigned to the Traditional Model

	N		Group Sessions		Individual Sessions		Hospital Days		Emergency		Perscript		Return Visits	
	Expl	Cntrl	Expl	Cntrl	Expl	Cntrl	Expl	Cntrl	Expl	Cntrl	Expl	Cntrl	Expl	Cntrl
ACOA	38	12	570	46	76	132	1	11	6	8	16	24	53	38
Agoraphobia	23	8	460	0	46	122	14	21	9	37	26	28	38	63
Borderline	42	29	840	109	5	609	3	145	0	289	38	87	22	493
Indep. Living	22	18	422	315	21	72	26	183	4	51	41	68	251	488
Perfectionism	26	17	390	0	24	401	0	19	0	23	14	39	13	208
TOTALS	151	84	2682	480	172	1336	44	379	19	398	135	246	377	1290
MEANS			17.8	5.7	1.2	15.9	0.2	4.5	0.1	4.7	0.9	2.9	2.5	15.4

Legend:
ACOA: Adult Children of Alcoholics 15-Session program
Agoraphobia and Multiple Phobias 20-Session program
Borderline Personality Disorder 20-Session program
Independant Living for Chronic Schizophrenics 25-Session program
Perfectionism Leading to Disabling Episodes 15-Session program
Note: Group therapy sessions for the control group were in traditional (i.e., nonpsychoeducational) groups, while group sessions for the experimental group were all in psychoeducational programs

Table 1

Data are from Cummings & Cummings, 1997

for each particular group. Because Center A was larger, there were 151 patients in the experimental group, while smaller Center B yielded 84 patients for the control group.

The results are shown in Table 1, which reveals that for these five categories, the average number of psychoeducational sessions (experimental group) was only two more than the average number of individual sessions in the control group. Not even taking into account the cost differential (individual therapy ratio 1:1 between patients and therapists, psychoeducational 1:8 to 1:15), this resulted in a 90% reduction in demand for individual therapy, a 95% reduction in hospital days, a 97% reduction in emergency services (including emergency room visits and drop-in sessions), a 70% reduction in prescriptions for medication, and an 85% reduction in return visits.

For illustrative purposes, these findings can be translated into economic terms. Assuming an hour of individual psychotherapy costs $100, the cost of a psychoeducational group program of one-and-half hours would be $150 divided by the average patient group of ten, which equals $15 per patient. What is startling, this $15 per patient unit then goes on to save between 70 to 97% in hospitalization, individual psychotherapy, emergency room visits, medication prescriptions, and return visits.

Behavioral Healthcare Integration in Medicare

Healthcare for older adults is far more costly than that for the younger population. With the growing numbers of older Americans, and with per patient costs steadily rising, the system is threatened with bankruptcy. The 1999 President's State of the Union address devoted a significant amount of time to saving Medicare. Yet little attention has been paid to reducing costs through behavioral interventions since the general consensus in government has been that older adults are from a generation that does not avail itself of psychotherapy. The fact is that most psychotherapists like to address issues pertinent to a younger generation (dating, marriage, divorce, parenting, step-parenting, career, job loss, etc.) Research demonstrates that when programs relevant to older adults are made available (widowhood, retirement, loneliness, alienation, feelings of uselessness, chronic or debilitating illness in self or spouse, etc.), these patients will seek help in greater numbers than their younger counterparts (Hartmann-Stein, 1997). This should not be surprising because the elderly are more at risk.

Appropriate behavioral interventions can not only save Medicare dollars, it can also spare the older adult from a great deal of stress and pain. Two such programs will be briefly described as examples of the impact that evidence-based programs can have in a population that has been neglected by most psychologists.

The author and his colleagues (Cummings, 1997) found themselves having to create a new managed behavioral program when Humana was awarded responsibility for the healthcare of the first large population of Medicare recipients, 140,000 such older adults on the West Coast of Florida in 1987. American Biodyne became responsible for the behavioral care component, and HCFA, expecting the usual elderly penetration of only 0.5% for psychotherapy, was determined to set the capitation rate accordingly. American Biodyne challenged this, projecting a penetration rate of 5 to 7% to be accomplished by outreach and by the creation of relevant programs. The government agreed, but only after it was assured their would be a proportional return of the prospective funding if American Biodyne fell short of that level. Not surprisingly, the elderly flocked to Biodyne at a rate exceeding 10%, threatening bankruptcy of the program. It was clear from the outset that effective programs had to be developed. This was accomplished, and among these were the Bereavement Program and the Early Alzheimer's Counseling Program. The first of these was imperative inasmuch as a 5% mortality rate in this population yielded nearly twenty widows or widowers every day.

The Bereavement Program

The year before the death of a spouse, the surviving spouse characteristically has a lower healthcare utilization rate because of the concentration on the dying spouse's care. After the death, however, the surviving spouse demonstrates a skyrocketing healthcare utilization rate. Some of this reflects pent up demand from the previous year, but the vast majority of this is the somaticized grief reaction. The Bereavement Study employed American Biodyne's familiar two centers design (proximal as well as demographically comparable). An early outreach program was instituted in which the patient was identified and contacted within two weeks of widowhood. In Center A (experimental) a Bereavement Program was created which treated patients in special groups after those with depression rather than bereavement were screened out. There were five to eight mourners in each group, depending on patient traffic. Fourteen two-hour group sessions were spaced as follows: four semi-weekly sessions followed by six weekly sessions, and then by four concluding sessions held monthly. Center B (control) addressed the widowed patient without outreach, and with traditional referral and individual psychotherapy. All patients were followed for two years after the death of the spouse.

The results are clear-cut. The patients who participated in the Bereavement Program showed some increase the first year after the death of the spouse, reflecting the lack of personal medical attention during the previous care-taking year. The second year after the death of the spouse healthcare returned to the rate of utilization expected of this age group. In contrast, the control group (traditional behavioral healthcare) demonstrated in the first year after the death of the spouse a healthcare rate twice that of the experimental group, and though it declined during the second year after the death, it remained 40% higher than that of the experimental

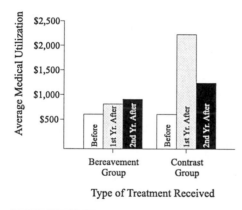

Figure 6

Average medical utilization for the year before and each of the two years after beginning the Bereavement Program, and for the same period for the contrast group that received individual psychotherapy rather than the Bereavement Program. Data are from Cummings, 1997.

group for that second year. After subtracting the cost of behavioral care the Bereavement Program resulted in a saving of $1,400 per patient for the two-year period, as shown in Figure 6. This amount, extrapolated to the general elderly population covered by this one health plan, translates to a potential saving of several million dollars. Even more importantly, however, this program can spare widowed older adults two years of avoidable suffering from physical symptoms and ill health.

Early Alzheimer's Counseling

During this same period a program focused on the caretakers of patients with early Alzheimer's dementia and on the patients themselves (Cummings, 1997). It has been noted for some time that the hardship imposed on the caretakers of Alzheimer's patients results in an increased rate of illness among the spouses or adult children caring for the person with dementia. The stress increases with both the length of the care-taking and the severity of the dementia, which is progressive and unpredictable, and is exacerbated by the patient's characteristic inability to show affection or gratitude.

The early Alzheimer's patient also experiences stress. Frequently disoriented when away from home, he or she soon experiences a characteristic "catastrophic emotional response" upon being disoriented in familiar surroundings. The response occurs before the dementia has damaged ego functioning; the patient is devastated by the experience, fears its recurrence, and is reluctant to leave home. There is a consequent narrowing of life space for both the patient and the non-afflicted spouse. The Early Alzheimer's Program patients were counseled to carry three telephone numbers of loved ones whom they were to call if they found themselves "lost," precluding the need for strangers to activate the emergency 911 systems with its consequent hospital involvement.

Ongoing counseling of care-takers on an as-needed basis, which included initial training in relaxation, guided imagery and meditation, along with education regarding the course of the Alzheimer's syndrome, proved highly successful in reducing the caretaker's incidence of illness and concomitant higher use of medical services. In addition, a hot-line with immediate advice not only reduced the number of emergency calls to physicians when the patient's behavior was baffling, but it also served as an emotional safety valve whenever the care-taker's stress became unbearable. The costs of this behavioral program were ongoing over several years rather than the relatively brief six and one-half month duration of the Bereavement Project, but so were the consistently significant medical savings which far more than offset these costs (see Figure 7).

CHARACTERISTICS OF POPULATION-BASED GROUP PROGRAMS

Most programs are verified expansions and modifications of the arthritis self-help course originally developed by Lorig and Fries (1990). In addition to an educational component tailored to the particular psychological or physical condition being treated, and the creation of a "buddy" support system, the protocols include the following objectives: (1) *Self-efficacy* (Bandura, 1977), which is a process of restoring selfconfidence by performance of discontinued tasks that were once part of daily life. (2) Defeating *learned helplessness* (Seligman, 1975), which is the sense of being crippled by overwhelming feelings that dictate, "I no longer can do this." (3) Restoring a *sense of coherence* (Antonovsky, 1987) that there is still meaning in life, but in a different way than previously.

THE INTEGRATED HEALTHCARE SYSTEM OF THE FUTURE

A number of large HMOs and regional group practices are making strides toward integrating behavioral health in primary care, among them Kaiser Permanente (Kent & Gordon, 1997), Healthcare Partners (Slay & McLeod, 1997), Group Health Cooperative of Puget Sound, now Kaiser Group Health (Strosahl, Baker, Braddick, Stuart & Handley, 1997), HealthPartners of Minnesota, and the Duke University Medical Center (Gunn, Seaburn, Lorenz, Gawinski, and Mauksch, 1997). Most primary care physicians, faced with the daily array of as many as 80% of their patients reflecting psychological problems, welcome collaboration with behavioral care specialists (Lucas & Peek, 1997), but caution that integration must proceed slowly to overcome formidable barriers. Their view is that separate departments of psychiatry and medicine perpetuate the notion that the mind and the body are separate, but this long-standing tradition is entrenched and will not pass easily. In addition, behavioral health specialists, and psychologists in particular, are reluctant to leave their private solo practice offices so that they may be on location with the primary care setting. Finally, the carve-out companies that have captured 75% of the insured behavioral healthcare market are fiercely opposed to giving up their domain by "carving-in."

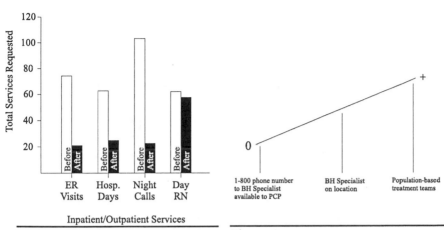

Figure 7	**Figure 8**

Reduction in outpatient (emergency room and drop-in clinic visits, night phone calls, and day advice nurse phone calls) and inpatient (hospital) services from the year before participating in the Early Alzheimer's Counseling Program to the year following. Data are from Cummings, 1997.

Intensity (degree) of integration on a continuum from a 1-800 telephone number, through the midpoint in which behavioral health specialists are on location, to the eventual obliteration of departments in favor of population/disease based treatment teams. Most programs (chemical dependancy, depression, life style, etc.) are before the midpoint

Fortunately, the integration of behavioral health with primary care can be accomplished in a continuum of steps, with a minimum of eighteen months required to reach the level of behavioral care practitioners being on location, and three to four years before there is an obliteration of traditional departments in favor of population/diseasebased teams. Figure 8 illustrates this continuum, beginning with a 1-800 number available to primary physicians for consultation with a psychologist 24-hours per day, proceeding to the midpoint in which psychologists are on location, and eventually reaching the level of departments being replaced by targeted teams. There is an appreciable increase in collaboration when the behavioral specialist is on location, permitting the primary care physician to walk the patient the few feet down the hall where the three (physician, psychologist, and patient) address the patient's problem. In such an arrangement, and even though the presenting complaint is regarded by the team as psychological in nature, the process is viewed by the patient as part of the totality of healthcare. It is precisely this lack of resistance by the patient that increases acceptance of psychotherapy from the national average of only 10% of referrals in the fragmented referral system, to 80% in the integrated model. The more the psychologist blends into the health system, the less will be the patient's feeling of having been abandoned by the physician only to be stigmatized as a "mental case."

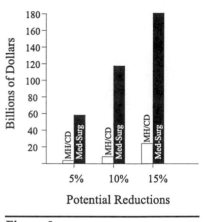

There are many examples of population-based teams (Cummings, Cummings & Johnson, 1997). In one setting a teen-age clinic (ages 13 to 19 with ongoing parental consent), is composed of pediatricians, nurse practitioners and

Figure 9

Reduction in billions of dollars potentially at the 5, 10, and 15% levels for the nation's mental health.chemical dependancy budget. Based on a total annual healthcare budget of $1.2 trillion in 1997. The estimates are from Cummings, 1997.

psychologists/social workers. These practitioners do not report to the departments of pediatrics, nursing or psychiatry, respectively, but rather to the teen-age clinic which has its own administrative staff and budget. This accords freedom from having to beg for resources (money, staff) from such departments, and results in highly effective programs. In this instance, teenagers being seen without having to be accompanied by their parents, were able to discuss freely issues of sex, drugs and other matters typical of this period. The findings over a four year period revealed significantly lower rates of drug abuse, teen-age pregnancy and venereal diseases. Another example of such teams functioning independently of departments are back clinics, composed of primary care physicians, behavioral care specialists and nurse practitioners who address one of the largest group of somaticizers, those with stress-related low back pain and who would not be benefited by surgery. Still other examples are rheumatoid arthritis clinics (which include the difficult patients with fibromyalgia), childhood asthma programs, and diabetes clinics.

Eventually economic considerations, pressed by large employers and third party payers will insist on the integration of behavioral health with primary care. All of the fat has been wrung out of mental health, whereas enormous savings are yet to be realized in the medical/surgical system. Figure 9 dramatically illustrates that a 5, 10, or even 15% saving in the mental health/ chemical dependency budget is scarcely a blip compared to such savings in medicine/surgery. Looking at the $1.2 trillion annual American health budget, a 10% saving through the appropriate treatment of the somaticizer,

would exceed the entire annual mental health/chemical dependency budget
for that year. Research has demonstrated that in an integrated system 5 to 10%
medical cost offset is modest, indeed. Before the integration of behavioral
health with primary care occurs, however, the policy makers will have to put
into place the required economic incentives. Current financial arrangements
perpetuate the status quo.

THE BEHAVIORAL CARE PRACTITIONER OF THE FUTURE:
A GOLDEN OPPORTUNITY

Doctoral level psychologists can no longer justify employment as psychotherapists as the trend among managed care companies and regional provider
groups is to hire masters level clinicians for that purpose. Any Ph.D. who
insists on competing as a therapist or counselor with M.A. psychologists will
have to accept fees commensurate with that lower level, and, indeed, many
doctoral psychologists are doing just that. The job market is grim for those
insisting on traditional psychotherapy employment or private solo practice.
At the same time, opportunities in health psychology are increasing. Several
of the nation's largest health systems are firing traditional doctoral psychotherapists as they hire, instead, doctoral level health psychologists who can
not only be on location with primary care, but are trained to perform outcomes
research, program planning, supervision of masters level therapists/counse-
lors, and other important activities. In some systems, health psychologists are
participants along with physicians in practitioner/equity plans (Cummings,
Pallak, & Cummings, 1996).

The psychotherapy of the future is much different from that for which most
psychologists have been trained. Only 25% of the practitioner's clinical time
will be in individual psychotherapy, which will be targeted and focused, and
based on empirically derived amalgams of all the techniques (behavioral,
cognitive behavioral, psychodynamic, strategic, systems). Another 25% will
be in group psychotherapy that is time-limited and closed. Open groups
where patients wander in for a year or two and wander out again are outdated.
In addition, 50% of the clinician's time will be in population/disease programs that will be both psycho educational and therapeutic. By adding the
number of patients involved in such a configuration in a national healthcare
system involving 14.5 million covered lives which employed such a ratio, less
than 10% of patients are seen in individual psychotherapy (Cummings, 1996).
The future doctoral practitioner in behavioral health will not only be (1) an
innovative clinician, but also (2) a trained researcher, (3) a creative program

planner, (4) a knowledgeable health psychologist, (5) a skilled manager, and (6) a compassionate, but astute business person (Cummings, 1996).

REFERENCES

Antonovsky, A. (1987). *Unraveling the mystery of health: How people manage stress and stay well.* San Francisco, CA: Jossey-Bass.

Bandura, A. (1977). Self-efficacy: Toward a unifying theory of behavioral change. *Psychological Review, 84,* 191-215.

Cummings, N. A. (1994). The successful application of medical offset in program planning and in clinical delivery. *Managed Care Quarterly, 2,* 1-6.

Cummings, N. A. (1996). The impact of managed care on employment and professional training: A primer for survival. In N. A. Cummings, M. S. Pallak & J. L. Cummings (Eds.), *Surviving the demise of solo practice: Mental health practitioners prospering in the era of managed care* (pp.11-26). Madison, CT: Psychosocial Press.

Cummings, N. A. (1997). Approaches in prevention in the behavioral health of older adults. In P. Hartman-Stein (Ed.), *Innovative behavioral healthcare for older adults: A guide-book for changing times* (pp. 1-23). San Francisco, CA: Jossey-Bass.

Cummings, N. A., (2000). The first decade of managed behavioral care: What went right and what went wrong? *Psychotherapy and Critical Issues in Managed Care, 1 (1).*

Cummings, N. A., & Cummings, J.L. (1997). The behavioral health practitioner of the future: The efficacy of psychoeducational programs. In N. A. Cummings, J. L. Cummings & J. N. Johnson (Eds.), *Behavioral health in primary care: A guide for clinical integration* (pp. 325-346). Madison, CT: Psychosocial Press.

Cummings, N. A., Cummings, J. L., & Johnson, J. N. (Eds.). *Behavioral health in primary Care: A guide for clinical integration.* Madison, CT: Psychosocial Press.

Cummings, N. A., & Follette, W. T. (1968). Psychiatric services and medical utilization in a prepaid health plan setting: Part 2. *Medical Care, 6,* 31-41.

Cummings, N. A., & Follette, W. T. (1976). Brief psychotherapy and medical utilization: An eight-year follow-up. In H. Dorken (Ed.), *The professional psychologist today* (pp. 126-142). San Francisco, CA: Jossey-Bass.

Cummings, N. A., Kahn, B. I., & Sparkman, B. (1962). *Psychotherapy and medical utilization: A pilot project.* Oakland, CA: Annual Reports of Kaiser Permanente Research Projects.

Cummings, N. A., Pallak, M. S., & Cummings, J. L. (Eds.), *Surviving the demise of solo practice: Mental health practitioners prospering in the era of managed care.* Madison, CT: Psychosocial Press.

Follette, W. T., & Cummings, N. A. (1967). Psychiatric services and medical utilization in a prepaid health plan setting. *Medical Care, 5,* 24-35.

Ford, C. V. (1983). *The somaticizing disorders: Illness as a way of life.* New York: Elsevier.

Ford, C. V. (1986). The somatizing disorders. *Psychosomatics, 27,* 327-337.

Gunn, W. B., Seaburn, D., Lorenz, A., Gawinski, B., & Mauksch, L. B. (1997). Collaboration in action: Key stratgies for behavioral health providers. In N. A.

Cummings, J. L. Cummings & J. N. Johnson (Eds.), *Behavioral health in primary care: A guide for clinical integration* (pp. 285-304). Madison, CT: Psychosocial Press.

Hartman-Stein, P. (Ed.), (1997). *Innovative behavioral health care for older adults: A guidebook for changing times.* San Francisco, CA: Jossey-Bass.

Jones, K. R., & Vischi, T. R. (1979). The impact of alcohol, drug abuse, and mental health treatment on medical care utilization: A review of the research literature. *Medical Care, 17* (suppl. 1), 43-13 1.

Jones, K. R., & Vischi, T. R. (1980). *The Bethesda Consensus Conference on Medical Offset. Alcohol, drug abuse, and mental health administration report.* Rockville, MD: Alcohol, Drug Abuse and Mental Health Administration.

Kent, J., & Gordon, M. (1997). Integration: A case for putting Humpty Dumpty together again. In N. A. Cummings, J. L. Cummings, & J. N. Johnson (Eds.), *Behavioral health in primary care: A guide for clinical integration* (pp. 103-120). Madison, CT: Psychosocial Press.

Kroenke, K., & Mangelsdorf, A. D. (1989). Common symptoms in ambulatory care: Incidence, evaluation, therapy, and outcome. *American Journal of Medicine, 86,* 262-266.

Lorig, K., & Fries, J. (1990). *Arthritis helpbook* (3 rd ed.). Reading, MA: Addison-Wesley.

Lucas, S. F., & Peek, C. J. (1997). A primary care physician's experience with integrated behavioral health care: What difference has it made? In N. A. Cummings, J. L. Cummings & J. N. Johnson (Eds.), *Behavioral health in primary care: A guide for clinical integration* (pp. 371-397). Madison, CT: Psychosocial Press.

Pellitier, K.R. (1993). Between mind and body: Stress, emotions and health. In D. Golernan & J. Gurin (Eds.), *Mind/body medicine* (pp. 19-38). Yonkers, NY: Consumer Reports.

Ross, E.C. (1998, December 7). Plans present mixed bag of results for providers, subscribers. *Tallahassee Democrat,* F1, 4.

Seligman, M.E.P. (1975). *Helplessness: On depression, development, and death.* San Francisco: CA: W.H. Freeman.

Slay, J. D., & McLeod, C. (1997). Evolving an integration model: The healthcare partners experience. In N. A. Cummings, J. L. Cummings, & J. N. Johnson (Eds.), *Behavioral health in primary care: A guide for clinical integration* (pp. 103-120). Madison, CT: Psychosocial Press.

Slay, J. D., & McLeod, C. (In Press). The Healthcare Partners Experience.

Sobel, D. (1995). Rethinking medicine: Improving health outcomes with cost-effective psychosocial interventions. *Psychosomatic Medicine, 57,* 234-244.

Strosahl, K. (1997). Building primary care behavioral health systems that work: A com pass and a horizon. In N. A. Cummings, J. L. Cummings, & J. N. Johnson (Eds.), *Behavioral health in primary care: A guide for clinical integration.* (pp. 37-59). Madison, CT: Psychosocial. Press.

Strosahl, K., Baker, N. J., Braddick, M., Stuart, M. E., & Handley, M. R. (1997). Integration of behavioral health and primary care services: The Group Health Cooperative model. In N. A. Cummings, J. L. Cummings, & J. N. Johnson (Eds.), *Behavioral health in primary care: A guide for clinical integration* (pp. 61-85). Madison, CT: Psychosocial Press.

Discussion of Cummings:

Medical Health Care and Mental Health Care: Integration and/or Partnership

Alan E. Fruzzetti
University of Nevada, Reno

In his "New Vision of Healthcare for America" Dr. Cummings provides a compelling description of the evolution of private mental health care reimbursement practices over the past 30 years. He also describes a number of important intervention and prevention innovations that benefit subscribers directly while significantly reducing costs (medical offset). He suggests that the reduction in medical utilization as a result of behavioral interventions will lead to a new evolution in service delivery, the integration of behavioral health and medical care, especially in primary care settings. A few comments in each of these areas follow.

HISTORICAL SHIFT IN REIMBURSEMENT PRACTICES AND TREATMENT DELIVERY

Dr. Cummings notes that significant changes have evolved in mental health care delivery, from reliance on inpatient hospitalization and long-term psychotherapies to much reduced inpatient hospital utilization and dramatically reduced reimbursement for extended, unfocused psychotherapy. He correctly notes the guild resistance to these changes, despite data on costs, outcomes, and utilization that suggest significant public benefits. His argument is likely to be provocative because rather than lamenting the changes that lead further away from general third-party reimbursement of long-term psychotherapy, he welcomes them.

His point is quite correct: decreasing reimbursement for very expensive services for a very small proportion of people has resulted in increased access to a broader array of services (toward a continuum of mental health care) for

Integrated Behavioral Healthcare: Positioning Mental Health Practice with Medical/Surgical Practice

many more people. Indeed, although he refers to this as an evolution, if access to mental health services continues to increase and historical barriers decrease, this may be seen in future decades as more of a revolution. The paradox is that the impetus for these changes (cutting costs, making money) may result in a more egalitarian system of access and resource allocation (cf. Albee, 1978).

However, as Dr. Cummings also notes, shifting funding within direct mental health services likely has already maximized efficiency. Thus, for access to mental and behavioral health and prevention services to continue to increase, medical utilization cost offsets must likely be demonstrated, and then embraced as the economic means to achieve broader access to mental health services.

MEDICAL AND BEHAVIORAL HEALTH CARE DELIVERY: INTEGRATION OR PARTNERSHIP?

Dr. Cummings notes that because "carve-out" systems (behavioral health care, separate from medical health care) likely have maximized efficiency within mental health care delivery, the only way to expand services and efficiency may be to re-integrate behavioral health care delivery with medical care delivery. This larger system (medical care expenditures being more than ten times those of mental health) would be able to provide significantly more behavioral health services (both intervention and prevention efforts) through significantly reduced medical utilization/cost offset. Indeed, Dr. Cummings provides several compelling examples of such offset. He concludes that only by "carving back in" (to the larger system), can system-wide cost savings, and increased services, be possible.

His pragmatic approach has many benefits. For example, problem-related treatment may be both more effective and more cost-efficient than diagnosis-based treatment (Fruzzetti, 1996; Hayes, Nelson & Jarrett, 1987), and would generally put more science into clinical practice (there would be more immediate incentives for providing effective treatment, and disincentives for not collecting data). Moreover, many mental health problems including ordinary life-development difficulties (e.g., bereavement, relationship problems, and high stress) have established links to higher medical care utilization. The consequent costs associated with "false positive" symptoms (e.g., ruling out heart problems when the person has stress-related chest pains or ruling out digestive disease in the presence of stress-related digestive problems) are enormous. Recovering even a modest fraction of these costs, as Dr. Cummings notes, could easily fund prevention and early intervention programs specific to life events or psychological difficulties. This approach targets specific behavioral interventions that have multiple, non-specific health consequences, rather than later paying for specific physical "symptom" or problem identification and/or amelioration. This later task, he notes, inefficiently allocates resources to expensive diagnostic procedures that do not identify treatable pathology.

Thus, the integration of medical and behavioral health care delivery systems (along with their administration and funding) may afford benefits to the vast majority of ordinary people: Most of us develop, at one time or another, either medical problems that are exacerbated by psychological and behavioral factors or medical problems that are in part caused by psychological and behavioral factors. For most people, then, integration could be a step forward toward improved behavioral and medical health. However, there are three issues that may, if not addressed, retard the success of full integration of behavioral and medical health care services, or inhibit the integration itself from progressing.

The first issue pertains to the group of persons with chronic mental health difficulties. For this relatively small segment of the population, medical cost offset for behavioral intervention is unlikely because mental health treatment costs may already exceed medical costs. For example, for a chronically mentally ill person who does not have high medical costs, but does have high outpatient mental health costs, there would be no medical cost savings for enhanced treatment or early intervention. However, several examples provided by Dr. Cummings argue for providing improved, data-driven interventions. This approach in general (system wide) could allow savings generated from one group to support programs, even expensive ones, for another group (if data demonstrate effectiveness). Ultimately, some programs are not inherently cost-effective, at least on an individual or collective cost basis. But when they are effective, some should be funded anyway because they are humane (Fruzzetti & Levensky, 2000).

The issue of how to fund services for people with chronic or serious (non-normative) mental health problems is generally less relevant to private systems than to public ones: Those with the most serious psychological difficulties are the least likely to work, have any kind of health insurance and are least likely to have access to effective mental health treatment programs in general. Thus, integration of behavioral health care delivery into primary medical care may be inhibited with this sub-population of chronically psychologically distressed individuals, primarily in the public sector.

The second factor to be considered involves the present zeitgeist with respect to the relationship between psychological and medical problems. Certainly, in recent years we have witnessed the increased medicalization of psychology (e.g., increased use of psychiatric diagnoses, movement toward prescription privileges for psychologists, adoption of more biological and less behavioral/psychological causal models). From a theoretical perspective, subsuming behavioral interventions into primary care may further reinforce this medicalization and associated reductionism. Although pragmatically more individuals may have access to psychological interventions, paradoxically they may view these interventions less as psychological or behavioral. This might result in diminished mind-body dualism, but could instead result in even further biological hegemony over behavioral science if the only relevant interventions and dependent variables in research are in the service of lowered medical utilization and enhanced medical care. Presumably, the development and testing of psychological models and treatments for psychological problems would suffer as a result, albeit only in small measure as a result of a change in mechanism (primary care) of mental health service delivery. Moreover, costs are not the only dependent variable: Intervening to alleviate some types of human suffering may be expensive, or at least may not offset by reduced medical expenditures.

Finally, for prevention efforts to be effective in the private sector the system funding the prevention must not lose money. Ultimately, either increased numbers of subscribers (more revenue) or reduced costs later on must fund prevention efforts. The problem for a private system is that many established effective prevention programs do not demonstrate lowered population problem incidence or prevalence within the number of years that subscribers stay with one insurer or managed care organization. For example, effective smoking cessation programs among young adults will not result in medical care cost offset for decades. By then, most participants will belong to other reimbursement or delivery systems. Thus, for many prevention programs even significant population-wide cost savings will not necessarily be cost effective for any one health care organization.

For the majority of people, an integrated model of medical and behavioral health care delivery in primary care settings likely will reduce system-wide costs for medical services and will simultaneously improve both access to services and the overall quality of available services. These are worthy goals. Nevertheless, a partnership model, wherein experts in behavioral and psychological health (for serious and chronic disorders that may show up in a small minority of the population) are available outside primary care may also be appropriate. Paying for these services, as well as those prevention programs without immediate medical cost offset remains a problem that can only be solved by attention to good science in the context of humane values.

REFERENCES

Albee, G. (1977). Does including psychotherapy in health insurance represent a subsidy to the rich from the poor? *American Psychologist, 32,*719-721.

Fruzzetti, A. E. (1996). Causes and consequences: Individual distress in the context of couple interactions. *Journal of Consulting and Clinical Psychology, 64,*1192-1201.

Fruzzetti, A. E., & Levensky, E. R. (in press). Dialectical behavior therapy with batterers: Issues and application. *Cognitive and Behavioral Practice, 7,* 435-447.

Hayes, S. C., Nelson, R. O., & Jarrett, T. (1987). Treatment utility of assessment: A functional approach to evaluating quality of assessment. *American Psychologist, 42,* 963-974.

3

The Integration of Primary Care and Behavioral Health: Type II Change in the Era of Managed Care

Kirk Strosahl, Ph.D.
Mountainview Consulting Group,
Moxee, Washington

Introduction
The integration of Primary Care and Behavioral Health
Mental Disorders, Psychological Distress and Medical Utilization
  Primary Care is the De Facto Mental Health System in the United States
  Health Care Seeking is a Complex Process
  Psychosocial Stress is a Major Cause of Medical Service Use
  Psychosocial Stresses Influence Health Status and the Course of Illness
  Health Care Decisions are Influenced by the Services Available
The Medical Cost Offset Effect
  The Magnitude of Cost Offsets is Considerable
  A Variety of Medical Populations Have Cost Offset Potential
  Cost Offsets are Observed in both Primary Care and Specialty Care
  A Range of Integrative Services can Address Behavioral Health Issues

Integrated Behavioral Healthcare: Positioning Mental Health Practice with Medical/Surgical Practice

INTRODUCTION

As managed care matures and evolves, the current emphasis on cost containment will give way to a focus on building quality oriented, cost effective delivery systems. One likely result of this trend will be the integration of behavioral services into primary care medicine. This article examines the empirical literature supporting the integration of services. One line of research suggests that there is a strong relationship between psychological distress and medical utilization. A second body of evidence indicates that significant medical cost efficiencies can be obtained by addressing the behavioral health needs of primary care patients through integrated services. A primary mental health model for integration is introduced, along with two essential program design strategies: horizontal and vertical integration. This model of care has been shown empirically to produce better outcomes, lower total health costs and produce more satisfied patients and providers. The nature of primary mental health care suggests that it is markedly different from traditional mental health specialty work. These differences are examined in detail. Finally, the roles of different mental disciplines in primary care are elaborated. It is clear that primary care integration represents a vast opportunity for the growth of the mental health industry. The ultimate challenge is whether mental health providers can adapt their service delivery philosophies, goals and strategies to fit the demands of the primary care environment.

THE INTEGRATION OF PRIMARY CARE AND BEHAVIORAL HEALTH: TYPE II CHANGE IN THE ERA OF MANAGED CARE

Managed care has had, and will continue to have, a profound impact upon the health and mental health delivery systems of the United States. While Generation 1 of managed care has been characterized by an excessive emphasis on supply side cost containment strategies, Generation 2 will be geared toward increasing both the efficiency and effectiveness of health care (Strosahl, 1996a, 1996b, 1995, 1994b). Many managed care prognosticators believe that the "floor" of cost containment achievable through cost cutting alone has been reached. Therefore, to continue the current downward trend in health care costs, a more basic re-engineering of systems, processes and financing models will be required. This is likely to lead to two pervasive themes in health care over the next decade. First, managed care will be pressured to equally weigh cost and quality, in response to increasing purchaser and customer dissatisfaction with what appear to be Draconian cost containment strategies. This will either be a "voluntary" process of reform or enforced through litigation and regulatory legislation. Second, the cumbersome and overlapping systems that provide health and behavioral health services will come under intense pressure to consolidate, as the marketplace seeks ways to reduce administrative redundancy by capitalizing on the economy of scale. A harbinger of these pressures is the unprecedented consolidation within the behavioral health industry over the preceding two years. At this point, two behavioral health care megaliths account for approximately 85 million covered lives!

From the perspective of system consolidation, there is already a movement underway to integrate services within fewer delivery systems (cf. Strosahl, 1998, 1996a, 1995, 1994a; Cummings, 1995). The merging of previously segregated systems can relieve much of the administrative cost burden associated with today's managed care while holding the promise of providing the "one shop stopping" that is so much in demand by consumers. Thus, the current climate of health care reform presents an historic opportunity to fully integrate health and behavioral health care. The arbitrary separation of mind and body, reflected in the segregation of the health and mental health service delivery systems, has not only had a destructive impact upon the health of the general population, but may be one of the primary factors underpinning the health care cost crisis (Strosahl & Sobel, 1996). Luckily, for the first time in five decades, financial pressures are driving a reconsideration of this badly misguided idea. It appears that the perspectives of medical and behavioral health experts, a hundred or more confirmatory research studies and several hundred thousand confirming anecdotal reports don't seem to sway the opinions of corporate, state, and federal decision makers nearly as easily as the smell of red ink! While many obstacles will need to be addressed before behavioral health and health services can be fully integrated (i.e., culture clash, turf issues, financing and benefit design), the most difficult challenge will be to develop an overarching framework for integration that can do justice to complexity of the task. Such a template should define the rationale for and mission of integrated services, how to build integrated services that can address the enormous unmet demand within the primary care population, lead to a model of integrated care that is feasible to implement in a cost neutral or cost negative environment and delineate the roles of the various mental health and health disciplines in a way that optimizes their overall impact on consumers. Without such a unifying template, the behavioral health industry is likely to institute a hodge-podge of poorly related strategies that will reflect negatively on the industry in the eyes of consumers, purchasers and regulators.

The purpose of this presentation is to propose an overall framework that addresses the important dimensions involved in developing, implementing and evaluating integrated primary care behavioral health programs. First, it will be useful to briefly review the compelling research literature that links mental disorders, psychosocial stresses with medical utilization. A foray into this literature must include a review of the medical cost offset and cost effectiveness research that is being generated to estimate the potential cost savings associated with integrated primary care. Second, it is critically important to examine the assumptions that will help define the overall mission of integration. The concepts underpinning population-based care will be briefly reviewed, with the belief that this approach to contemporary primary care medicine will easily generalize to integrative behavioral health service delivery as well. Horizontal and vertical integration, two distinct but complementary population care approaches, will be examined to provide the structural framework for building integrated services. The "primary mental health care" model developed by this author and others at Group Health Cooperative of Puget Sound will be introduced. This approach to integrated services has been shown to be clinically effective, popular with consumers and primary care providers, inexpensive to implement and general enough in scope to fit the demands of almost any primary care delivery setting. To conclude, we will examine a topic of increasing controversy and importance, namely, the roles and functions of different behavioral health provider disciplines. Given the increasing emphasis in managed behavioral healthcare on using the lowest cost provider possible, there is a need to articulate what functions can appropriately be discharged by a masters level provider in primary care, and which functions seem to require the expertise of a psychiatrist, prescribing nurse specialist or a psychologist.

Mental Disorders, Psychological Distress and Medical Utilization: Basic Concepts

There is a significant mismatch between the reasons that stimulate a request for medical care and the traditional medical services that are offered. The result is many missed opportunities to identify and manage the true drivers of the demand for health services. Consequently, contemporary primary care medicine is awash in red ink from wasted resources, poor quality, unsatisfied patients, and frustrated providers. Understanding the basic processes which influence health care seeking as well as provider and delivery system factors that drive up the "controllable" aspects of medical utilization can lead to well conceived efforts to build integrative services that actually address the needs of the health care consumer.

Primary Care is the De Facto Mental Health System in the United States

The Epidemiological Catchment Area project, a large multi-site study of over 18,000 households in the United States, provides a sobering picture of the delivery of behavioral health services in the United States. The approximate one year incidence of diagnosable mental disorders, including substance addiction, is approximately 17% (Regier et al., 1990). Of such patients, only half seek any form of mental health care. Of the half that do seek mental health care, 50% receive it solely from their general physician. This means that half of all the mental health care in the United States is provided by general medical providers (Narrow et al., 1993). A very similar service utilization picture emerged in the more recent National Co-Morbidity Study (Kessler et al., 1994). To Compound the problem, these addressed the service use characteristics of the bewildering number of patients with life stress, losses, conflicts and illnesses requiring lifestyle adjustment that are routinely seen in primary care. For example, 50% of randomly sampled primary care patients have clinically elevated depression or anxiety levels (VonKorff et al., 1987). The magnitude of the behavioral services provided overall becomes more obvious when we consider that fully 70% of all psychotropic medications are prescribed by general physicians (Beardsley et al., 1988), including 80% of all antidepressants. The continuous deluge of patients presenting with behavioral health needs makes it nearly impossible for the busy primary care physician to effectively address behavioral health concerns.

Health Care Seeking is a Complex Process

Whether or not people are physically ill, and even how ill they are, is *not* the primary determinant of whether they decide to seek medical care. Studies have suggested that only a quarter of the decision to seek health care is explained by disability or morbidity alone (Berkanovic, Telesky & Reeder, 1981). As Lynch (1993) suggests, the demand for health care may be triggered by health morbidity (the patient is vomiting blood), the patient's sense of need (the patient has a bad cold and just wants it "checked out"), the patients preference regarding specific types of health care (the patient wants only a doctor to look at a particular medical problem) and psychosocial motives (the health care visit is the patient's only social activity of the week).

Psychosocial Stress is a Major Cause of Medical Service Use

Nearly 70% of all health care visits have primarily a psychosocial basis (Fries et,. al., 1993; Shapiro et al., 1985). A recent study of the 10 most common complaints encountered in primary care among a large population sample revealed that less than 16% had a diagnosable physical etiology during a three year follow up period (Kroenke & Mangelsdorff, 1989). The most frequent psychosocial drivers of medical utilization are mental disorders, alcoholism/drug addiction, deficient social support, lack of coping skills, and a stressful home/work environment (cf. Friedman et al., 1995). To make matters worse, these factors frequently occur in combination among the highest utilizers of medical services (Katon et al., 1992). For example, a recent study suggests that, on average, primary care patients with even mild levels of depression use two times more health care services annually than their non-depressed counterparts (Simon, 1992).

Psychosocial Stresses Influence Health Status and the Course of Illness

Many seminal studies show that psychosocial factors are positively related to poor general health status, functional disability and long term health morbidity and mortality. Not surprisingly, each of these outcomes is strongly related to elevated medical costs. Self-perceptions of health status are related not only to the decision to seek health care, but also predict eventual objective health status (Sobel, 1995). Many patients respond to psychosocial stresses by developing vaguely defined, distressing physical symptoms that have no organic basis. Such patients can have very negative perceptions of their general health and are strongly motivated to seek health care to determine what the problem is (Smith, Monson & Ray, 1986).

Functional disability, a major aspect of quality of life and health status, is the loss of adaptive physical, social or occupational role functioning in response to a physical or mental illness. The negative impact of psychosocial distress on functional health status can be greater than most common chronic medical conditions. In terms of physical, role and social functioning, the Medical Outcomes Study revealed that depressive symptoms are more debilitating than diabetes, arthritis, gastrointestinal disorders, back problems, and hypertension (Wells et al., 1989). Functional disabilities are not only expensive to manage in the medical system, but are a primary concern for employers because of the pernicious effects of absenteeism and reduced productivity that often accompany functional disabilities.

Psychological distress, whether it contributes to or is the result of medical illness, can complicate medical treatment and increase medical costs. The risk of early morbidity, mortality and relapse among patients with chronic illness such as heart disease or cancer is strongly associated with depression, elevated psychological stress and deficient coping skills (Frasure-Smith, 1991; Fawzy et al., 1993). Compliance with prescribed medical treatments is directly and negatively effected by psychosocial variables such as depression, alcohol abuse and patient expectations and evaluations of care (Robinson, Wischman & Del Vento, 1996).

Health Care Decisions are Influenced by the Services Available

Ignoring the psychosocial needs of the patient often invites uncontrolled escalation in medical visits, hospitalizations and/or consumer dissatisfaction. Yet these needs must be responded to in a "15 minute" hour work environment that ordinarily lacks on-site, integrated behavioral health services (Strosahl, 1996a, 1996b). Many patients may present with masked symptoms of distress and instead be treated as if they had serious health problems, often with the effect of exponential increases in health care costs (Yingling et al., 1993).

If the time-pressured primary care physician cannot address these psychosocial needs, what options are open? Referral to an offsite behavioral health provider is essentially the only option a physician has other than to accept the additional time demands of managing the patient in toto. Even when the referral option is exercised, it is anything but a certainty that the patient will follow through. Discussions about seeking mental health services are often viewed as stigmatizing ("It's all in your head"). Referrals studies have consistently shown that only 1 in 4 patients sent to a behavioral health provider will actually show up for the initial appointment. More often than not, the primary care physician ignores the problem, reaches for the prescription pad to satisfy the patient or refers the patient to another medical specialist. The potential cost consequences of these actions are significant and often do not result in appreciable improvements in health care outcomes. At Group Health, Seretonin Re-uptake Inhibitors (SRI's), the vast majority prescribed by primary care providers, account for 1/7 of total pharmacy costs. At the same time, studies in the GHC system have shown that less than 50% of depressed primary care patients who are prescribed anti-depressants meet diagnostic criteria which establish suitability for anti-depressant therapy (Katon, et al., 1996). In a study of emergency room patients with chest pain, nearly 41% met criteria for either an anxiety or depressive disorder as a primary medical diagnosis (Yingling et al., 1993). Patients with psychosocial needs will continue to "travel" in both primary and specialty care medicine as long as there are no behavioral health services available at the point of contact.

The Medical Cost Offset Effect:
How Integrated Services Can Reduce Medical Costs

The term medical cost offset refers to a reduction in medical costs that occurs as a result of a patient receiving appropriately designed behavioral health services in lieu of medical services. There are two distinct types of medical cost offsets. One is a direct cost offset, in which more expensive medical services which would have been directed to an identified patient or immediate family members are defrayed by the provision of alternative behavioral health services. It is important to remember that cost offsets can be robust among immediate family members of an identified patient as well (McDonnell Douglas, 1986).

The second type of cost offset is indirect, in which the provision of behavioral health services produces cost savings through a general increase in system efficiency. A classic example of indirect cost offsets is the concept of "productivity leveraging." Here, the goal of integrated behavioral health care is to remove patients with basic psychosocial needs from physician schedules (instead such patients are seen by a behavioral health provider), so that patients with more acute medical needs have improved access. Theoretically, getting to these acutely ill patients earlier reduces the medical costs associated with treatment, while producing increased revenues from billable services due to the medical complexity of the patient. Thus, the money saved is not directly accrued from providing behavioral health services to the index patient, but rather is saved by increasing access to services for the seriously ill.

Many proponents of integrated care argue that potentially huge direct and indirect medical cost savings can be obtained through the integration of medical and behavioral health services. The purpose of this section is to review several important components of the contemporary cost offset literature. The reader interested in a much more detailed analysis of this literature should be aware that there are several excellent recent review articles available (Chiles, Lambert & Hatch, 1999; Friedman et al., 1995; Sobel, 1995; Strosahl & Sobel, 1996).

The Magnitude of Cost Offsets is Considerable

While the amount of cost savings varies, many studies suggest that provision of behavioral health services may be a major medical cost containment strategy. Cost savings in the vicinity of 20-40% are not uncommon for well-designed programs. For example, an intervention program targeting elderly patients hospitalized with hip fracture cost $40,000 in psychological and psychiatric consultative services, but reduced in-patient lengths of stay and associated medical expenses by $270,000, resulting in a net savings of roughly $1300 per patient (Strain et al., 1991). A targeted psychosocial intervention with "high utilizing" Medicaid outpatients found that medical costs declined by 21% at 18-months compared to a rise of 22% in those not receiving any mental health treatment (Pallak et al., 1995). This latter study is revealing because it demonstrates that providing brief therapy that is targeted to address a patient's most pressing life problems can have an immediate impact on health care seeking.

Many psychosocial interventions can produce better quality of care while simultaneously reducing overall medical costs. These savings are often substantial, as evidenced in a study which showed that a consultative intervention supporting primary care providers reduced annual medical charges by $289 (33%) for somaticizing patients while simultaneously improving their physical functioning (Smith et al., 1995). Integrated care can also impact the outcomes and costs associated with mental disorders in primary care. A recent randomized clinical trial testing the Integrated Care Program for Depression (Robinson, Wischman & Del Vento, 1996) found that depressed primary care patients treated in this model were nearly twice as likely to achieve clinical recovery, compared to their untreated depressed counterparts

(Katon et al., 1996). An associated cost effectiveness analysis revealed that, although the absolute costs of integrated treated were higher than "usual care", the aforementioned improvements in clinical response produced a net incremented cost effectiveness of $491 per patient (Von Koff et al., 1998).

A Variety of Medical Populations Have Cost Offset Potential

Cost offsets have been demonstrated for a wide variety of populations within primary care: parents with sick children, patients with chronic illness, arthritis, asthma, coronary artery disease, poor health habits (i.e., smoking, obesity, sedentary lifestyle), mental disorders (i.e., depression, anxiety/panic, somatization) and chronic pain syndrome. The types of interventions that have produced these effects include individual and family psychotherapy, groups, educational classes and reading materials, as well as systems for providing assessment and treatment information from behavioral health providers to primary care physicians. Interestingly, the largest medical cost offsets to date occur with pre-surgical preparations and basic behavioral medicine interventions. Both place less emphasis on "Traditional" psychotherapy and instead focus on patient education and self management strategies (

Cost Offsets are Observed in Both Primary and Specialty Care Populations

While most medical cost offset programs have been implemented in hospital based behavioral medicine settings, a new wave of cost offset research with primary care patients suggests this population may also be an important intervention target. Primary care based programs typically work with patients on stress management (relaxation, exercise, daily scheduling) and problem solving strategies for addressing life stresses (parenting a hyperactive child, reducing social isolation, addressing a marital conflict). Such programs also educate the patient in how unresolved stress can produce a variety of physical symptoms and a feeling of poor general health. One study of a program for high utilizing patients with distressing physical symptoms and significant psychosocial problems showed that, after six months, patients reported less physical and psychological discomfort while averaging two fewer health care visits than a control group of patients who did not participate in the program. The estimated net savings of the intervention were $85 per participant (Hellman, et al., 1990).

A Range of Integrative Services Can Address Behavioral Health Issues

Most of the early cost offset research involved measuring the impact of individual psychotherapy in reducing medical costs (Cummings & VandenBos, 1981). More recent studies suggest that a variety of interventions targeting psychosocial and informational needs can also reduce overall healthcare costs. These include brief behavioral health consultation (Smith et al., 1995, Drisbow & Bennett, 1993), videos (Robinson et al., 1989), printed materials and "bibliotherapy" (Kemper et al., 1993) classes and groups (Wilson et al 1993., Caudill et al., 1991) as well as support groups (Lorig, et al., 1993, Kennell et al., 1991). All of these approaches involve giving the patient the information and direction needed to solve life problems without seeking unneeded medical services.

Cost Offsets Vary Among Populations and Service Settings

The potential for cost offset is heavily dependent upon the population that is targeted and the types of medical services that will be offset. For example, a meta-analysis of the cost offset literature suggested that maximum cost offset potential exists among the elderly and primarily is accrued through a reduction of in-patient costs (Mumford et al., 1984). In contrast, cost offsets for younger adults are likely to be smaller and are obtained through a reduction in out-patient medical services.

The First Fork in the Road: Type I or Type II Change?

Before going further with this discussion, it is may be useful to recall the old Chinese saying: "If we don't figure out where we are going, we're bound to end up where we are headed." Inherent in the primary care integration movement is the risk that the mental health industry will fail to see the important differences between primary health care and the traditional speciality mental health model. Rather than engaging in Type II change (i.e., re-engineering), the natural tendency will be to simply apply the traditional concepts of specialty mental health to primary care settings, whether they fit or not. Proponents of the latter approach emphasize the importance of providing specialty mental health care in collaboration with interested physicians (Doherty & Baird, 1983; McDaniel, Campbell & Seaburn, 1990). In this perspective, the mental health provider operates as the "house shrink" within the primary care clinic, taking troublesome patients into therapy and essentially providing the medical team better access to specialty mental health care. This approach is easy to sell and has the feel of "god, mother and apple pie" to many mental health providers, because it requires only a small refinement of the existing mental health specialty model (i.e., Type I change).

Practical experience suggests that following this approach is a formula for failure. Addressing the formidable needs of the primary care patient population is not simply a matter of applying old mental health philosophies, skills and interventions in a new setting. Providing behavioral health services in primary medicine requires fundamentally different philosophies and skill sets than is the case in specialty mental health work. The work pace is faster, the needs of the patient population are more heterogenous, the team context of primary care is dramatically different and the amount of demand for behavioral health services far exceeds the capacity of a mental health specialty approach. At Group Health, providers who adopted the specialty mental health role in primary clinics were quickly overwhelmed with demand and were effectively inaccessible to the majority of physicians. Once physicians discovered that access was a problem, referrals dried up. In those clinics where behavioral health providers promoted collaborative treatment sessions involving the behavioral health provider, physician and patient, a very small minority of primary care physicians engaged the service. The uninvolved physicians cited the negative effects of lost practice time for the remainder of their patients and a general skepticism about the need for conjoint visits. Perhaps more importantly, providing mental health specialty services in primary care quickly marginalized the behavioral health providers. They were not viewed as primary care providers, but rather as visiting mental health specialists. This had a dramatic impact on the types of patients referred for behavioral health services. Generally, those patients with serious mental disorders or who were disruptive to the normal flow of daily practice were referred. While these patients certainly required care, the opportunity was lost to effect the lives of hundreds of other patients with less flagrant mental health issues.

In contrast, providers trained in behavioral medicine and health psychology concepts were much more successful in their attempts to integrate. These providers specifically avoided the role of "house shrink" and instead engaged physicians around the value of brief patient centered behavioral health consultations and the temporary co-management of certain patients. These providers developed and led patient education classes for at risk populations, participated in group care clinics with members of the primary care team and used the forum of consultation and co-management to improve the psychosocial interventions of primary care team members. As a rule, these providers had few problems with access, were utilized by nearly every primary care provider and were generally viewed as core members of the medical team. In conclusion, there is no guarantee that the integration movement will succeed, and the risk of eventual failure will exponentially increase if mental health providers refuse to "think out of the box."

Population-Based Care: The Underpinning of Integrative Care

The population based care model is an enormously flexible and powerful framework for sorting through and resolving the key issues regarding the most workable structure of an integrated care system. Population based care is grounded in public health concepts that are unfamiliar to most behavioral health providers. Briefly, the public health "mission" is not just to address the needs of the "sick" patient, but to think about similar patients in the population who may be at risk, or who are sick and do not seek care. A population based planning process starts with the following questions: What percentage of the population have conditions like this? How many seek care? Where do they seek care? Are there variations in the services provided that can be linked to differential clinical outcomes? Are there interventions that can prevent the occurrence of this condition in patients who have similar risk factors?

When developing a planning and implementation framework for integrated behavioral health services, focusing on population based care concepts is critical. For example, what types of behavioral health service needs exist in the primary care population of interest? What service delivery model can increase penetration into the whole population? What services can be efficiently provided for the "common causes" of psychological distress? When are more intensive clinical pathway interventions appropriate in the primary care setting? When is a patient more likely to benefit from a referral for specialty mental health care? These are just a few of the critical planning questions that must answered to permit an integrated service to function properly in general medicine.

Horizontal and Vertical Integration:
Two Complementary Integration Models

In the population care approach, there are two distinct but complementary approaches to providing integrative primary care: horizontally and vertically organized programs.

Horizontal integration is the most basic form of integrative service, because almost any behavioral health concern can benefit from a well conceived general behavioral health service. Horizontal integration programs are built to penetrate as much of the primary care population as possible. The goal is to deliver a large volume of brief, targeted psychosocial services with the result that the behavioral health of the entire population is systematically improved. Traditional primary care medicine is largely based upon the horizontal integration approach. As many as 80% of all patients in a primary care catchment will receive at least one medical service annually; however, few patients will receive highly specialized care. Patients who truly require medical specialists are referred to hospital based consultation and treatment centers. Similarly, in the horizontal integration approach, medical patients with severe disorders that cannot be managed in primary care are referred for specialty mental health care.

Vertical integration involves providing targeted, specialized behavioral health services to a well defined sub-population, for example, primary care patients with major depression. This deployment of vertically organized care pathways is a major theme in contemporary medical practice and is variously referred to as chronic disease or chronic condition management. Typically, vertical integration programs are designed to systematically provide care for high frequency and/or high cost patient populations such as depression, panic disorder, chemical dependency and somatization. With respect to frequency, a complaint that is represented frequently in the population (like depression) is a good candidate for a special process of care. With respect to cost, some rare conditions are so costly that they require a special system of care, for example, patients with chronic back pain.

Primary Mental Health Care:
The Service Philosophy of Integrated Care

Several recent publications have described a primary mental health care approach to integrated services (Strosahl, 1998, 1997,1996a, 1996b, 1994b, Strosahl et al., 1997, Quirk et al., 1995). While the term may imply that the focus is primarily on providing mental health services, the model itself carries a very broad definition of what constitutes effective integrative care. Managing the psychosocial aspects of chronic and acute diseases (i.e., behavioral medicine), using behavioral concepts to address lifestyle and health risk issues (i.e., health psychology) and providing consultation and co-management in the treatment of mental disorders and psychosocial issues all fall within the purview of this approach. In this sense, primary mental health is consistent with the philosophy, goals and strategies of primary care medicine. Specifically, there is an emphasis on early identification and treatment, long term prevention and "wellness". Primary mental health services are designed to support and increase the effectiveness of primary care providers. There is no attempt to take charge of the patient's care, as would be the case in a specialty mental health approach. Rather, the goal is to manage the patient within the structure of the primary care team, with the behavioral health provider functioning as a core team member.

Structurally, the primary mental health model is designed to meet the great demand for behavioral health services existing in the primary care population. As discussed in a previous section, this model of care involves providing direct consultative services to primary care providers and, where appropriate, engaging in time limited collaborative management of patients who require more extensive services. Consultations and brief targeted interventions are delivered as the first level of care for patients with behavioral health needs. If a patient fails to respond to this level of intervention, or obviously needs specialized treatment, the patient is referred on for specialty mental health care (Strosahl, 1994b). Typically, consultation visits are brief (15-30 minutes), limited in number (1-3 visits), and are provided in the general medicine wing. Often, patient contacts occur in exam rooms or in offices nested within the medicine unit. This makes referrals from primary care team members seem routine and "seamless". As far as the patient is concerned, a behavioral health consultation is just another routine primary care service. Done properly, a team referral completely removes the stigma associated with receiving a behavioral health service and, consequently, many populations that are notoriously resistant to receiving specialty mental health services (i.e., the elderly, ethnic and cultural minorities) will readily accept a primary mental health referral.

Relationship of Horizontal and Vertical Integration Strategies

Generally, a properly designed integrative care system must respond to a) the severity and complexity of the identified behavioral health needs within the population to be served and b) provide services in a way that can address the heightened percentage of the primary care population that will access services. Whereas a certain percentage of patients obtain benefit from consultation and very brief intervention visits, patients with more complicated problems are better addressed in "critical pathways", where fairly sophisticated services can be delivered in a cost effective manner. To be fully integrated, a system needs to have a combination of highly accessible general behavioral health services, as well as targeted clinical pathways capable of addressing the needs of high frequency and/or high impact sub-populations.

As mentioned previously, many primary care patients can be managed using a horizontally integrated general consultation approach. Even patients who otherwise might be good candidates for a critical pathway program can still benefit from a basic services that focus on personal problem solving and the effective use of coping skills. In addition to helping the patient, an implicit goal of consultation is to raise the skill level of the primary care team members so that "routine" problems are more effectively address within the context of the 10 minute medical visit. Primary care providers learn best through consultation and shared co-management. By sharing hundreds of cases, it is possible to improve the general level of care provided during medical visits, even if the behavioral health provider is never involved.

Within general medicine, there is a sub-population of patients with multiple psychological and, often, concurrent physical health issues who consume inordinate amounts of health care resources. Often, these services are delivered without appreciable clinical benefit. High utilizing patients are frustrating for medical providers because they can easily disrupt daily practice schedules, tend to elicit unnecessary medical tests and procedures, as well as create a sense of failure in the provider. The behavioral health provider must be able to provide consultation and co-management services over time for this troublesome patient group. This form of itegrated care is described as **specialty consultation**. The goals of this approach are threefold: 1) create effective team based utilization management plans that curtail unscheduled and unnecessary medical visits; 2) shift the burden of services from the medical providers to the behavioral health provider (i.e. "funneling the patient"); 3) create a behavior change plan that focuses on basic functional outcomes (rather than symptom elimination) that can be monitored and reinforced by every member of the medical team. Often, multi-problem medical patients will be managed within the specialty consultation model over several years.

This integrated program level of primary mental health is designed for high frequency and high impact primary care populations such as major depression, panic disorder, somatization and alcohol abuse. Integrated programs use condensed evidence based interventions that are tailored for the fast work pace of primary care. The intent is for the behavioral health provider to temporarily co-manage the patient with various members of the primary care team Typically, more behavioral health services are provided in vertically integrated programs than is true for horizontal programs. This fact notwith-standing, the emphasis of the clinical interventions is quite similar: patient education, self management skills, compliance with medication and creating a context where primary care team members can reinforce and build upon each other's interventions. An excellent example is the Integrated Care Program for Depression, in which a primary care provider and behavioral health consultant work together in a structured program which combines cognitive behavioral and/or pharmacotherapy treatments for patients with major depression or depressive symptoms secondary to life stress (Robinson, 1996; Robinson, Wischman & Del Vento, 1996). Research indicates that, compared to the usual care available in general medicine settings, the Integrated Care Program produced superior clinical outcomes, better medication compliance, increased use of coping strategies by patients, more satisfied patients and primary health care providers (Katon et al., 1996; Robinson et al., 2001). Interestingly, the remission rates and overall effect sizes obtained in these studies compare very favorably to those reported in specialty field trials examining the effects of cognitive behavioral and medication treatments for depression. This occurred, despite the fact that the Integrated Care Program only required 3-4 total hours of behavioral health services, a quarter of the session time normally required to achieve the same result using a mental health specialty approach.

Building Successful Integrated Care Systems: From Design to Implementation

The lessons learned at Group Health and other systems I have consulted with over the past decade suggest that there are many potential barriers to implementing a sound integrative care system. From the planning perspective, the most important obstacle is the lack of an accepted model of care. In many systems, programs as diverse as off site behavioral medicine classes, conjoint therapy sessions with physicians and general health promotion classes will all be swept under the rubric of integrated care. In a sense, it is better to describe such efforts as part of a incomplete patchwork quilt. The pieces are there, but there is no overall scheme that helps put the pieces in the right place. The perspective of population based care can do much to create a picture of what the quilt should look like, while the threads of horizontal and vertical program planning tie the system together.

Our experience does indeed suggest that there are certain rules of the road for building integrated systems that work. *In general, the main "mileposts" involve three core areas: Co-location of services, addressing the full spectrum of need and affirming the basic mission of primary mental health care.*

Providing on site services is an absolutely essential component of an integrated care system. The most effective integrated programs have a behavioral health provider "nested" in the medicine practice area. This creates an ongoing presence for behavioral health services, provides countless opportunities for "curbside consultations" with primary care providers and eliminates most of the resistance patients have about seeing a behavioral health specialist. Even having a behavioral health pod on-site, but in a separate wing of the medical facility, creates a sense of separateness, reduces spontaneous consultations and increases the resistance level of patients. When co-locating a behavioral health provider, make sure that sufficient hours are made available to guarantee access for newly referred patients. In the typical case, this will require between 2-6 hours weekly for every 1000 primary care patients; depending upon the health care system.

The decision to fully co-locate ultimately boils down to the reallocation of precious office/exam room space (i.e., turf), and is a good test of the resolve of higher level medical and behavioral health leaders. In most systems, behavioral health providers are viewed as "non-sink" team members, that is, they don't require medical technology to do their work. Thus, when space gets tight, the behavioral health providers are the first to be off-loaded to a separate wing, a mobile office trailer in the parking lot, etc. Addressing this problem at the system level is at least a ten-year process, the usual time frame for new facility planning and construction. During the interim, sponsoring an integrated care system involves a commitment not to physically separate the behavioral health provider from the rest of the primary care team.

Several behavioral health companies now offer on-demand phone consultation to primary care providers. While this is a nice ancillary service, emergency consultative services are infrequently used, have limited impact on overall population health and are fundamentally disconnected from the process of routine primary care. In general, these types of programs reflect a half hearted commitment to integration, where keeping the carve out model intact and costs low are the ultimate objectives. In reality, integrated care and carved out services are at fundamental odds, both philosophically and structurally.

A second milepost in implementing an integrated care system is to assure that services are available to address the full spectrum of behavioral health needs within the primary care population. This requires implementing both horizontal and vertical integration programs that are carefully interconnected to ensure seamless patient flow. When resources are limited, it is possible to use the population based planning framework to determine which vertical programs (critical pathways) are likely to have the largest impact on the population. Similarly, our experience suggests that implementing an easily accessible consultation/brief intervention program makes sense when resources are tight or when the integration initiative is expected to be cost neutral.

A third milepost is the degree to which behavioral health services are consistent with the philosophies, goals and strategies of primary care. This is a subtle but powerful determinant of successful integration. For example, many systems have placed psychotherapists on site in primary care clinics, to provide specialty mental health care to physician referred patients. Physicians may receive intake reports, copies of session notes and may even participate in a conjoint session, when the occasion demands it. While the collaboration between mental health and primary care providers is certainly admirable, this approach essentially involves operating a mental health specialty service in a primary care clinic. Responsibility for care shifts to the mental health provider, who operates as a specialist. Paradoxically, falling into this approach reactivates the decades old marginalization of the mental health function in primary care. Managing the behavioral health needs of primary care patients is the responsibility of every provider on the primary care team, not just the behavioral health professional. Thus, even co-location of services and a collaborative care model do not guarantee that behavioral health services are integrated.

In a properly constructed integrative care system, behavioral health is not a specialty service, but is a routine component of medical care. A patient is just as likely to see a behavioral health provider as any other member of the primary care team. Primary mental health ideally showed me part of the patient's basic medical benefit. At the process of care level, behavioral health plays a significant part in evidence based medical practice algorithms and guidelines. For example, the patient who presents to urgent care with benign tachycardia is first evaluated for panic disorder before being referred on to cardiology. The patient who experiences a major life stress such as divorce is immediately referred for coping skills support. The patient's behavioral health goals are recorded in the medical chart, so that core coping strategies can be reinforced during routine medical visits. The patient who recovers from a major depression is monitored over time using a relapse prevention plan supported by the nurse, physician and behavioral health provider. At the primary care team level, preventing the occurrence of another depressive episode takes on the same importance as assuring the patient's general health. The advantages of a fully integrated approach are obvious: better coordination of care, better clinical outcomes, reduced medical costs and increased customer satisfaction. Most importantly, practicing side by side would allow primary care and behavioral health providers to learn from each other and form a thorough appreciation of the sublime interdependence of the psyche and soma.

The Roles of Different Mental Health Disciplines

In today's cost conscious environment, behavioral health administrators are facing a question of fundamental significance for the future of behavioral health. Specifically, they must attempt to determine what the unique roles of the different mental health disciplines will be in the care giving system of the future. How should psychiatrists, psychologists and master's level providers be used and what should the provider mix be? This question is also confronting the architects of integrated delivery systems, usually in cost neutral environments where the issue is what resources need to be shifted to the primary care setting without dismantling the capacity to provide mental health specialty care. Given the obvious disciplinary survival issues at stake, it is no accident that this hotly contested issue elicits the worst in self serving guild based rhetoric. Attempts to homogenize all mental health providers ignore the fact that there are huge differences both in the intensity and philosophical orientation of gradute training for each of the major provider groups. On the other hand, reifying a particular group because of its degree or type of training ignores the fact any provider from any training background can be a superb primary behavioral health provider. Correspondingly, even the most advanced degree does not guarantee success in primary care. To sort through this maze of politically charged issues, it will be useful to examine what the unique contributions of each discipline can be. This approach assumes that all the mental health disciplines are needed and can have a value added impact in an integrated care system.

Psychiatry and other prescribing medical disciplines such as Physicians Assistants and Advanced Practice Nurses generally have special expertise in psychopharmacology and are well grounded in the medical aspects of psychological disorders. This makes them ideally suited for managing medically complicated patients who require psychotropic medicines and consulting with primary care providers with the goal of improving general prescription practices. Indeed, this consultation liaison approach has been shown to readily improve anti-depressant prescription practices (Katon et al., 1995). At the same time, the increased expense involved in using prescribing providers mandates that they not act as "front line" primary care providers. Rather, they should see the most difficult types of patients (i.e., medically ill, medication non-responders, chronically mentally ill) while at the same time being available to provide on demand consultation on medical and prescribing issues to non-medically trained behavioral health providers.

Psychologists receive in-depth training in the application of behavioral principles to psychological disorders, medical illness, and health risk factors. As such, psychologist can readily develop and implement behavioral medicine and health psychology interventions, both at the individual, class and group levels. In addition, psychologist are expected to be proficient in all aspects of program design and evaluation, including the creation of treatment manuals, constructing research designs and analyzing research data. Psychologists are more likely to have exposure to and training in evidence based procedures for complicated conditions such as chronic pain, major depression, obsessive compulsive disorder and so forth. Consequently, the optimal use of psychologists is to have them focus on building behavioral medicine and health psychology "pathways", provide training and consultation in the use of effective clinical procedures and help manage high utilizing multi-problem patients within the primary care team environment. Similar to psychiatrists, psychologists cost more to deploy in the field and, for that reason, may not be used as "front line" providers in every system.

Masters level providers, particularly social workers, tend to receive in-depth training in the social, systems and familial aspects of psychological and medical conditions. They often have training in medical social work principles and can provide case management and linkages with community programs and resources. This unique training background allows the master's level provider to fit well into the primary care team setting, with its overall emphasis on gatekeeping and effective triage. Equally important, master's level providers are capable of providing basic consultation and intervention services. The fact that masters level clinicians tend to be the least expensive licensed providers means that they may be the "backbone" of many integrated delivery systems. They typically will be used to manage "garden variety" behavioral health problems, implement manualized integrated care programs and provide case management services when the need arises.

SUMMARY

Without doubt, the next era of managed care will be oriented toward improving the overall quality of care to consumers by integrating services within fewer settings. This provides an opportunity to re-connect medical and behavioral health services in a way that could dramatically increase the public health. This is not something that should be recklessly pursued. Instead, there is a need to develop a sound, cost effective approach that can generalize across rural and urban settings, network and staff delivery systems and a wide variety of health insurance plans. The primary mental health model articulated in this presentation has been implemented successfully in a number of different settings. It appears to be cost effective, maximizes the unique contributions of the various provider groups and has significant empirical support in the outcome literature. Clinicians, administrators and researchers may find this approach intriguing and worthy of further exploration.

REFERENCES

Beardsley, R, Gardocki, G, Larson D., & Hidalgo, J. (1988). Prescribing of psychotropic medication by primary care physicians and psychiatrists. *Archives of General Psychiatry, 45,* 1117-1119.

Berkanovic, E., Telesky, C., & Reeder, S. (1981). Structural and social psychological factors in the decision to seek medical care for symptoms. *Medical Care, 21,* 693-709.

Caudill M., Schnabel R., Zuttermeister P., Benson H., & Friedman R. (1991) Decreased clinic use by chronic pain patients: Response to behavioral medicine interventions. *Clinical Journal of Pain, 7,* 305- 310.

Chiles, J., Lambert, M. J., & Hatch, A. L. (1999). The impact of psychosocial interventions on medical cost offset: A meta-analytic review. *Clinical Psychology: Science and Practice, 6(2),* 204-220.

Cummings, N. (1995). Impact of managed care on employment and training: A primer for survival. *Professional Psychology: Research and Practice, 26,* 10-15.

Cummings, N., & VandenBos G. (1981). The twenty years Kaiser-Permanente experience with psychotherapy and medical utilization: Implications for national health policy and national health insurance. *Health Policy Quarterly, 1,* 159-175.

Drisbow E., Bennett H., & Owings J. (1993). Effect of preoperative suggestion on postoperative gastrointestinal motility. *Journal of Western Medicine, 158,* 488-492.

Doherty, W., & Baird, M. (1983). Family therapy and family medicine. New York: Guilford.

Fawzy, F., Fawzy, N., & Hyun, C. (1993). Malignant melanoma: Effects of an early structured psychiatric intervention, coping, and affective state on recurrence and survival six years later. *Archives of General Psychiatry, 50,* 681-689.

Ferguson, T. (1996). *Health online.* Reading, MA: Addison-Welsey.

Frasure-Smith, N. (1991). In-hospital symptoms of psychological stress as predictors of long-term outcome after acute myocardial infarction in men. *American Journal of Cardiology, 67,* 121-127.

Friedman, R., Sobel, D., Myers, P., Caudill, M., & Benson, H. (1995). Behavioral medicine, clinical health psychology and cost offset. *Health Psychology, 14,* 509-518.

Fries, J., Koop, C., & Beadle, C. (1993). Reducing health care costs by reducing the need and demand for medical services. *The New England Journal of Medicine, 329,* 321-325.

Hellman, C., Budd, M., Borysenko, J., McClelland, D., & Benson H. (1990). A study of the effectiveness of two group behavioral medicine interventions for patients with psychosomatic complaints. *Behavioral Medicine, 16,* 165-173.

Katon, W., Robinson, P., Von Korff, M., Lin, E., Bush, T., Ludman, E., Simon, G., & Walker, E. (1996). A multifaceted intervention to improve treatment of depression in primary care. *Archives of General Psychiatry, 53,* 924-932.

Katon, W., Von Korff, M., & Lin, E., Bush, T., Lipscomb, P., & Russo, J. (1992). A randomized trial of psychiatric consultation with distressed high utilizers. *General Hospital Psychiatry, 14,* 86-98.

Katon, W., Von Korf, M., Lin, E., Walker, E., Simon, G., Bush, T., Robinson, P., & Russo, J. (1994). Collaborative management to achieve treatment guidelines: Impact on depression in primary care. *Journal of the American Medical Asociation, 273,* 1026-1031.

Kemper, D., Lorig K., & Mettler, M. (1993). The effectiveness of medical self-care interventions: A focus on self-initiated responses to symptoms. *Patient Education and Counseling, 21,* 29-39.

Kennell, J., Klaus, M., McGrath, S., Robertson, S., & Hinkley C. (1991). Continuous emotional support during labor in a United States hospital: A randomized controlled trial. *Journal of the American Medical Association, 265,* 2197-2237.

Kessler, R., Nelson, C., McGonagle, K., Liu, J., Swartz, M., & Blazer, D. (1994). Lifetime and twelve month prevalence of DSM-III-R psychiatric disorders in the United States. *Archives of General Psychiatry, 51,* 8-19.

Kroenke, K., & Mangelsdorff, A. (1989). Common symptoms in ambulatory care: Incidence, evaluation, therapy and outcome. *American Journal of Medicine, 86,* 262-266.

Lorig, K., Holman, H., Sobel, D., Laurent, D., Gonzalez, V., & Minor, M. (1994). *Living a healthy life with chronic conditions.* Palo Alto, CA: Bull Publishing Company.

Lorig, K., Mazonson, P., & Holman, H. (1993). Evidence suggesting that health education for self-management in patients with chronic arthritis has sustained health benefits while reducing health care costs. *Arthritis and Rheumatology, 36,* 439-446.

Lynch, W. (1993). The potential impact of health promotion on health care utilization: An introduction to demand management. *Association for Worksite Health Promotion Practitioner's Forum, 8,* 87-92.

McDonnell-Douglas Corporation. (1989). *Employee Assistance Program Financial Cost Offset Study,* 1985-1988.

McDaniel, S., Campbell, T., & Seaburn, D. (1990). Family-oriented primary care: A manual for medical providers. New York: Springer-Verlag.

Mumford, E., Schlesinger, H., & Glass, G. (1984). A new look at evidence about reduced cost of medical utilization following mental health treatment. *American Journal of Psychiatry, 141,* 1145-1158.

Narrow, W. Reiger, D., Rae, D., Manderscheid, R., & Locke, B. (1993). Use of services by persons with mental and addictive disorders: Findings from the National

Institute of Mental Health Epidemiologic Catchment Area Program. *Archives of General Psychiatry, 50,* 95-107.

Pallak, M., Cummings, N., Dorken, H., & Hanke, C. (1995) Effect of mental health treatment on medical costs. *Mind/Body Medicine, 1,* 7-12.

Quirk, M., Strosahl, K., Todd, J., Fitzpatrick, W., Casey, M., Hennessey, S., & Simon, G. (1995). Quality and customers: Type II change in mental health delivery within health care reform. *Journal of Mental Health Administration, 22,* 414-425.

Reiger, D., Narrow, W., Rae, D., Manderschied, R., Locke, B., & Goodwin, F. (1993). The de facto US mental and addictive disorders service system: Epidemiologic catchment area prospective one-year prevalence rates of disorders and services. *Archives of General Psychiatry, 50,* 85-94.

Robinson, J., Schwartz, M., & Magwene, K. (1989). The impact of fever health education on clinic utilization. *American Journal of Disabled Children, 143,* 698-704.

Robinson, P., Katon, W., Von Korff, M., Bush, T., Ludman, E., Simon, G., Lin, E., & Walker, E. (*Manuscript under review*). Effects of a combined treatment for depressed primary care patients on behavioral change and process of care variables.

Robinson, P., Katon, W., Von Korf, M., Bush, T., Ludman, E., Simon, G., & Walker, E. (*Manuscript under review*). Psychologists treat depression in primary care: What changes when depression scores improve?

Robinson, P. (1996). *Living life well: New strategies for hard times.* Reno, NV: Context Press.

Robinson, P., Wischman, C., & Del Vento, A. (1996). *Treating depression in primary care: A manual for primary care and mental health providers.* Reno, NV: Context Press.

Shapiro, S., Skinner, E., & Kessler, L. (1984). Utilization of health and mental health services: Three epidemiologic catchment area sites. *Archives of General Psychiatry, 41,* 971-978.

Simon, G. (1992). Psychiatric disorder and functional somatic symptoms as predictors of health care use. *Psychiatric Medicine, 10,* 49-60.

Simon, G., VonKorff, M., & Barlow, W. (1995). Health care costs of primary care patients with recognized depression. *Archives of General Psychiatry, 52,* 850-856.

Smith, G., Rost, K., & Kashner, T. (1995). A trial of the effect of a standardized psychiatric consultation on health outcomes and costs in somatizing patients. *Archives of General Psychiatry, 52,* 238-243.

Sobel, D. & Ornstein R. (1996). *The healthy mind, healthy body handbook.* Los Altos, CA: DRx Publishing.

Sobel, D. (1995). Rethinking medicine: Improving health outcomes with cost-effective psychosocial interventions. *Psychosomatic Medicine, 57,* 234-244.

Spitzer, R., Kroenke, K., Linzer, M., Hahn, S., Williams, J., deGruy, F., Brody, D., & Davies, M. (1995). Health related quality of life in primary care patients with mental disorders. *Journal of the American Medical Association, 274,* 1511-1517.

Strain, J., Lyons, J., Hammer, J., & Fahs, M. (1991). Cost offset from a psychiatric consultation-liaison intervention with elderly hip fracture patients. *American Journal of Psychiatry, 148,* 1044-1049.

Strosahl, K. (1998). Integration of primary care and behavioral health services: The primary mental health care model. In A. Blount (Ed.), *Integrative primary care: The future of medical and mental health collaboration* (pp. 43-66). New York: Norton.

Strosahl, K. (1997). Building primary care behavioral health systems that work: A compass and a horizon. In N. Cummings, J. Cummings & J. Johnson (Eds.), *Behavioral health in primary care: A guide for clinical integration* (pp. 37-68). Madison, CT: Psychosocial Press.

Strosahl, K. (1996a). Primary mental health care: A new paradigm for achieving health and behavioral health integration. *Behavioral Healthcare Tomorrow, 5,* 93-96.

Strosahl, K. (1996b). Confessions of a behavior therapist in primary care: The odyssey and the ecstasy. *Cognitive and Behavioral Practice, 3,* 1-28.

Strosahl, K. (1995) Behavior therapy 2000: A perilous journey. *the Behavior Therapist, 18,* 130-133.

Strosahl, K. (1994a). Entering the new frontier of managed mental health care: Gold mines and land mines. *Cognitive and Behavioral Practice, 1,* 5-23.

Strosahl, K. (1994b). New dimensions in behavioral health primary care integration. *HMO Practice, 8,* 176-179.

Strosahl, K., Baker, N., Braddick, M., Stuart, M., & Handley, M. (1997). Integration of behavioral health and primary care services: The Group Health Cooperative Model. In N. Cummings, J. Cummings, & J. Johnson (Eds.), *Behavioral health in primary care: A guide for clinical integration* (pp. 61-86). Madison, CT: Psychosocial Press.

Strosahl, K., & Sobel, D. (1996). Behavioral health and the medical cost offset effect: Current status, key concepts and future applications. *HMO Practice, 10,* 156-162.

Von Korff, M., & Simon, G. (1996). The prevalence and impact of psychological disorders in primary care: HMO research needed to improve care. *HMO Practice, 10,* 150-155,

Von Korff, M., Shapiro, S., Burke, J., Teitlebaum, M., Skinner, E., German, P., Turner, R., Klein, L., & Burns, B. (1987). Anxiety and depression in a primary care clinic: Comparison of diagnostic interview schedule, general health questionnaire and practitioner assessments. *Archives Of General Psychiatry, 44,* 152-156.

Wells, K., Steward, A., Hays, R., Burnam, M., Rogers, W., Daniels, M., Berry, S., Greenfield, S., & Ware, J. (1989). The functioning and well being of depressed patients: Results from the medical outcomes study. *Journal of the American Medical Association, 262,* 914-919.

Yingling, K., Wulsin, L., Arnold, L., & Rouan, G. (1993). Estimated prevalences of panic disorder and depression among consecutive patients seen in an emergency department with acute chest pain. *Journal of General Internal Medicine, 8,* 2315.

Discussion of Strosahl:

Take Me to Your Leader!

Linda J. Hayes
University of Nevada, Reno

The experience and accomplishments of Kirk Strosahl in bringing about needed changes in systems of managed behavioral health care makes him a leader in this field. My aim in this commentary, therefore, is not to contest his analysis of these complex issues, but rather to further the discussion of one aspect of his exposition, namely, the unique roles of different mental health disciplines in the care giving system.

Strosahl outlines the appropriate responsibilities of three classes of professionals for the delivery of mental health services in accordance with the skills they are assumed to have, and given the costs of their involvement in this process. His suggestions in this regard are briefly reviewed in the following section.

Professionals' Roles in Caregiving

Psychiatrists and other prescribing medical professionals are regarded as having special expertise in psychopharmacology and the medical aspects of psychological disorders. As such, they are well suited to the management of medically complicated patients who require psychotropic medications, as well as to the improvement of prescribing practices of primary care providers. The salaries of professionals in this class prohibit their participation as front line care providers, however.

Psychologists are regarded as having expertise in the application of behavioral principles to the management of psychological disorders and medical conditions, as well as in program design and evaluation. They are said to be suited to the role of assuring the use of effective clinical procedures,

Integrated Behavioral Healthcare: Positioning Mental Health Practice with Medical/Surgical Practice

particularly with high-utilizing multi-problem patients. As with medically trained professionals the salaries of these professions prohibit their deployment as front line caregivers.

Finally, Masters' level providers are regarded as having expertise in case management and community service linkages, as well as are held capable of executing manualized interventions for patients with less complicated behavioral health problems. These are, thereby, the appropriate roles of these professionals; and given their lower salaries; they are most appropriately employed as front line care providers.

Strosahl's arguments are compelling with one exception; namely, he fails to specify which of these professional classes most appropriately assumes the responsibility of the team leader. My commentary focuses on this issue.

TREATMENT EFFECTIVENESS

To determine which of these professions is best suited for leadership in these circumstances, we may examine their qualifications as they apply to the responsibilities of this role; and to do so, we must first delineate these responsibilities. Generally speaking, leadership is observed in the outcomes achieved by the group led. In the present context, thereby, the leader's primary responsibility is to assure *continuous improvement in treatment effectiveness*, as measured in the *quality* of treatment outcomes achieved in relation to the *efficiency* with which they are achieved. Assuring continuous improvement in treatment effectiveness is a complicated issue, though, as neither quality nor efficiency is readily documented such as to claim its demonstration.

Treatment Effectiveness as the Quality of Treatment Outcome

With regard to the quality of treatment outcome, both definitional and measurement problems must be acknowledged. Measures of treatment outcome tend to be rather primitive. For the most part, they amount to decontextualized verbal reconceptualizations of one's own well-being, garnered under conditions of rather powerful demand, and in the absence of corroborating evidence of change in related acts in context.

Despite the limitations of such measures, they continue to be adopted, and there are several reasons why this is so. Among them are the assumptions that verbal behavior is referential in nature, such that what one says about a circumstance mirrors that circumstance; and secondly, that an individual has special advantage with regard to describing circumstances in which he or she participates. Both of these assumptions are questionable. Verbal behavior is not profitably regarded as a tool to communicate one's experience of the world. It is, itself, behavior; and it is multiply controlled. Moreover, not all of its controlling variables are found in the circumstances it is purported to mirror. Secondly, self-knowledge is of social origin, as Skinner (1957) has so eloquently explained, and its elaboration varies across a wide range in concert with the verbal community to which an individual has been exposed. Even a description of one's own *behavior* tends to be compromised by motivational factors, let alone descriptions of its *controlling variables* or, more commonly, the reasons for it.

More objective measures of well-being are not typically collected, in part because the behaviors indicative of them necessarily occur in contexts other than those in which treatment is ongoing, making the costs associated with collecting them prohibitive. In general, providers are aware of these problems with self-reports, as indicated by their tendency to corroborate the evidence of self-report by other, more indirect measures of treatment outcome.

Among the latter is service utilization. The logic here is that if utilization decreases, the need for treatment must have declined, such that the decrease in utilization is taken to provide support the evidence of well being gleaned from client satisfaction. The problem with this logic, though, is that both service utilization and client satisfaction are multiply determined. Decreased utilization, for example, is not only less likely if services are effective, but also less likely if they are ineffective, or are difficult to access, regardless of their effectiveness. Moreover, given that the life-long circumstances giving rise to even "garden variety" behavior heath problems are unlikely to be reconfigured, over the course of the increasingly brief interventions characteristic of managed behavioral health care, as to provide a magnitude of relief sufficient to constitute treatment success, any relief actually experienced may predict greater utilization to "finish the job."

The real problem here is not so much the measurement of treatment outcome but rather the nature of the treatment. That is to say, the inadequacies of outcome measurement are predicated on the assumptions underlying the practices employed to produce such outcomes in the first place. The practices of psychotherapy are founded on the same questionable assumptions concerning verbal behavior and self-acknowledge as guide the selection of treatment outcome metrics, with one important addition. The additional assumption is that changes in a person's decontextualized verbal behavior, should this occur in therapy, will produce changes in their verbal and nonverbal behaviors in relevant real-life contexts. Mental health problems are years in the making, though, and they are engaged by life circumstances that continue to prevail after the discontinuation of the treatment. These problems are not likely to be impacted substantially as a function of verbal discourse in even fifty units of such discourse, let alone four.

I do not mean by this to imply that extending the course of treatment is a solution to the problem of treatment effectiveness. Even if extending the course of treatment were to achieve a slightly higher quality of treatment outcome, it would, at the same time, serve to undermine efficiency metrics sufficiently to undermine treatment effectiveness overall; and, hence, would not solve the problem at hand.

In summary, I am not convinced that the job of assuring continuous improvement in treatment effectiveness will be accomplished by developing more adequate measures of the quality of treatment outcome. Better measures of treatment outcome are not worth the cost of their development until treatment practices have undergone a similar development.

The most often cited development of the latter is what has been called the "manualizing" of therapy. I am not convinced that this movement constitutes a development in the direction of improved therapeutic practices. The manualizing of therapy means only that more providers, without the training required to make independent treatment decisions, and whose involvement in the therapeutic process is thereby less expensive, are able to conduct the same sorts of verbal discourse, in roughly the same ways. It is the practice of discourse therapy itself that is the problem, not the rigidity with which it is conducted.

Having taken this stance, let me back up just a little by acknowledging that the manualizing of therapy movement is being fostered by those practitioners who are most inclined to conduct outcomes-based research on the therapeutic process. Hence, despite what I believe to be fundamental problems with both the practice of discourse therapy as well as the measures of its outcomes, the practices that *are* being manualized are more likely to produce a better quality of treatment outcome, however measured, than those that are not.

Manualizing treatment eliminates the need for decision-making on the parts of practitioners, and this circumstance prevails in many other professions with good effect. For example, all of the decisions regarding medical treatment, including those pertaining to psychotropic medications, are made by scientists in medical research facilities, not by practicing physicians and psychiatrists in medical clinics. The practice of medicine is fully manualized in other words, and the quantity of its achievements over the past hundred years or more greatly outstrips those of the undisciplined practice of psychotherapy.

Finally, whatever might be the long-term effects of manualization for the *quality* component of treatment effectiveness, its impact on the *efficiency* aspect of effectiveness cannot be underestimated. Manualizing is necessary to take advantage of the opportunity afforded by the participation of less costly care providers at the front lines of service delivery, and it will continue to be fostered for this reason.

Treatment Effectiveness as Measured in Efficiency

Efficiency is not accomplished solely by providing the tools needed to take advantage of masters' level participants in the delivery of *therapeutic* services, however. Cost savings are also available by way of their participation in *diagnostic* services. Diagnostic decisions impact the extent to which more expensive care providers are engaged in service delivery, and the adequacy of these decisions is thereby a critical determinant of the efficiency aspect of treatment effectiveness. Decision making of this sort is not regarded as one of the areas of expertise associated with lower cost providers, however; hence they are not typically engaged at the front lines of this aspect of treatment delivery.

It would seem to me that this is a problem that might also be solved by manualization. Again, the field of medicine provides an example of the beneficial effects of "manualization." Great strides have been made in the development of computerized diagnostic programs, and a comparable emphasis on the development of computerized psychological assessment would seem to be a source of tremendous savings in the managed care environment.

CONTINUOUS IMPROVEMENT IN TREATMENT EFFECTIVENESS

Returning to the issue of leadership, I suggested that this capacity was best measured in the outcomes achieved by the group led, and that the most significant outcome, for the leader of a behavior health care team to pursue, was continuous improvement in treatment effectiveness as it pertains to behavioral health. Treatment effectiveness, in turn, was argued to be measurable in the quality of the treatment outcome achieved and the efficiency with which it was achieved. As argued above, I believe that we have a long way to go with respect to the issue of quality. The opportunity to achieve a much higher standard of efficiency is available, though, and efficiency is no less important than quality in the make-up of treatment effectiveness.

Continuous improvement in treatment effectiveness is a different issue altogether, though, and one about which I have said very little. The success of a leader in assuring continuous improvement in treatment effectiveness depends on a set of skills that are assumed, by Strosahl, to be peculiar to only one class of professionals involved in the behavioral health care team, namely, the psychologist (and undoubtedly only a subdivision of this class.) These are the only professionals assumed to have the research skills necessary to assess whether or not the services rendered were the services needed to alleviate the problem presented (i.e., diagnostic effectiveness); and if so, whether the services rendered had this effect (i.e., therapeutic effectiveness.) The psychologist is the only member of the treatment team who is capable of making these decisions in a rigorous way, and for this reason, the psychologist is the only one capable of serving as an effective leader of a behavioral health care team. The highest paid professionals on teams typically assume the responsibilities of leadership, however. The higher salary is regarded as fair compensation for the burden of decision-making, as well as the discomfort of blame, in the case of wrong decisions. This is a legitimate argument so long as the burdens and discomforts of leadership are the issue. The history of behavioral health care suggests that this argument has held sway. In short, it has been the psychiatrist, not the psychologist on the mental health team, who has been willing to bear the burden and suffer the blame, and who has received the higher salary for doing so.

We are talking about the *future* of behavioral health care, though, not its history. The responsibilities of an effective leader in the managed behavioral health care environment do not include a willingness to bear the burden of decision making, nor to suffer the blame for wrong decisions, because decision-making is based on scientific data, for which no one is to blame, including the leader. It is the capacity to collect and interpret such data that constitutes the primary responsibility of the leader in this new and developing system of care. And if these responsibilities warrant a higher salary for the leader, so be it!

References

Skinner, B. F. (1957). *Verbal behavior*. New York: Appleton-Century-Crofts.

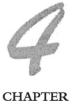

CHAPTER

Programmatic Approaches to Care and Outcomes: The Medical Co-Management Group Appointment

Jaylene Kent, Ph.D.
Division of Behavioral Medicine

Malcolm Gordon, M.D.
Kaiser Permanente, San Jose

Integrated Behavioral Healthcare: Positioning Mental Health Practice with Medical/Surgical Practice

BACKGROUND

The ushering in of a new era of healthcare not only has brought us demands for accountability, cost containment, and quality outcomes, but also an incentive for healthcare innovation to meet these demands. Perhaps there has never been a better climate for appreciating the innovations and cost savings offered by behavioral medicine, health psychology, and integrated approaches to health care, particularly in the primary care arena. As a practicing health psychologist and Subchief of the Division of Behavioral Medicine at San Jose/Kaiser Permanente, the first author and her colleagues have been in the forefront of developing innovative, cost effective clinical behavioral medicine programs for primary care patients for the past ten years. Two of those management programs, one for asthma and one for hypertension, both called "Medical Co-management Group Appointments" (MCGP) will be the focus of this chapter.

DEFINITION OF TERMS

Before further discussion, clarification of terms is necessary. On occasion, "behavioral medicine" has been used interchangeably with "behavioral health" or what has historically been known as "mental health". For the purposes of this chapter, "behavioral medicine" refers to a broad, interdisciplinary approach to health, not just mental health, and is the clinical application of psychoneuroimmunology. Often, clinical psychologists working in behavioral medicine are specialists called "clinical health psychologists". They are clinical psychologists with advanced training in medical settings who use cognitive, behavioral, and traditional psychological interventions to treat medical patients. They often have specialized knowledge in the nonpharmacologic management of particular medical illnesses, a focus on health rather than pathology, and an understanding of stress and its impact on health and illness.

DIVISION OF BEHAVIORAL MEDICINE AT KAISER PERMANENTE MEDICAL CENTER/SAN JOSE

It is within the framework described above that the Division of Behavioral Medicine at San Jose Kaiser has evolved. In general, the services of the Division focus on reducing physical and emotional symptoms related to illness or stress through group programs with: 1) an emphasis on both nonpharmacologic and traditional medical approaches to care, 2) skill building, self management, and lifestyle change, (building self efficacy), 3) improving quality of life, and/or, 4) identifying, treating, or referring psychiatric problems of the medically ill to specialty psychiatry when appropriate. Nearly all of the services in the Division are delivered in a group format by integrated teams of providers (health psychologists, physicians, social workers, and R.N.'s).

A Brief View of Group Approaches to Care

Group approaches to care are not a new idea. Psychological practitioners, health educators, and lay leaders have been meeting with patients/members for psychotherapy, education, skill building, and support for many years. Group psychotherapy has been identified as the treatment of choice for certain psychological disorders such as panic and chemical dependency and the successes of Alcoholics Anonymous, a lay led group, have been well established for many years (Cummings, et.al., 1997). In the medical arena, psychoeducational classes for medical patients taught by health educators and lay led chronic disease self-management groups have also demonstrated positive outcomes (Cumming, et.al., 1997). In summary, group care is associated with: 1) improved quality of care, 2) improved clinical efficacy, 3) improved patient/member satisfaction, 4) improved provider satisfaction, and 5) increased cost effectiveness (Cummings, et.al, 1997).

Integrated Group Treatment Comes to Primary Care

Building on both the long tradition of groups and skill building as a viable, cost effective model for delivering care and the belief that integrated care is better care, the medical co-management group appointment (MCGA) has evolved at San Jose/Kaiser. This appointment type has been used to treat nearly all populations with chronic medical conditions in both primary care and subspecialty arenas. A general description of this model is presented below.

An Integrated Approach to Care:
The Medical Co-Management Appointment (MCGA)

The goals of the Medical Co-Management Group Appointment (MCGA) are to deliver medical care equivalent to that of an individual medical appointment with a physician, but with the additional benefits of a peer support group, focused education, skill building, and the expertise of a health psychologist. This appointment type is a hybrid of group psychotherapy, a psychoeducational class, and an individual medical appointment.

In this model, ten to fifteen medical patients come together for a one and a half hour long group, which is co-led by a physician and a health psychologist. The meeting is often organized around a diagnostic theme, such as hypertension, irritable bowel syndrome, cancer, or asthma. During this time, not only is traditional medical care delivered by the physician (clinical interviews, focused clinical examinations, tests ordered, lab results discussed), psychological and behavioral expertise is delivered by the health psychologist. Genuine collaborative care happens in "real time" with the patients.

In addition to what is described above, a specific educational topic may be presented by the group leaders and skills particular to the illness may be taught, e.g., how to take your own blood pressure, to use a peak flow meter, or to use deep breathing for managing stress. All of this occurs in the milieu of group support.

An Overview of the MCGA Structure

Group format. Two different group formats may be used for the MCGA: "drop-in"/"open" or "closed", similar to traditional group psychotherapy.

Drop-in/open format. In this format, patients may "drop-in" to the group medical appointment without scheduling the visit. The M.D./Ph.D. team leaders accept "all comers" and the composition of the group often varies with each meeting. MCGP's with this format often meet weekly. The patients may or may not be specific to the physician co-leader's practice. Programs at San Jose/Kaiser using this format include those for asthma, congestive heart failure, irritable bowel syndrome and subspecialty care.

Closed format. In this format, patients are clustered into closed cohorts, much like a traditional, ongoing psychotherapy group. In other words, the same patients come together regularly for their medical group appointment. The periodicity for the meetings may be much greater in the closed format than the open format. For instance, the group may convene only once every four months rather than every week, which is often the case with the "drop in" groups. The patients may or may not be specific to the physician co-leader's practice. Programs at San Jose Kaiser using this format include those for hypertension and chronic benign pain management with long-term opiate use.

How to select a format. The key variable to consider when selecting a group format is access. If the clinical course of a disease is characterized by intermittent flare-up of symptoms or if there is subjective distress associated with symptoms, a drop-in/open format would be recommended as it allows for weekly treatment for those conditions. If access to the provider is difficult, e.g., the provider has a very busy practice; the creation of a group with a drop-in format might be very beneficial.

Co-Management Team Composition and Roles

The MCGA takes the traditional skills and roles of the health care team, physicians, psychologists, medical assistants, and patients, and brings them together in a new and synergistic way.

Primary Care M.D. One of the most notable challenges for the physician co-leader is being in the room with ten to fifteen medical patients at the same time. Although daunting initially, all physicians to date (approximately 15) have achieved some comfort level with this aspect of the model. A second major learning for the physician is working in tight collaboration with a psychologist. This is a new experience for most primary care practitioners. Generally, the psychologist can provide mentoring and cross training to the physician in both of these areas.

The additional tasks associated with the physician's role in the GCMA include:

> Recruiting patients into the program (i.e., screening for medical appropriateness, "selling the program", and inviting patients to join).
> Offering a broad range of typical medical interventions including focused physical examinations, ordering

lab tests, writing referrals, and discussing test results
during the group.
Providing preventative health care (immunizations,
health screening tests, counseling regarding risky
lifestyle behaviors, etc.).
Supporting non-pharmacological interventions which
may be introduced by the health psychologist.
Educating members/patient.
Charting.
Collaborative treatment planning with the psychologist
and patient.

Many of the tasks for the physician in the group appointment remain
similar to those of the individual appointment, but the emphasis on education,
life style change, and self efficacy is greatly enhanced.

Primary Care psychologist/health psychologist. A primary challenge for
the health psychologist is co-leading a group with a physician who has no
experience or training in this area. As in any successful co-therapist relationship, mentoring, communication, patience, and cooperation are key to developing a smooth co-leadership team. Another major challenge for the health
psychologist is becoming knowledgeable in the pathophysiology, medical,
and nonmedical management of a wide variety of medical conditions. Generally, the physician co-leader can provide cross training in this area.

Other specific responsibilities for the health psychologist include:

Facilitating group process.
Treatment goal setting in collaboration with the
physician and patient, generally including a
behavioral as well as medical component.
Identifying and treating/referring psychological
morbidity as appropriate.
Clinical interviewing, facilitating compliance,
enhancing self efficacy.
Educating/teaching members/patients.
Sharing expertise in the non-pharmacologic and
behavioral aspects of the medical condition
Charting.

Medical assistant. Most group appointments benefit from the support of a
medical assistant. Their role may most accurately be viewed as one of program
assistant. Many of the logistical and patient flow issues are the medical

assistant's responsibility, along with the execution of usual medical assistant and clerical functions. The tasks include:

> Scheduling the group appointments.
> Telephoning members/patients to remind them of the appointment.
> Ordering medical charts.
> Taking vital signs when patients arrive to the program.
> Managing patient flow (ensures there are at least ten to fifteen members per meeting).
> Maintaining group charts.
> Triaging telephone messages.
> Stocking group room with consults, laboratory slips, etc.
> Preparing patient information handouts and other member materials.

Member/patient as active participant. Perhaps the most radical shift in this approach to medical care is the active recruitment of the member/patient to the health care team. Nothing is more vital in the management of chronic illness than having the patient collaborating with the other members of the health care team to optimize wellness and to minimize symptoms and disease on quality of life. The MCGA's:

> Increase focus on self-care.
> Enhance self-efficacy and confidence in managing symptoms and health needs.
> Improve matching between type of provider and member need.
> Encourage participation in the treatment plan from development to implementation to monitoring and follow-up.

An enthusiastic attitude toward the program by the group co-leaders and medical assistant are key to programmatic success and engaging the member.

What Medical Conditions Respond Well To the MGCA?

The majority of chronic diseases can be handled in a MGCA. Those with the following characteristics may be especially responsive to this model:

> Chronic, usually lifelong medical conditions.

Conditions which demonstrate sub-optimal clinical
control despite utilization of considerable
healthcare resources.

When lifestyle and behavioral factors in combination
with medications are the accepted treatment.

When member/patient participation is critical to optimal
control.

If educational information helps members/patients
understand the disease process.

When there is high prevalence in the healthcare
membership.

Program Evaluation of MCMA's

Program evaluation data have been collected across a number of the
Medical Co-Management Group Appointments offered at San Jose/Kaiser. In
nearly all cases, each patient has served as their own control when looking
at clinical efficacy and health care utilization patterns. The specific areas of
interest for program evaluation included: 1) clinical efficacy, 2) medical/
pharmacy utilization, 3) patient satisfaction, and 4) provider satisfaction. One
trend are clinical efficacy programs, which are ssociated with:

Improvement in symptoms and clinical markers of
disease.

Reduction or optimization of pharmacological treatment.

Improved functional status/quality of life.

Another trend are medical/pharmacy programs, in which it is not a
surprise to see:

More appropriate and/or reduced use of medications.

More appropriate utilization of health care services.

The trend is improved member/patient satisfaction. Member satisfaction
surveys from programs consistently yield high scores. The majority of the
participants found the programs to be:

Convenient, as they had all of their medical needs met in
one visit and ready access to their provider.

Satisfying, as they often enjoyed the more extended time
with the providers.

A superior way to care for their illness.

A fourth trend Improved provider satisfaction. Both M.D. and Ph.D. providers found the model to be satisfying. It allows for:

> Broadening the skill set of providers through cross-fertilization.
> Professional stimulation.
> Diversity/variety in the workday.
> Convenient access to appropriate colleagues/teammates for consultation.
> Getting to know patients in a more complete way.
> True collaborative care.

Innovative MCGP'S: Hypertension and Asthma

Hypertension Medical Group Co-Management Program

Rational for program development. Traditional medical care for hypertension has mainly emphasized pharmacological treatment with less emphasis on behavioral factors and self-efficacy. However, research has clearly demonstrated that lifestyle modification including weight control, low sodium diet, regular aerobic exercise, and stress reduction can be important factors in blood pressure control (JNC, 1993). Additionally, traditional care for hypertension has largely relied upon blood pressure readings obtained in the medical clinic, even though clinic readings are well-known to be influenced by anxiety and stress related to the medical setting (white coat hypertension). White coat hypertension syndrome can often overestimate the level of hypertension, where as there is now ample evidence that home blood pressure recordings obtained by the patient are more reflective of overall hypertension control and the risk of developing end-organ damage.

The authors believed that an integrated group program utilizing home blood pressure readings might be a superior model for delivering care to these patients. To this end, they developed and continue to pilot a hypertension MGCP with a closed format for patients with uncomplicated hypertension.

Group membership and referral. Members were eligible to join the group program if they:

> Were in the primary care physician's panel of patients (the second author).

Had minimal or no complicating disease (hyperlipidemia, mild diabetes mellitus, and mild coronary artery disease were acceptable).
Were willing to participate.

Program structure. Patients come into the clinic in cohorts of ten to fifteen for three consecutive, weekly, one and a half hour sessions. In these meetings, they learn behavioral aspects of care relevant to hypertension including stress management, nutrition, and exercise. Additionally, they learn to monitor their own blood pressure and maintain home logs. During these three weekly sessions, group members develop their own treatment goals and hypertension management plan with both a behavioral and medical component. The group leaders function as consultants to this process.

After completing these three consecutive weeks, members return to the clinic as a group every four months for a follow-up meeting. This is a similar frequency with which they would have otherwise been seen for the monitoring of their high blood pressure. Follow-up care at these meetings focuses on their home logs, compliance with their treatment plan, goals, and their successes. During the follow-up sessions, a health related topic might be discussed in addition to reviewing progress in blood pressure management. Often, selected topics are linked to the season of the year. For instance, during flu and cold season, the self-treatment of upper respiratory infections is discussed. During the allergy season, allergy symptoms and their management are discussed. Group members are also encouraged to obtain any other medical care they might need at this time in the group appointment, e.g., refills on medications for other conditions, prevention, etc.

Program evaluation. Outcome data showed significant findings for improved systolic and diastolic blood pressure control for both home and clinic readings even while medication use was reduced. Patients appeared to maintain good blood pressure control over at least 2 years time, the current length of the program.

Patient satisfaction was very high. Of the seventy-one patients who completed the satisfaction survey, 96.5% believed this approach to hypertension management to be a more effective approach for managing hypertension than the 1:1 care they had been receiving from their physician.

The program also appeared to reduce demands for individual visits with their physician by almost fifty percent, even though patients in the program were free to schedule an individual visit with their physician at any time. A preliminary cost analysis indicates that this program is cost neutral in the first year and will reduce costs subsequently, assuming there are 12 members at each group meeting.

Variables	Mean Diff.	N	P Value
Mean Home Systolic Reading	6.15	40	.030
Mean Home Diastolic Reading	4.25	40	.037
Mean Clinic Systolic Reading	3.01	40	.041
Mean Clinic Diastolic Reading	3.02	40	.011
Medication Burdens	4.49	40	<.0001

Figure 1

Clinical Efficacy of the Hypertension Management Program (2 years).

Summary. Our program evaluation data suggest this may be a superior treatment approach for some patients when compared to traditional care. At the time of this writing, three other M.D./Ph.D. teams at San Jose/Kaiser have adopted this model for their patients.

Asthma Self Management MCGA

Rational for program development. Traditional medical care for asthma has largely emphasized pharmacological and educational management of this disease. Non-compliance is one of the major factors resulting in increased healthcare utilization by individuals with asthma. Research has clearly demonstrated that educational information alone is necessary but not sufficient to insure behavioral change (Wyka-Fitzgerald, et. al., 1984), which is important for improving care to this population. In order to meet the needs of this population, the asthma MCGA, with a drop-in group format was developed by an M.D./Ph.D. team for the management of poorly controlled asthma.

Program structure. In this program, patients may "drop in" at any time the group meets, although their initial visit must be triggered by a referral from a primary care provider. Patients come to the clinic for weekly, 2 hr sessions where they learn to monitor their peak flow readings, to adjust their preventative medications (most commonly inhaled steroids) for maintaining good control, and to learn other behavioral aspects of care relevant for asthma. Often there is a need to diagnose and differentiate anxiety and panic attacks from asthma attacks with these patients.

Members participate in the creation of their own asthma management plan and identify their own treatment goals. They are encouraged to come into

■ N = 71

■ 96.5% believed this approach to hypertension management is more effective approach than prior care.

Figure 2

Patient Satisfaction with Hypertension Management Program

the group until their asthma is in good control and then come to a yearly follow-up meeting. They are also encouraged to "drop in" to the program for a "tune up" if they feel their asthma is out of control, rather than the Emergency Department or the After Hours Clinic. Prevention issues are covered as well as seasonally appropriate information during the flu and allergy season.

Group membership. Eighty percent of the group members were classified by the program physician with severe asthma based on inhaled beta-agonist drug use and spirometry readings.

Outcome data. Program evaluation data on patients who had attended the group seven times showed significant findings for improved asthma control based on spirometry readings and more appropriate medication use. Quality of life as measured by the "Asthma Quality of Life Measure" (Marks et.al, 1992) was significantly improved.

There was reduced utilization of the Emergency Department as well as individual visits in the outpatient clinic.

Summary. This program evaluation data suggest the GCMA approach for the management of poorly controlled asthma may be superior for some patients when compared to care as usual.

CONCLUSION

The Group Co-management Medical Appt (GCMA) offers significant benefits to medical patients, providers, and health plans. In this model, patients enjoy the benefits associated with an integrated approach to clinical evaluation and treatment, a peer support group, increased time with their physician, focused education, and skill building. Teaming the skills of the primary care physician with the expertise of the health psychologist broadens

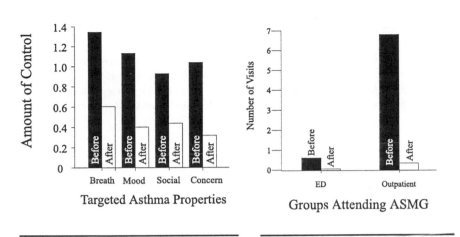

Figure 3

Asthma Quality of Life Measure. (N = 51), (P < 0.0001). From Bertagnolli & Charlu, unpublished data, 1999.

Figure 4

ED and Outpatient visits, 6 months prior (black columns) and 6 months after (white columns) attending ASMG (N = 30). From Bertognolli & Charlu, unpublished data, 1998.

the range of services and clinical interventions that can be offered and suddenly, there is the opportunity for "one stop shopping" in primary care. These programs are not for everybody, nor intended as a substitute for traditional one on one care. It is probably best suited for capitated, organized health care delivery systems such as HMO's and managed care networks with large memberships to serve. However, the findings do suggest that for some individuals and some medical conditions, this approach may well be the treatment of choice. They can meet the range of clinical care needs from treatment, prevention, and management. Equally important, they can lower costs by reducing demands for care, matching member needs to provider, improving clinical outcomes, and providing health care in "one stop shopping".

REFERENCES

Cummings, N., Cummings, J., & Johnson, J. (1997). *Behavioral Health in Primary Care: A Guide for Clinical Integration*. Madison: Psychosocial Press.

Joint National Committee on Detection, Evaluation, and Treatment of High Blood
    Pressure: The Fifth Report (JNCV) (1993). *Archives of Internal Medicine, 153,* 154-
    183.

Marks, G., Dunn, S., & Woolcock, A. (1992). A scale for the measurement of quality
    of life in adults with asthma. *Journal of Clinical Epidemiology, 45*(5), 461-472.

Wyka-Fitzgerald, C., Levesque, P., & Panciera, T. (1994). Long term evaluation of
    group education for high blood pressure control. *Cardiovascular Nursing, 20*(30),
    13-18.

Discussion of Kent and Gordon:

Reinventing the Team Model: Can Quality and Lower Cost Go Hand in Hand?

Gregory Hayes, M.D., M.P.H.
University of Nevada, Reno

The experience of the still-underway, managed health care revolution has too often been negative. Professionals have decried the restrictions on their ability to diagnose and treat. Doctoral-level professionals have complained bitterly about the loss of quality they feel is inherent in farming out tasks they have traditionally done to lesser-trained individuals.

Consumers have complained about a lack of services, sometimes fatal delays in decision-making, and an unwillingness on the part of some managed care organizations to "do the right thing" for the patient. Both the president and Congress have felt the need to push forward some version of a patients' bill of rights to empower individuals to fight back against what they perceive to be an unfeeling emphasis on profits first. Organizationally, HMOs have folded, leaving large blocks of people with fewer and fewer choices, or choices have been restricted by organizations merging and merging again into faceless mega-corporations seemingly fixated on the bottom line. The current upheaval is far from over, but is it all doom and gloom within the health care industry? Not really. There are also many hopeful signs that counterbalance the horror stories so loved by the media.

No one can discount the unsettled nature of the current state of affairs in the health care. No doubt it will take decades to find a workable path through the confusion. But meanwhile, examples abound that show the opportunities embedded in crisis. The long-term goal underlying the changes in health care is to maximize efficiency so that the most benefit is produced for every dollar spent. Can we squeeze more out of a dollar while keeping our primary focus

Integrated Behavioral Healthcare: Positioning Mental Health Practice with Medical/Surgical Practice

on the quality of the result achieved? From one program at Kaiser Permanente, one of our oldest HMOs, comes a strongly affirmative response (lest some believe that HMOs and managed care are a product of only the last 20 years, let me emphasize that when I say old I mean *old* – the first incarnation of the future Permanente structure began pre-World War II to serve Kaiser employees building the Grand Coulee Dam; the modern Kaiser Permanente system began following its successful use during WWII. With such experience come s the ability to teach many lessons.) Their work on finding better ways to address the common ailments of hypertension and asthma provides us all with hopeful sign for the future of health services. It *is* possible, at least sometimes, to find a new way of addressing a medical problem that shows improved outcome, improved patient satisfaction, *and* saves money.

As many of us have experienced both personally and professionally, it is painful to operate within a budget. It can be challenging to make decisions knowing our professional efforts will be carefully scrutinized for the benefits they do or do not produce. But this focus on efficiency need not mean an unavoidable decrease in quality. Rather, quite the opposite may be true.

A new incarnation of the team model is at the root of the special management programs addressing high blood pressure and asthma at Kaiser's San Jose facility. As the authors point out, there is nothing new about using teams. And yet somehow, at least for many of us, there is. In this case, what is very new for most professionals is the particular way in which psychologists and physicians directly address the multiple levels of problems at work in these two common health problems. Previously, if physicians even considered the possibility of a mental health component in treating hypertension and asthma, they either took on the task of counselor themselves (an area in which they have little or no training) or turned to a psychiatrist, a specially trained physician who tended to be similar to the primary care physician in his or her orientation to solutions through medication. The Kaiser model, however, places non-physicians, doctorally trained psychologists with special training in behavioral medicine in a direct, working relationship with the primary physician. Even for physicians who have worked with psychologists on such problems in the past, the Kaiser model takes things a step further. In this case, the working relationship between professionals is truly face-to face—a tightly woven interaction which finds primary care physicians working with psychologists in groups of up to 15 medical patients at a time. While a group approach to problem solving may not be new, this in-the-trenches, hands-on, "real time" approach to team work is thoroughly unfamiliar territory for most physicians. It is a far cry from the more familiar relationship of referring patients to some other place – down the hall or across town – to deal with the mental aspects of their disease in the absence of the physician. As the authors point out, this unfamiliarity represents a real challenge to making the model work. But work it does. Physicians learn from psychologists. Psychologists learn from physicians. One measure of success of the model would be the positive response from physicians and psychologists alike, but, more important in this managed care world of working within budgets are the striking changes in outcome: less medication used, fewer hospital visits, improved symptoms, and, strikingly, patient satisfaction ratings that reached 96.5% during this study (of those participating, this percentage of patients found the new model more effective than the traditional one.) In health care it is almost unheard of to see such high ratings. While the sample is small and the results are preliminary, the evidence does suggest that sometimes there really may a better way to the get the job done and done right.

The authors hedge their bets in telling us that innovative programs such as this are only for certain individuals and never to be seen as a substitute for traditional care. While certainly it is true that one size never fits all, I have to wonder whether we should not at least consider the possibility that we are indeed looking at a substitute for the traditional treatment method. In managed care environments, especially those that are truly capitated systems, the need to focus on "most bang for the buck" means we really do need to find efficiency everywhere we can. In this case, the data so far show that Kaiser Permanente/San Jose has created a model that works. It improves outcomes and patient satisfaction (no need for patients to demand their rights to fight back in this case!). It brings professionals of different disciplines together in an effective way that teaches them the value of each orientation. It helps physicians find the data necessary to dampen their almost unthinking tendency to throw more pills at the problem. And to the delight of those hoping to find a sane and workable answer to the managed care crisis it also saves money. What could be better? It is creative efforts such as this that help to teach physicians (the biggest stumbling block to any such innovation) the value of more intimate team approaches (especially non-pharmacologic approaches). With each such success – documented by data and replicated in multiple facilities – more becomes possible. My vote is to further develop the management model Drs. Kent and Gordon described by using it throughout the Kaiser system. If success continues, it should become as widespread as resources allow for it is in efforts such as this that the hope of the future lies.

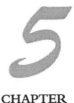

CHAPTER

Organizing a Collaborative Health Care Delivery System in a Medical Setting

James D. Slay, Jr., Rel.D.
Caroline McLeod, Ph.D.
John N. Johnson, M.D.
Health Care Partners

Integrated Behavioral Healthcare: Positioning Mental Health Practice with Medical/Surgical Practice

INTRODUCTION

For the last two decades there has been growing interest in the strategies and processes required to successfully integrate behavioral health and primary care. This book is about the application of these strategies and processes as a means of revitalizing behavioral health care.

The point has been made by others throughout this book that what we are proposing is not only necessary but it is something that is achievable. Achievable, we believe, in an organization whether it is composed of three persons or three thousand. Consider these examples: In Atlanta, a young primary care physician entered her practice some 10 years ago and found immediately that most of her patients were overwhelmed by psychosocial issues that had been unnoticed and unattended to. Her practice grew at such a rate that she decided to add to her professional staff. Her choice was to add another primary care physician or to add someone to work to meet her patients' psychosocial needs. She chose the latter, a Licensed Clinical Social Worker. The success of this integrated service is now known throughout her community and across the land.

In Minneapolis, we have observed at Health Partners C.J. Peek, Ph.D., Richard Heinrich, M.D., and others involving themselves year after year in developing an integrated model of care within a medical group of several hundred thousand patients. Integrated behavioral health and primary care has become their regular and ongoing way of doing business.

Looking at the work of Kaiser Permanente in Northern California, we learn that their patients are now being divided into groups of 20,000. Transdisciplinary teams of providers are trained to care for these groups of patients. Each team includes physicians, psychologists, social workers, and nurse practitioners. It is being proposed that this integrated service be used throughout the Kaiser system.

It is timely that a book on revitalizing behavioral health care be written. The expectation for more relevant and appropriate service for behavioral health is now being required by health plans and employer groups. Their request is for higher quality, better service and at lower costs. Assembly Bill 88 in California, which becomes effective July 1, 2000, requires that mental health services be given parity in the delivery of service and in the fair and equitable definition of health care benefits. NCQA has for several years been increasing requirements for combined and coordinated care between behavioral health and biomedical providers.

This dynamically changing health care environment has and will continue to provoke many responses. One prominent and disturbing response is provided by major carve-out companies advancing the "carve-out" as a solution to coordinated care and equal access to behavioral and biomedical services. Further fragmentation of the delivery system will prevent a solution to the very problem that we are being asked to solve. It has been well documented that when medical and psychological services are separated and fragmented, access to and utilization of behavioral health is severely limited, coordinated care is almost non-existent and utilization of medical services remains high. Our research at HealthCare Partners confimrs this finding.

We have chosen to see NCQA requirements as doors of opportunity and propose that the model best able to respond to these increasing requirements is one of an integrated medical and behavioral health care system of delivery. The question is no longer what should we do? What we should do has been documented in the literature for the last 45 years. We agree with Kurt Kroenke, M.D., Nicholas Cummings, Ph.D., and others who have said that the time has come to demonstrate how to do it. The cry is for a model of care that is carefully and systematically organized and provides a roadmap that will enable us to create an integrated health care service.

In this chapter we will use our experience with Collaborative Care at HealthCare Partners to answer the question: *How to do it*. We will describe how created an integrated system that depends upon biomedical providers and behavioral health providers working together side by side. We will describe how we merged two different professional disciplines so that these providers are able to accomplish together far more than they could ever accomplish apart. In short, we will describe the development of a transdisciplinary body of caregivers. Through these descriptions, we intend to impart to the reader not only how our system was developed, but how it can be *created, implemented, transported*, and *sustained* in other organizations with the result of improving patient health status, patient satisfaction, and provider satisfaction while reducing unnecessary healthcare utilization.

BECOMING A LEARNING ORGANIZATION :
A BRIEF HISTORICAL PERSPECTIVE

In the mid to late 70's, Bay Shores Medical Group, a multispecialty group in the South Bay area of Los Angeles County with 80,000 members was among the first medical groups in Southern California to enter into a new world called managed care. Throughout the 80's and the early 90's, Bay Shores was challenged to respond to a rapidly changing health care environment. The leaders of Bay Shores observed that medical groups began to become polarized. Some became managers of costs, while others were steadfastly developing the skills of managing care. Bay Shores made an intentional decision to maintain its integrity and stay the course in managing care. It was in the early 90's that the group also decided that it could maintain this integrity only by becoming a "learning organization" (Senge, 1990).

Two characteristics emerged from this decision. The first was a leadership model that was team-based. The second was a philosophy of inclusion rather than exclusion. Instead of administering benefits in a restrictive manner, the group decided to deliver services based on patients' needs. While other groups were operating in the traditional top down leadership model, Bay Shores chose to operate from a bottom up perspective that included ideas and innovations from the very front line of patient service. Infused into this organizational structure were members of the medical leadership as well as those who had administrative responsibilities. An unusual feature of this structure was the inclusion of leadership from those in behavioral health care. The resulting multidisciplinary team culture had as its focus, the integration of all clinical, financial, and operational systems. This notion of involving all levels of the organization proved to be both valuable and significant and a major reason for our success. We found that whenever we abandoned this principal, that negative outcomes were felt immediately.

An Innovation in Integrated Care

In 1993, the first author described this organizational principal in an article entitled *Carving In and Keeping In Mental Health in the Managed Care System*. The effort became one of the group's major program emphases.

> "To enable integration of mental health care delivery, we
> developed an organizational structure that would en-
> courage interdependence among senior managers and
> foster collaboration among service providers in the pri-

mary care setting. The group president, who is a physician, the administrator, the medical director, and the director of the behavioral health department spent a significant portion of their time working together on plans for meeting these goals. Senior managers encouraged implementation of the philosophy of integrated health care by being directly involved in meetings of the various primary care departments, in quality assurance and utilization review activities, ... " (Slay & Glazer, 1995 p. 1119)

The organization determined to apply this philosophy in the development of an integrated system of delivery in primary care. Three steps were taken at this time. The first was an experiment to place part-time behavioral health staff in the Pediatric and Family Practice settings. The major resistance at this point was the fear that Behavioral Health would be overwhelmed and over-utilized by the need for their services. What happened instead was an immediate move towards a shared and balanced care approach with brief and timelier interventions involving medical and behavioral providers working together. A second was the decision to employ a naturalistic study of ten patients presenting in these primary care settings to determine what therapeutic affect the integrated service was having on them and what were the financial costs and benefits of such interventions. There were positive clinical results and...

"... All ten patients followed in the study had reduced claims after implementation of the integrated model of care. Even the two noncompliant patients had slight reductions in claims. Total claims for medical and mental health care decreased form $8,001 during the six months before implementation to $5,022 during the six months after implementation for patients in the chemical dependency group and from $9,150 to $5,898 for patients in the panic disorder group, for a total savings of $6,231." (Slay & Glazer, 1995 p. 1119)

The third decision we made was the formation of an Integration Health Care Task Force which was developed in 1993 and is a working model of the philosophy which we are describing.

". . .a task force to explore ways of implementing the integration of mental health care. Task force members were appointed by the medical director. They were, in addition to the medical director, the group's administrator, the director of behavioral health department, the staff psychiatrist and other clinicians form the behavioral health department, including the group's addition specialist, four physicians, one each from the group's four primary care departments-family practice, internal medicine, obstetrics and gynecology, and pediatrics-and two nurse practitioners. This task force, which is now a standing committee, addressed three areas of interest: developing more accurate mental health screening tools for primary care clinicians, developing more specific and less labor-intensive treatment modalities through use of patient psychoeducation, and fostering more collaborative involvement of mental health clinicians within primary care settings." (Slay & Glazer, 1995 p. 1119)

Peripheral Vision: We Learned From Others

At that time in our organizational history, we observed that other medical groups like ours were emphasizing these same operational and clinical principals. They too were deciding to keep internal the services of behavioral health and were attempting to integrate them into all medical services. We observed that their groups were being very successful. Some contemporaries of ours were Mullikin Medical Group, Bristol Park Medical Group, Palo Alto Medical Group, Harriman Jones, Scripps, HealthCare Partners, Magan, and others. What we learned ourselves and later saw as a common phenomenon, that not only were the skills of the behavioral health staff used for treating patients directly, but their skills were used to manage change and develop leadership through their respective organizations.

Bay Shores' Merger With Healthcare Partners

In 1994, Bay Shores Medical Group merged with Huntington Medical Group and California Primary Physicians. With the merger came the consolidation of over 48 years of combined managed care experience, along with expertise in programs applying psychosocial intervention. From the combined experience has come a vision of an integrated health care delivery system that bridges the traditional fragmentation between psychological and biomedical providers. The new organization known as HealthCare Partners is a larger multispecialty group now serving over 350,000 patients in 37 medical sites.

A Global Mission and Purpose

The leadership of the new organization set as a top priority creative ways of delivering quality medical care within a managed care environment. It is committed to designing clinical care operational innovations that fulfill the promise of managed care.

Our vision and mission statement reflects this commitment:

> "We are dedicated to the well being and the respectful, compassionate healing of our patients and our communities. We will achieve this vision by: partnering with our patients to excel in the healing arts; partnering with our staff to continually improve our systems and services and to build a work environment grounded in dignity, trust, accountability, and collaborative teamwork; partnering with our clients and customers to provide the best value in health care and to be a recognized leader in our industry; and partnering with our community to work for the common good. As a physician/provider-led organization, we believe that we are best able to clearly align quality outcomes for our patients with our business objectives."

Our vision and mission form the framework in which we have set four ongoing objectives: to improve patient satisfaction, provider satisfaction, clinical outcomes, and to provide cost-effective service. The programs we choose to embark upon must not only match our vision, but also achieve these quality improvement objectives. As managed care experts, it was clear to us that the fragmentation of medical services was a major obstacle in improving these areas of concern. In 1996, the Board of Directors initiated the Collaborative Care Research and Development Project. A Senior Medical Director, the Director of Behavioral Health, and a Ph.D. researcher recruited for this project were given the responsibility to give direction and oversight.

THE COLLABORATIVE CARE PROJECT: BACKGROUND RESEARCH

One important study that greatly influenced our commitment to integrated care was published by Kroenke and Mangelsdorff (1989). (See Figure #1). Examining the incidence of the 14 most common symptoms within a population of 1,000 internal medicine outpatients, the authors found that up to 84% of the time no organic etiology could be found for the symptom. They concluded that unresolved psychosocial stress was one reason for these unnecessary primary care visits.

The financial cost associated with the utilization by those who had no organic etiology was high; Figure #2 shows comparison of the costs for patients who had diagnosable medical conditions with those whose symptoms had no organic etiology. And those individuals who had no diagnosable

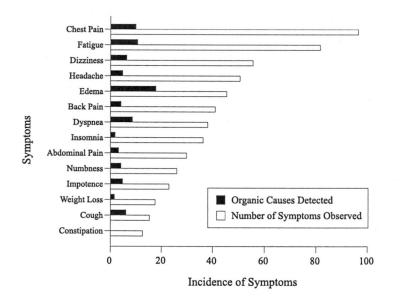

Figure 1.

The incidence of 14 common symptoms (lighter shading) in 1,000 internal medicine outpatients, compared with those in which an organic disorder was detected (darker shading). Data are from Kroenke & Mangelsdorf, 1989

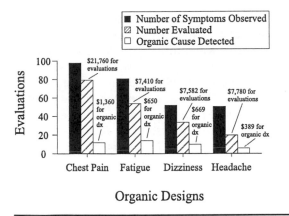

Organic Designs

Figure 2

Evaluations and the cost per organic diagnosis for five symptoms in 1,000 internal madicine outpatients in 1988 dollars. Data are from Kroenke and Mangelsdorf, 1989.

medical or psychiatric illness were likely to report no improvement in symptoms at follow-up. So, in short, it seems that the needs of a majority of patients seen in primary care remained unaddressed in spite of substantial financial expenditures.

Other studies also support the notion that emotional distress and psychosocial issues play a strong role in the course of illnesses that present in primary care:

> Rather than the acute illnesses prevalent fifty years ago, a large percentage of illnesses presenting for   treatment today are related to lifestyle and stress (Wickramasekera, 1989).
>
> A high percentage of mental illness shows up in primary care (Blacker & Clare, 1987; Nielson & Williams, 1980), where it is not well recognized or treated (Perez-Stable, Miranda, Munoz, & Ying, 1990; Katon, 1995).
>
> A high percentage of visits in primary care are due to distress without organic or psychiatric basis (Kroenke & Mangelsdorff, 1989; VandenBos & DeLeon, 1984).
>
> Increased morbidity and mortality is associated with depression in patients with medical illness (Friedman & Booth-Kewley, 1987; Wells, Golding, & Burnham, 1988; Carney et al., 1988).
>
> Functional status in patients with depression is as low or lower than in patients with chronic disease (Wells, Stewart, & Hays, 1989).
>
> Individuals reporting depression and/or stress incur more health care costs than individuals who do not report these risk factors (Goetzel, Anderson, Whitmer et al., 1998).

Discussions with primary care physicians across our company revealed that their experience was similar to that described in the literature. As a result, we decided that while it is important that we continue to provide appropriate treatment to those patients with clear medical problems, we must simultaneously pay better attention to the substantial number of primary care patients seeking help for stress-related illness. External research coupled with a recognition of our own clinical experience provided the impetus we needed to invest in a careful examination of our own system of delivery and the development of a more integrated system. We decided to create an integrated system of care that would manage the biopsychosocial needs of our patients at the primary care level. Importantly, this system would need to deliver care at equal or decreased cost when compared to a fragmented care system. This integrated system of care we called "Collaborative Care."

DESCRIPTION OF THE COLLABORATIVE CARE PROJECT

The Collaborative Care Project is a pilot program developed to redesign the primary care delivery system to resolve the problems created by the traditional fragmentation of care. It refers to a model of service that relies on the sharing of clinical assessment, planning, and treatment between health care providers trained in behavioral health and biomedicine. The program was designed to:

1. Develop key collaborative skills between behavioral and medical providers that result in increased quality of care for the patient.
2. Increase satisfaction in patients and providers.
3. Decrease inappropriate and ineffective medical utilization among primary care patients with psychosocial distress.

Because behavioral and medical providers have traditionally been trained in settings that treat mind separately from body, patients who suffer from illnesses that require attention to both components receive less than optimal care. Collaborative Care is a model designed to identify and treat patients with depression and other biopsychosocial issues in the primary care setting. It is different from usual clinical care in that:

1. Behavioral Health (BH) providers are co-located with physicians in the primary care site, thereby

providing patients with an opportunity for immediate and timely attention.

2. Both Primary Care (PCP) and BH providers are sensitized to the role that emotional distress (i.e., anxiety, depression, life stress) plays in illness.

3. Medical and behavioral health providers are provided with a forum to educate one another and to design collaborative treatment plans for those patients who need them.

4. Communication and combined interventions between providers are the norm, rather than the exception.

The Collaborative Care pilot provided for the development of systems and skills that support the integration of appropriate behavioral and medical services. It also measured the effects of this integration in pilot sites. The information gathered formed the basis for a system-wide implementation of Collaborative Care throughout our organization. In the next few pages we provide an overview of the phases of the project.

Phase 1: Development of a Cross-Disciplinary Body of Experts

Collaborative Care involves a fundamental intervention into the way that clinical care is provided at primary care sites. In the process of attempting to create an integrated system, it became clear that the strong, separate identities and practices of the Behavioral Health and Family Practice Departments created difficulties for patients trying to find their way from one specialty to another. Critical to the ability to meet these patients' needs was the development of interdepartmental bridges and connections made with the advice and assistance offered by the Health Care Integration Task Force. The Task Force was selected from HealthCare Partners staff and was formed for the purpose of redesigning and rethinking our delivery system. This group was established as a team of independent, transdisciplinary experts, and included administrators, medical directors, psychologists, psychiatrists, primary care doctors, physical therapists, counselors, and nurse practitioners.

The Health Care Integration Task Force provided a foundation for the Collaborative Care Project in several important ways. Initially, the team of experts provided comments about noteworthy literature and discussed how these findings were relevant to clinical care at HealthCare Partners. Later on, they provided advice and consultation regarding the training process for behavioral health and primary care providers. They helped to determine the feasibility of evaluation processes and procedures. Administrative staff were able to identify needs for the support of this new and developing program, Clinical staff provided knowledge about patient and provider behaviors within the system. Most importantly, the Task Force worked collaboratively to identify key ideas related to the Collaborative Care Project, then disseminated these ideas to their colleagues and support staff. The lines of separateness between specialties began to diminish as these professionals experienced the opportunity of working together to develop a collaborative system.

Important objectives for Collaborative Care were identified as follows:

> To improve the ability of biomedical providers to detect psychosocial needs.
> To improve the rate of intervention in patients identified with psychosocial needs (including the appropriate use of psychotropic drugs).
> To improve clinical outcomes.
> To improve patient satisfaction with clinical services.
> To improve healthcare providers' assessments of their ability to meet patient needs.
> To decrease inappropriate and ineffective medical utilization.
> To achieve these objectives at similar or decreased cost to the medical group when compared to a fragmented system.

Phase 2 -Data Collection Under Fragmented Care

Clinical care was studied at two sites, Site 1 and Site 2. The sites were chosen because of the similarities in patient population and the willingness of the providers to assist us in the project.

Survey data were collected from primary care patients at Site 1 and Site 2 in January and February of 1997, prior to the implementation of Collaborative Care. This model is designated the "Fragmented Care model," since behavioral health treatment, if it occurs, is applied in such a way that the primary care physician is unaware of it. The term "Fragmented Care" refers *to any health care that relies on single practitioners' knowledge, where treatment plans are developed in the absence of information exchange between specialists*. Fragmented care occurs in situations where specialties are separate or carved out to separate health care companies, or where specialists practice without established clinical/administrative systems for communication.

As part of the survey process, reports on patient health status, including emotional distress, were provided to physicians directly before patient visits. Under Fragmented Care, physicians were able to make little use of the information.

Phase 3- Collaborative Care Training and Data Collection at the Pilot Site

Collaborative Care training and the co-location of behavioral health providers began at Site 2 in March of 1997. As part of the initial training, information collected under Fragmented Care was provided to the health care providers. The survey data collected from consecutive primary care patients acted as a training tool, since it identified for clinical discussion a target patient population that needed improved intervention. At semi-monthly meetings in the pilot site, researchers, physicians, nurse practitioners, behavioral health specialists, and administrators discussed findings and worked to find collaborative solutions to meet problems identified by the data.

In addition, patient satisfaction data were collected from consecutive patients seen in Collaborative Care in Site 2. Then, follow up data from previously surveyed patients were collected in September and October of 1997 under Collaborative Care in Site 2. Finally, in January of 1998, Collaborative Care was instituted at Site 1. Providers at both Site1 and Site 2 completed surveys describing their satisfaction with Collaborative Care.

Phase 4 - Analysis of Pilot Data

Working with consultation from primary care and behavioral health providers, data from fragmented and collaborative care conditions were analyzed.

Phase 5 - System-Wide Implementation

Upon determination that the Collaborative Care process achieved significant measurable positive results; leadership approved the implementation of the process at 16 other medical clinic sites. Collaborative Care is now in place in 18 of our organization's 30 sites.

Central to the implementation of Collaborative Care is the development of a team culture. Long-term training and education among providers is critical to the process, so structured forums to facilitate communication were developed and implemented. Thus, monthly Collaborative Care Forums were initiated (see timeline) for the participating primary care physicians who received feedback about their patients from their behavioral health colleagues. During these meetings, clinical case studies are reviewed and discussed among all of the participating providers, providing mutual education about clinical issues and creating a foundation for a culture that encourages transdisciplinary problem solving.

Examples of Forum topics include:

> From Fragmentation to Collaborative Care
> Somatization Disorders
> Detection of Depression in Primary Care
> Treatment of Depression in Primary Care; including guidelines for antidepressants
> Adult Attention Deficit Hyperactivity Disorder
> Pervasive Developmental Disorder
> Battered Persons, Victims, Adult Abuse
> Personality Disorders
> Chemical Dependency

The Collaborative Care Forum continues to be used as the major tool for developing collaborative care service as a core competency for our providers. It is used throughout our organization.

COLLABORATIVE CARE EVALUATION

Measures

The Collaborative Care Project utilized four measurement tools-the SF-36 and three surveys:

> **The SF-36** (Short Form 36) is a standardized instrument designed to measure a patient's functional status. Of particular interest to our study are the Mental Health and Physical Functioning scales.
> A **Service Satisfaction Questionnaire** was designed by evaluators and providers to provide fast feedback about whether the collaborative care system was, indeed, meeting patient needs.

A **Stress Intervention Survey** was designed to help us
understand the perceived need for counseling
services among patients utilizing primary care. It
also measures satisfaction with behavioral health
services and overall satisfaction with the medical
group.

Providers filling out a brief **Provider Satisfaction Survey**
evaluated how well Collaborative Care was working
and what impact it had on their practice.

Procedures

Using these tools, we collected information in three related studies: a) the
Collaborative Care Pilot; b) patient satisfaction with the collaborative care
system; c) provider satisfaction with the collaborative care system. The
methodology for each are described next.

Collaborative Care Pilot

A sample consisting of 666 consecutive patients presenting for treatment
at both sites during the months of January and February 1997 under Fragmented Care were compared to a sample of 463 patients presenting in
September and October of that year. The sample represents 87% of all patients
seen by specified providers over the targeted time of data collection.

Primary care physicians were contacted to participate in an on-site health
status survey of their patients. After a particular provider agreed to participate, patients making a primary care appointment were mailed a survey with
a letter that requested that they bring the completed survey with them to the
clinic. The survey consisted of the SF-36 and the Stress Intervention Survey.

Patients were informed that the survey was part of a pilot program that
involved providing additional information to the primary care provider at the
time of the visit. The completed survey data was entered into the computer at
the time of the appointment; a report was generated for the primary care
provider prior to the time that the patient was seen. In those few instances
where the patient was late and the report could not be provided before the
patient was seen, the report was given to the primary care provider after the
visit.

Six months after initial data collection, patients were mailed follow-up surveys. Telephone calls were made to encourage patients to return the surveys. Surveys were mailed again to persons who did not make an initial return, but who were willing to fill the survey out later. Patients who did not return a survey were contacted only once after the mailing; patients who could not be contacted by telephone were mailed a second survey.

The electronic medical records of those individuals participating in the survey were examined for provider practices related to Collaborative Care. The records were reviewed for notes made one year prior to the date of the survey, and two months after the survey had been completed. The following information was collected from the record:

> Patients were identified as being in distress by medical record note if mention was made that the patient was under stress, was anxious, or depressed.
> All mention of referrals to behavioral health was noted.
> All mention that the patient was already in behavioral health treatment was noted.
> All prescription of psychotropic medications by the primary care provider was noted.

Administrative data were collected for all visits to medical group and all referrals made for the period of one year before the survey to two years later. Using Access, the encounter level data was aggregated by patient, then aggregated by quarter, such that the last day of the fourth quarter began with date of health status survey. The data were exported into SPSS for statistical analysis.

As the project progressed, the participating primary care physicians received feedback about their patients in the structured Collaborative Care Forums. During these meetings, clinical case studies were reviewed and discussed among all of the participating medical and behavioral health providers, providing on-going education to the providers.

Collaborative Care Patient Satisfaction

Starting in April 1997, 105 consecutive patients who were seen by behavioral health providers in the collaborative care setting were asked by the provider to fill out the Service Satisfaction Questionnaire. The request was made at the end of the first session. Eighty-seven percent of these patients complied with this request.

Patients were told that the survey was anonymous, and that it would be used to evaluate whether having a counselor on site (rather than at a designate behavioral health site) was useful to the patients. Patients were free to decline, although few did. Clinicians did not make this request of patients who were distraught or of those whose clinical care might in any way be jeopardized. The data was entered into the Statistical Program for Social Sciences (SPSS) and analyzed.

Provider Satisfaction

The 16 providers at both sites completed an anonymous survey after the implementation of the Collaborative Care program. The survey requested information about how the providers responded to Collaborative Care. The survey data were entered in SPSS and analyzed.

Summary of Findings

Outcomes and Response to Outcomes

The Collaborative Care Project had significant impact on primary care and behavioral health provider practices, in that more patients were correctly identified, more patients were treated and communication between behavioral health and primary care providers improved.

A significant number of primary care patients report emotional distress. One-third of primary care patients scored 45 or below on the SF-36 Mental Health scale. These individuals were more likely to report having a chronic illness such as arthritis or diabetes, were less educated, were more likely to have been out of work, were more likely to report that stress plays a role in their illness, and were less likely to be satisfied with HealthCare Partners services.

Under fragmented care, emotional distress predicts high utilization and medical costs. After controlling for the Physical Functioning scale of the SF-36, the Mental Health scale predicted high health care utilization and costs.

Primary care physicians tended not to recognize, document, or address issues involving emotional distress under fragmented care. Discussions with physicians providing care under a fragmented system revealed reluctance to address emotional distress that was related to: 1) a lack of information about how to discuss emotional issues and how to make a referral to Behavioral Health without jeopardizing the relationship with the patient; 2) an inability to envision how things might improve for patients in high-stress situations;

and 3) a lack of recognition of how such information might be useful to other providers treating the patient.

Access to behavioral health services is poor under Fragmented Care. Even when psycho-social needs were recognized and patients were referred to counseling, patients did not access behavioral health services under Fragmented Care. (See Figure #3.) About one quarter of those referred ever accessed our behavioral health services.

A high number of patients report stress plays a role in their illness. We were surprised that almost 40% of the patients in our study perceived that stress played somewhat of a role in their illness. (See Figure #4.)

Improvement in the identification of distress under collaborative care. Under Collaborative Care, primary care physicians identified and were more ready to document distress. The increased documentation seems related to improved understanding of the range of Behavioral Health interventions available as well as the importance of sharing this clinically relevant information.

Improvement in treatment practices under Collaborative Care. Under Collaborative Care, medical records reflected an increased willingness on the part of the primary care provider to recommend behavioral health services or pharmacotherapy to their patients in distress.

Improving behavioral health access through the "hallway handoff." Under Fragmented Care, about one quarter of the few patients referred to behavioral

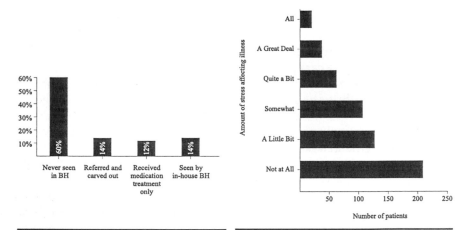

Figure 3	Figure 4
Percentage of referred patients who actually accessed Behavioral Health services	Patients' response to the question "To what degree do you think that stress is playing a role in your illness?"

health was actually seen in the Behavioral Health Department. Initially, under Collaborative Care, about 80% of patients who were "handed off" by the primary care physician to the behavioral health specialist on site were actually seen by the behavioral health clinician. At the beginning of the study, patients were seen almost immediately by the clinician, or were able to quickly make an appointment due to the ready availability of administrative staff. As the behavioral health clinician's time became filled with appointments, and as administrative staff became more busy with other work, patients were more likely to have to call to make an appointment. With this delay, about 50% of patients with a behavioral health recommendations were seen by BH clinicians. From this experience, we learned that immediacy of contact with administrative staff and/or the clinicians at the primary care site is critical to providing access to care for the distressed patient.

Improved treatment rate in the target population. The proportion of the target population (those with emotional distress as reflected by low Mental Health scores) seen in behavioral health in the six month period after the reference visit significantly increased from 13% under Fragmented Care to 27% under Collaborative Care. Current treatment rates are expected to be higher since improvements in administrative systems involving support staff have been implemented.

Increase in the number of collaborative conversations. Primary care providers reported an increase in the number of collaborative conversations under the collaborative care system. This is an important change in practice because Collaborative Care works to foster increased sensitivity and skill related to psychosocial issues for primary care providers. At the same time, the program works to foster increased knowledge and sensitivity to medical issues for behavioral health providers. Thus, even though patients may never be seen directly by a behavioral health provider, they will still received improved care.

Improved clinical outcomes under Collaborative Care. Under Collaborative Care, a higher proportion of patients improved, moving from distressed status to no longer in distress. Of the patients who scored below 45 on the mental health scale, only 38% under Fragmented Care improved, while 57% improved under Collaborative Care (See Figure #5).

Decreased medical utilization under Collaborative Care for patients reporting low mental health scores. In the groupo of distressed patients with initial mental health scores below 45, Collaborative Care was associated with decreased primary care visits and fewer referrals to medical specialists when compared to Fragmented Care. After the reference visit, overall utilization in primary care dropped markedly and significantly under the collaborative care model.

The reduction in primary care visits can be expected to drive decreases in overall visits because primary care is the gatekeeper for all specialty care. Appropriate care at the primary care site can be expected to decrease all other visits because further help seeking beyond primary care arena is no longer needed.

Under the fragmented care condition, analyses show increasing trends for referrals made to specialists outside of our organization after the reference visit. In contrast, under the collaborative care condition, there was a decreasing trend for these referrals. This result supports the notion that Collaborative Care is helping our providers meet patient needs more effectively, utilizing medical resources within our organization.

High patient satisfaction with Collaborative Care. Patients reported high satisfaction with the collaborative care system (See Figure #6).

High provider satisfaction with Collaborative Care. Providers report high satisfaction under Collaborative Care related to their ability to better meet the needs of their patients (See Figure #7).

This pilot of Collaborative Care has been extremely successful. It has identified problems in health care delivery under Fragmented Care, has demonstrated improvements in quality of care, provider satisfaction, and patient satisfaction, and has shown evidence of utilization reduction that should result in decreased costs to the organization. Most importantly, the program has developed a basis for knowledge in a group of skilled providers that can be disseminated throughout the organization as a core competency.

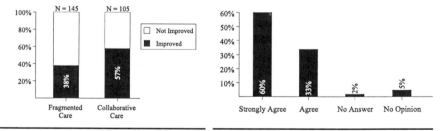

Figure 5

Percentage of patients with low mental health scores who improve under collaborative and fragmented care.

Figure 6

Under Collaborative Care, 93% of patients agree with the statement: "I am more satisfied with my overall health care because this new system allows medical providers and counselors to work as a team to support me."

We believe that Collaborative Care, along with other clinical innovations, is successfully differentiating our organization from its competition, even allowing us to attain national recognition for foresight in improving patient care. We believe that the model of care we are developing can be *implemented* in any size medical organization, that it can be *transported* from one part of an organization to another, that it can be *sustained* and that it will reduce the total cost of health care delivery.

Discussion

Most health care providers were trained in an old paradigm that prepared them to treat major mental illness or a major medical illness focusing on either severe psychiatric needs on one hand, or severe medical needs on the other. The emphasis was to master technology, and patients were treated as if they had discrete medical or psychiatric illnesses. Under Collaborative Care, providers treat patients in a setting that addresses human vulnerability to both medical and behavioral concerns. In addition to treating individuals with readily identifiable physiological disorders (and related psychosocial issues), the new paradigm addresses the needs of the 60-85% of patients who have no organic illness but who seek medical help.

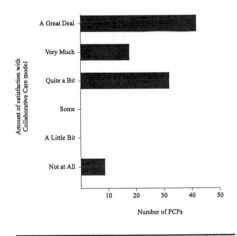

In our work, we have learned that Collaborative Care offers solutions to many of the difficult issues encountered in the primary care medical setting. We have been able to identify serious problems in the medical system under Fragmented Care. Patients with moderate distress are typically not identified or treated effectively, in spite of a high number of visits to their physician. This population is often frustrating for the physician to care for, as no ready solutions are available under Fragmented Care.

Under Collaborative Care, clinicians were able to reach those patients with a result of decreased utilization of medical services. These patients, met in a timely fash-

Figure 7

PCPs response to the question "To what degree has Collaborative Care supported you in your efforts to provide quality care?."

ion, were amenable and responsive to treatment. These patients do not usually access behavioral health services under a fragmented care system, due to distance to the clinic and to the fact that the emotional distress is not great enough to overcome reluctance to share concerns to unknown providers. Because of co-location and the "hallway handoff," Collaborative Care represents a real solution to the problem of caring for these patients, who are usually dissatisfied with the quality of their care.

Under Collaborative Care, medical providers are able to expand their detection of undiagnosed and untreated patients with depression, anxiety, and somatization. And, patients seen by behavioral health counselors are better supported in their compliance with medical treatment plans. Thus, Collaborative Care increases quality of care and reduces the number of unnecessary outside medical referrals, primary care encounters, and related services.

As we plan for the future development of Collaborative Care, we recognize that clinicians must pay special attention to the steps necessary to change primary care and behavioral health patterns of practice. Investment in educating the providers themselves is needed in order to develop practices that allow colleagues to work together in real time on real time patient problems, planning together, and combining skills for appropriate assessment and intervention. Understanding how primary care patients differ from patients who would ordinarily access care through behavioral health clinics needs to be developed further. There is a need for innovation in treatment for this population. Group medical treatments and short-term intervention for seniors are other promising options that can be implemented in our organization.

Experience with Collaborative Care has shown that there is also a need for a better system of administration; a need for training of receptionists and medical assistants; a need for the inclusion and integration of clinical records to facilitate timely sharing of information among providers; and a need for a more effective system to measure and analyze costs to the organization.

As a leader in the development of Collaborative Care, we believe that our organization has a market advantage. Future plans include further extension and implementation of Collaborative Care throughout our company. Another innovation currently underway is increasing the use of group treatments. We are planning to increase the number of brief, focused psychotherapy groups and add a number of psychoeducational groups to treat special patient populations. We will also profit by aligning ourselves with agencies such as the newly formed University Alliance for Behavioral Care and The Collaborative Care Task Force of the California Association of Physicians Organizations to continue research but more the development of Collaborative Care in discussion with several agencies that have expressed interest in such partnerships.

Achieving the Medical Cost Offset

Don Berwick of the Health Care Improvement Institute offered important guidance for those of us invested in the redesign of the health care delivery system. He writes:

> "Without a clear focus on the needs and experiences of individual patients, much of the financial and structural reorganization now rampant in health care will be unlikely to yield improvements that matter to the patients we serve. As we change the system of care, five principles can help guide our investment of energy:
>
> 1. Focus on integrating experiences, not just structures.
> 2. Learn to use measurement for improvement, not for judgment.
> 3. Develop better ways to learn from each other, not just to discover best practices.
> 4. Reduce total costs, not just local costs.
> 5. "Compete against disease, not against each other" (Berwick, p. 839).

This statement summarizes well the focus of our work in our redesign at HealthCare Partners. It is in this way, we believe that our delivery system will remain both clinically viable and financially sound.

The medical cost offset phenomena, says William Glazer "is an example of how cost savings and improved treatment can occur concurrently. It represents the best aspect of the managed care movement" (Glazer, 1992, p. 20). He says the "offset occurs when the appropriate and effective treatment of psychological distress reduces the total health care costs for the individual, the family, the payer and the managed care organization. (Glazer, 1992, p. 20). We believe that integrated primary care and behavioral health services represent an excellent opportunity to improve quality of patient care in a medical environment that has become increasingly financially restricted.

Three criteria have to be met before medical groups can profit from the offset:

1. Collaborative Care is in place and delivered preferably in the primary care medical setting.
2. Behavioral treatment is targeted on disease states and is delivered from a brief focused psychotherapy philosophy. Most of the therapy to be delivered in time limited and psychoeducational groups.
3. That the clinical, operational, and financial systems be integrated so that there is bottom up and top down involvement support and accountability.

Continuing as a "Learning Organization"

We began this writing by outlining the philosophy of a team-based, integrated culture involving all elements of the health care system. As this philosophy has been implemented, several things came forward that we believe are important to impart to the readers. First, we learned that our patients know what it is they need when they come for health care. Over 40% as indicated in the earlier writing knew that stress was an important factor in their illness. As we attend to those stress factors, we not only give satisfaction to the patient, but we go away as providers feeling that we have made a full, true, and complete contribution to those who come to us for help.

We learned that even in this time of dramatic and tumultuous change in health care, when behavioral health providers and primary care providers are placed in a learning environment that fosters exploration of new alternatives

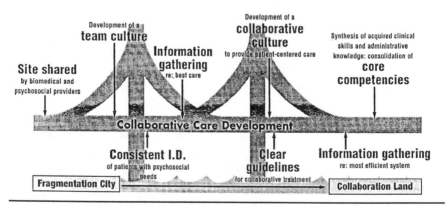

Figure 8

The development of Collaborative Care.

for the sake of the patients to whom they are committed, these providers are able to change deeply entrenched treatment practices.

We learned that no matter what new treatment protocols and practice guidelines are presented for appropriate treatment, that a learning environment has to be in place before new practices will be realized.

We learned that no matter how carefully we work to make fragmented systems of delivery effective, very few patients who are referred to behavioral health ever reach the destination for service. In the collaborative care environment, we are able to provide care to the majority of patients needing assistance.

We learned that by carefully disciplining ourselves as health care leaders, and by refusing to succumb to the temptation to be lost in outmoded systems of care, that we can bridge the chasm between mind and body medicine and that will keep us moving from fragmentation to collaboration. In Figure 8 we have outlined the steps required to move to the new system of delivery, or how to move from, what we call, Fragmentation City to Collaboration Land.

REFERENCES

Berwick, D. M. (1996). Quality comes home. *Annals of Internal Medicine, 125,* 830-843.

Blacker, C. V. R., & Clare, A. W. (1987). Depressive disorder in primary care. *British Journal of Psychiatry, 150,* 737-751.

Carney, R. M., Rich, M. W., Freedland, K. E., Saini, J., TeVelde, A., Simeone, C., & Clarke, K. (1988). Major depressive disorder predicts cardiac events in patients with coronary artery disease. *Psychosomatic Medicine, 50,* 627-633.

Friedman, H. S., & Booth-Kewley, S. (1987). The "disease prone" personality": A meta-analytic view of the construct. *American Psychologist, 42*(6), 539-555.

Goetzel, R. Z., Anderson, D. R., Whitmer, R. W., Ozminkowski, R. J., Dunn, R. L., & Wasserman, J. (1998). The relationship between modifiable health risks and health care expenditures. *Journal of Environmental and Occupational Medicine, 40*(10), 1-12.

Katon, W. (1982). Depression: Somatic symptoms and medical disorders in primary care. *Comprehensive Psychiatry, 23*(3), 274-287.

Kroenke, K., & Mangelsdorff, A. D. (1989). Common symptoms in ambulatory care: Incidence, evaluation, therapy, and outcome. *American Journal of Medicine, 86,* 262-5.

Nielson, A. C., & Williams, T. A. (1980). Depression in ambulatory medical patients. *Archives of General Psychiatry, 37,* 999-1004.

Perez-Stable, E. J., Miranda, J., Munoz, R. F., & Ying, Y. (1990). Depression in medical outpatients: Under recognition and misdiagnosis. *Archives of Internal Medicine, 150,* 1083-1088.

Senge, P. (1990). *The Fifth Discipline.* New York: Doubleday Press.

Slay, J. D., Jr., & Glazer, W. H. (1995). Best practices: 'Carving in' and keeping in mental health care in the managed care setting. *Psychiatric Services, 46*(11), 1119.

VandenBos, G., & DeLeon, P. (1984). The use of psychotherapy to improve physical health. *Psychotherapy, 25*(3), 335-343.

Wells, K. B., Golding, J. M., & Burnham, M. A. (1988). Psychiatric disorder in a sample of the general population with and without chronic medical conditions. *American Journal of Psychiatry, 145,* 976-981.

Wells, K. B., Stewart, A., & Hays, R. D. (1989). The functioning and well-being of depressed patients: Results from the medical outcome study. *Journal of the American Medical Association, 262,* 914-919.

Wickramasekera, I. (1989). Somatizers, the health care system, and collapsing the psychological distance that the somatizer has to travel for help. *Professional Psychology: Research and Practice, 29*(2), 105-111.

Discussion of Slay, McLeod, and Johnson:

Collaborative Care Evaluation: Report to Healthcare Partners

Martin E. Gutride, Ph.D.
Reno, Nevada

This review has been written by a Licensed Psychologist whose 32 year professional career has primarily involved clinical work. He has been in full time private practice for the last 15 years. Prior to that he had approximately five years experience as Director of two inpatient psychiatric facilities, and twelve years of experience working with severely mentally ill institutionalized patients in state facilities. More than 50% of the reviewer's current clinical work is with medically hospitalized patients in area hospitals. This, of course, involves close collaborative relationships with physician and other health care provider colleagues. It is therefore with great interest that the reviewer undertook this critique of McLeod et al's chapter.

There can certainly be little question that the work of McLeod et al is the type of undertaking which will be necessary to promote a , major change in our current health care delivery system. Nicholas Cummings, Ph.D. (1995) first identified integrated health care as a long overdue correction to our current fragmented system which primarily reflects the mind/body dualism formulated by Renee Descartes centuries ago.

This dualism has been a significant factor in the success of our now "industrialized" managed care approach to health care. Managed care was able to carve out behavioral health from physical health followed by decimating behavioral health benefits in order to save costs. Mind/body dualism makes it easy to sell the notion that psychological problems are unrelated to medical problems and perhaps just not as important. McLeod et al do an excellent job in the initial pages of their chapter challenging this dualistic notion and creating the rationale for carving back in. The most exciting aspect of their work, to this reviewer, is their demonstration of the benefits in following a fundamental premise in health care: treatment of the whole

Integrated Behavioral Healthcare: Positioning Mental Health Practice with Medical/Surgical Practice

person. Collaborative or Integrated care naturalistically responds to that premise. It will be no easy task for our current health care system to move toward the collaborative model. The authors allude to their efforts in this regard in the section "Intervention." It seems to this reviewer that this section should have been the first section of the chapter and significantly more detailed. Practitioners reading this study would be extremely interested to learn how potentially willing professionals from the various disciplines were identified , pulled together, trained and otherwise encouraged to change "business as usual".

A different organization to the Chapter is part of a more general concern as to "who is the intended audience?". It appears that the authors may have tried to write for a variety of audiences including practitioners, research scientists, administrators, etc. While there are no intrinsic problems in doing so there must be significant attention paid regarding how material is organized and presented. It is easy for one audience to become lost while reading material which may be most interesting to another audience.

Since this chapter is an outgrowth of a research endeavor, the quality of the research and its findings must certainly be addressed. "Field" research, with all of its problems, is the type of research which ultimately will be necessary to convince our society that collaborative care is the future of health care. McLeod et al are to be commended for bringing a research orientation to "real world" changes. There are of course many "classical" research critiques which can be applied to this study but these will undoubtedly be addressed by the author's academic colleagues. This reviewer will focus on some of the conclusions and statements made by McLeod et al which raise questions as to the potential usefulness of this study in promoting meaningful change in our health care delivery system.

McLeod et al. accurately reflect the thrust of future work and concerns which must be addressed. The most important of these concerns from this reviewer's perspective, is the development of "a more effective system to measure and analyze costs to the organization." Managed health care in today's society too often overlooks concern for "what is best" for the patient. It is primarily governed by Wall Street economics. McLeod et al have demonstrated with this initial study that collaborative health care clearly has the potential for promoting human welfare in a way our current system could never achieve. Future studies must demonstrate that it makes economic sense to develop the collaborative approach or the status quo will prevail.

6

CHAPTER

Behavioral Technologies in Disease Management: A New Service Model for Working with Physicians

Robert Dyer, Ph.D.
Criterion Health, Inc.,
Bellvue, WA

Definition of Disease Management
The Need: Incidence and Impact of Chronic Illness
    Diabetes
    Chronic Obstructive Pulmonary Disorder
    Pain
    Hypertension
    Pediatric Impulsivity and Depression
Current Systems: Pressures on Primary Care
Acceptance of Disease Management
Lifestyle Modification: Medical Non-Compliance
What we know about Primary Care Need and Want

Integrated Behavioral Healthcare: Positioning Mental Health Practice with Medical/Surgical Practice

DEFINITION OF DISEASE MANAGEMENT

The concept of disease management is quite young and currently evolving. The two most common definition's which seem to capture the essential efforts around disease management are as follows:

Disease management is a systematic approach designed to minimize degenerative symptomatology in patient's suffering from chronic diseases requiring significant lifestyle related accommodations.

Or:

Disease management is an integrated system of interventions and assessments designed to optimize quality of life, clinical and economic outcomes with specific disease states.

The essential elements seem to include:

Targeted disease syndromes; most often chronic lifestyle related syndromes
Organized approach to intervening; implies multi-disciplinary approach- physician, educator, pharmacy, etc.

Desired results that improve quality of patient life and
functioning; implies less invasive or expensive medical resources utilized.

The Need: Incidence and Impact of Chronic Illness

Traditionally, behavioral health treatment has been associated with
syndromes such as anxiety, depression and substance abuse, areas commonly fitting under the headings of mental disorders. All the while the growth
and common deployment of technologies has been occurring in these areas
additional efforts have been underway in the traditional venue of physical
medicine.

Individuals suffering from chronic lifestyle related illnesses have much
to gain by receiving behavioral technologies directed at helping them manage
their symptoms. Efforts to assist changes in diet, lifestyle, activity, developing
habits of compliance on appropriate pharmacy dosing and cognitive restructuring are all the domain of the behavioral technologies. Successful programs
impacting these necessary lifestyle modifications of people suffering chronic
debilitative illnesses represent reduced symptomatology, decreased pain and
suffering, increased functioning abilities, decreased work absences, fewer
hospitalizations and less overall medical expenses. It would seem everyone
would wish our medical interventions to strive for these goals.

Specific syndromes representing the interface of requiring lifestyle changes
in order to minimize symptomatology (or improve quality of life) are the targets
for behavioral disease management initiatives. While a case can be made for
very broad applications of the technology this paper suggests focusing on a
few, high incidence illnesses which directly benefit by disease management
efforts. The syndromes targeted are: adult onset diabetes, chronic obstructive
pulmonary disorders, hypertension and chronic pain conditions such as
arthritis.

A sense of the magnitude of disease management can be obtained by
comparing the monthly treatment costs of our target syndromes paid by
insurers:

$266	Hypertension
$491	Diabetes
$585	Asthma

This data is from a 1998 Price Waterhouse study. For comparison, the
average monthly commercial treatment cost for chronic behavioral health
disorders is $180.

The magnitude of the problem is exemplified in the numbers:

Diabetes

While only slightly more than three per cent of the population are diagnosed with diabetes it represents 14 per cent of all health care costs. Forty per cent of that is estimated to be inpatient costs associated with difficulties in lifestyle management. (Also note that the American Diabetes Association estimates one person with diabetes undiagnosed for every one diagnosed.)

Chronic Obstructive Pulmonary Disorder (COPD)

Asthma and emphysema impact five per cent of the population and represent ten per cent of all health costs. Pediatric asthma difficulties represent 40 per cent of all pediatric inpatient admissions. Episode costs of care are among the highest of all disorders and significantly need for inpatient care is related to unstable lifestyle.

Pain

Pain related issues significantly impact the functioning (absenteeism, disability) of twelve per cent of the population. Arthritis alone accounts for twelve per cent of all office visits by the elderly.

Hypertension

Fifteen per cent of the population is diagnosed with hypertension. This is the single most frequent diagnosis; over 27 million in 1996. Over fifty per cent of people diagnosed are medically out of care within twelve months. Of those in care, less than fifty per cent are following the medical plan as prescribed.

Pediatric Impulsivity and Depression

A syndrome the author adds to this list of chronic lifestyle related issues is one that impacts pediatricians and family physicians in a worrisome way;

attention deficit disorder syndromes. The U.S. Office for drug Enforcement notes that one in seven children are receiving prescription medication for behavioral or psychiatric reasons. Over seven per cent of latency age boys receive medication for attention deficit disorder alone. Five per cent are medicated for depression. We know the majority of children identified with ADHD or depression will be treated for these disorders for many years, i.e. they are "chronic" conditions. The most common stolen and illegally sold prescription drug is Ritalin. The need for an organized supportive system to educate and encourage appropriate utilization

Financial Impact of Chronicity Need: People who use Medical Services vs. Cost of Services

Lives Covered	Medical Expenses
5%	60%
45%	37%
50%	3%

Figure 1

Reviewed medical claims. From Value Health Sciences (1995).

is obvious and strongly supported by pediatricians and family physicians.

A survey of HMO plans found four per cent of plan members who utilized care accounted for over thirty per cent of all health care costs (Terry, 1998). COPD, diabetes, pain and hypertension accounted for approximately half of that total amount. Over 43 million Americans suffer from chronic lifestyle related diseases.

According to Figure 1, five per cent of all covered lives cost sixty per cent of all expenses paid for care. Clearly, targeting resources to assure maximum success for this five per cent has the greatest potential for impact.

By comparison all mental and addictive disorders *combined* (over 300 diagnoses) result in eight per cent of the population receiving care in one year and medical expenditures accounting for eight per cent of all healthcare costs.

Current System: Pressures on Primary Care

We are at a point in healthcare where the funding is once again creating (and limiting) what interventions are available.

The sad fact is funding systems, more than technology, have been the impediment to behavioral interventions in physical medicine (and conversely, the motivator of growth of traditional mental health services). Biofeedback and self- control regimens have a long and rich tradition of providing assistance to individuals with physical symptomatology. Biofeedback receives little or no reimbursement from major insurers. Similarly the use of health educators or office assistants for skill building or medical compliance regimens has received little financial support. The lack of support by insurance companies has resulted in little broad application of the technology. Most current disease management initiatives are driven by HMOs or pharmaceutical companies who have direct financial benefits. Insurance executives acknowledge the need and even the results of existing programs, but voice concerns of "opening" funding categories for fear of being "exploited" by providers. Most major coordinated disease management programs are separately funded and identified as exceptions by insurers (See Figure 2).

Percent of HMOs with
Disease Management Programs

75% offer at least one disease management program
60% offer two to four programs
57% offer Asthma programs
50% offer Diabetes programs
50% offer High Risk pregnancy programs
23% offer Congestive Heart Failure programs
20% offer Breast Cancer programs
17% offer Depression programs
17% offer Cholesterol programs
15% offer HIV/AIDS programs

Figure 2

Percent of HMO's and Disease Management programs available.

Capitation payments in managed care contracts change the traditional incentives to providers. In traditional fee for service payment systems incentives are placed on seeing the most expensive providers and procedures possible (i.e. those with the largest profit margins). No financial incentives exist for "curing" people- providers only get paid for seeing patients and get paid more if the patients need more.

Capitation pays a fixed amount with minimal regard to how much care is accessed. This has led to problems of undertreatment, i.e. "drive- by deliveries", etc. but it also encourages the patient's health. Physicians have a financial stake in doing whatever makes people be as healthy as possible to minimize their overall need for care.

The dominant model of managed care involves insurance plan members accessing all care though a primary care physician. This "gatekeeper" delivers basic care and "prescribes" specialty care as needed. Physician groups are managing financial resources at their own financial risk. They want the most cost- effective solutions, as they get to keep the savings.

Acceptance of Disease Management

The acceptance of disease management in the era of managed care is best exemplified by the utilization of disease management programs by Health Maintenance Organizations (HMOs).

HMOs are taking the overall financial risk for delivering care to broad populations. They want integrated systems that insure cost effectiveness. They have embraced the concepts of disease management.

Of 282 HMOs, seventy five per cent offered at least one disease management program. Sixty per cent offered disease management programs for up to four conditions. The beneficiaries of programs offered are moderately to severely ill plan members.

Lovelace Health systems of Albuquerque, NM identified thirty conditions that accounted for 80 per cent of their total costs. They targeted sixteen of those as having significantly improved episodes with disease management programs:

> Diabetes
> Low back pain
> Pediatric asthma
> Birth episode
> Breast cancer
> Stroke care
> Depression
> Knee injuries
> Chronic cardiac illnesses
> Peptic ulcer disease
> Congestive heart failure
> Hysterectomy
> Attention deficit disorder
> Hypertension
> Adult asthma
> Alzheimer's disease

Consistently, disease management programs post from twenty- five to forty per cent medical savings results. A list of sample results finds a boring consistency in the decreased overall medical savings of disease management participants (see Padgett, 1997 for representative sampling of programs and their results for a wide diversity of syndromes). The results most often extend beyond simple financial savings, for example; Value Health, in conjunction with Eli Lilly has created a diabetes disease management program. Their site patient impact targets are:

> 50% reduction in lower extremity amputations
> 70% reduction in episodes of ketoacidosis
> 50% reduction in end- stage renal disease
> 60% reduction in diabetes related blindness
> 40% reduction in lost work days

As can be seen, significant financial savings accrue to such programs, but additionally these results mean very impressive gains for a patient's quality of life.

Lifestyle Modification: Medical Non-Compliance

Physicians have long recognized that their recommendations to patients about changes in diet, activity and basic cognitive approaches to illnesses have not resulted in much success though the years. Human nature just doesn't allow easy replacement of long- standing, well- practiced maladaptive habits with unfamiliar new behaviors just because someone suggests it would be a good idea. Thirty years of research suggests medical non- compliance rates for medication taking, diet and activity prescriptions exceed fifty per cent across many diverse syndromes. For example, patients seen by primary care doctors stop taking their antidepressant medication at a rate exceeding sixty per cent within six months of initial prescription(Katon et.al., 1992).

What We Know About Primary Care Need and Want

The American Medical Association abstracts medical practices in the United States (AMA, 1999). We know the following about the over 250,000 independently practicing primary care physicians:
Time spent:

> 89% Office based
> 2% Other
> 9% Hospital based
> 2 house calls
> 7 nursing home visits per week
> 16 hospital visits per week
> 107 office visits per week
> 47 billed hours of care per week
> 9 uncompensated/ discounted services per week

How organized:

> 12% one partner
> 34% 3 or 4 partners

36% practice solo
17% practice in settings with over 4
(AMA Survey does not count employee physicians,
    which is around one third of total physicians.)

Why people see primary care physicians:

Respiratory issues (15%)*
Blood pressure/ hypertension (8%)*
Exams/ progress reports (3%)
Pain (2%)*
Skin related (2%)
Gastric (2%)
Cardiac (1%)

Age impacts visits significantly. What follows are most frequent reasons people over 75 years old saw their physician:

Blood pressure (12%)*
Arthritis (12%)*
Respiratory (8%)*
Cardiac (5%)
Diabetes (4%)*
Gastric (2%)
Skin related (1%)
* = target syndromes of this paper.

Average visits to physician per person in a year:

2.8 visits per year

Primary Care Disposition of office visits:

72% prescribed medication
49% leave with return visit planned
29% referred for internal "counseling"
15% for diet
10% exercise counseling
4% cholesterol reduction
3% smoking cessation
5% referred to other physician
4% referred to other non-medical personnel
2% for physiotherapy

2% for family / personal- **This is traditional referral out
  for Mental Health!**
<1% for alcohol / drug counseling
<1% for family planning

Thirty per cent of office visits believed by PCPs to be "psychological" in
nature. The Medstat Groupä, of Ann Arbor, MI reviewed medical claims in
1995 and found the following:
The most frequent outpatient billings were for:

Allergic rhinitis
Essential hypertension*
Back disorders*
Respiratory symptoms*
Joint dislocations
Abdominal and pelvic symptoms
Neurotic disorders*
Lipid disorders

The outpatient care episodes with the most expensive episode costs were:

Respiratory symptoms*
Abdominal and pelvic symptoms
Neurosis*
Back and disk disorders*
Hypertension*
* = target syndromes of this paper.

In 1997, Spectrum Health, Inc. of Bellevue, WA conducted a survey with
Seattle area primary care physicians. Highlights include:

71% of office visits were for follow up to chronic
conditions.
Over 70% stated the preferred mode of treating chronic
pain would include lifestyle management.
Over 70% stated the preferred mode of treatment for
asthma would include lifestyle management.
Almost 90% stated preferred mode for treating diabetes
would include lifestyle management.
Well over 80% stated the preferred mode for treating
hypertension would include lifestyle management.

Less than 30% of the time in all follow- up visits were patients suffering these disorders seen by anyone other than a physician.

Over 70% did not offer lifestyle management services in their practices

Relative to the use of physician extending personnel, Physicians wanted:

57% someone to process charts for them

43% someone to see chronic patients in prescribed protocols

43% someone to process prescriptions.

43% someone to verify managed care benefits.

29% someone to process lab results.

21% someone to process referrals out of practice.

14% someone to help follow- up with patients.

86% would like to add revenue to their practice by providing lifestyle management services.

60% stated internal revenue generation would result in increased utilization.

Over 80% were interested in adding a "qualified health educator and care coordinator" to their practice (Yurdin, 1997).

Physician Extending

An hour of primary care time costs an average of $196. The need for lower cost solutions to service common issues is widely known. Patient education, functional assessments, skill building, prompting, etc. can and are often performed by "physician extenders".

36% of all office- based care procedures performed were delivered by physician extenders (Over 264,000,000 visits in US in 1996- AMA).

The use of physician extenders seems directly related to size of setting and amount of capitated payment in the revenue mix of the setting.

64% of physicians in staff model HMOs have physician extenders.

23% of physician groups contracting for risk have extenders.

16% of medical groups with no risk contracts have extenders.

6% of solo practitioners have extenders.

Overall, 28% of PCPs employed extenders (Grandinetti, 1999).

A Behavioral Model of Disease Management

As can be seen the demand from patient needs and physician desire is strong to have an organized approach to assisting lifestyle modification to accommodate minimizing the symptomatology of chronic illnesses. What follows are the essential features of an organized approach embracing the best findings of today's behavioral technologies.

Business Model

What is proposed is a model where behavioral providers organize a systematic approach that is offered as a contract to medical groups, in much the same manner as many medical groups purchase medical laboratory services or physical therapy.

The essential business exchanges are the behavioral health entity will deliver a trained health educator who will perform a set of services approved by the physicians, document those services and report performance results of those interventions in exchange for payment.

The value additions to the physician include state of the art information about improving medical compliance and lifestyle accommodation to the target syndromes.

This implies the health educator will document in the physicians medical record; working as a practice extender to the physician.

The target practice for purchasing such a contract will probably have four or more primary care physicians in a single location. This size will support a full time presence for a "physician extender" (henceforth called a "health educator").

Make no mistake, the business model must directly attend to how contracting for the services will either:

> Make revenue for the practice,
> Decrease expenses for the practice; or
> Decrease financial risk for the practice (and therefore
> decrease expenses).

Targeted Syndromes

The target syndromes that align themselves for a common approach include:

Adult onset diabetes
Attention deficit disorder
Chronic obstructive pulmonary disorder (especially
     asthma and emphysema)
Chronic pain (especially arthritis)
Depression
Hypertension

Note: a pediatric subset of ADHD, depression and pediatric asthma bundle nicely to fit adequate demand for full time relevance to any multiple pediatrician or mixed pediatric/ PCP practice.

The scope of offerings must bundle similar systemic approaches for at least three syndromes to achieve impact worthy of contracting in an outpatient practice. In an open full time medical practice it must be assumed that only around twenty per cent of all easily identifiable eligible patients would be referred to the on site program. A significant volume must be available to create the ongoing demand for the services.

Packaging

In order to train and assure consistency in application by the health educators it is necessary to make a common system in which the processes and resources have a common "look and feel" across syndromes. Intervention protocols and patient education materials must be non- controversial and subject to editing by the practitioners to reflect the standards of the physician.

Any inserted intervention must be compatible with the practice. Finding an efficient way to communicate between the physician educator and physician is essential. Since we are proposing "selling" this model to physicians a brief way to show the relevance as well as essential features of the "product" are also essential. Written, editable materials are necessary. At least the following materials should be available to the interested physician:

> Indications for and contraindications for the disease
>   management program.
> Intervention protocols for each syndrome.
> A set of "prescriptions" for each decision point in care, i.e.
>   points where care significantly increases in inten-
>   sity.
> Functional lifestyle assessments for each syndrome.
> Patient education materials.
> Health Educator training materials.

While many interesting and potentially powerful findings are emerging from the field of alternative medicine it is strongly recommended that all materials initially presented reflect the least controversial aspects of attending to the syndrome as possible. All necessary materials can be generated from primary American Medical Association sources (J.A.M.A., New England Journal of Medicine, etc.) or the major trade associations representing the syndromes (American Diabetes Association, American Lung Association, American Heart Association, etc.). Modifications reflecting the experience of the physician or health educator can be modified into the interventions later as jointly identified and agreed.

It is imperative that the health educator not surprise the physician by saying or doing significant interventions without those being disclosed and approved. The health educator works under the auspices of the physician-they must be in sync with each other. (Also, it is important to note that behavioral health professionals are stereotyped as liberals, "soft and fuzzy"-in order to overcome potential stereotypes it is wise to insure your materials reflect science and a logical, linear approach to assisting the physician.)

Intervention Essentials

The essential services being sold reflect the major finding's from research on improving medical compliance, replacing maladaptive habits and adult learning. The model for a potent behavioral intervention that emerges includes at least the following components:

Functional Assessment

Assessment tools need to exist for at least three separate purposes:

Initial lifestyle assessment. Questionnaires need to sample how diet, activity, medication taking habits and current syndrome symptoms (frequency and intensity) impact level of functioning. This provides structured feedback about appropriateness for services as well as benchmarks for later comparison.

Skill building assessment. As specific issues are identified performance samples need to occur to chart progress toward (new) habit acquisition or to identify behavior chains impeding progress.

Evaluation/impact sampling. At pre-set times the results of the intervention need to be globally sampled. This is both critical symptom and patient perceptions of services monitoring. Frequency and intensity of key symptoms along with perceptions about services received need to be taken to develop population trends that can be reviewed to improve overall offerings.

Patient Education

Participants need reference material. The patient education materials present basic information about the disease; major symptoms, course of illness, common treatment regimens and realistic expectations for life changes with the progress of the illness.

Materials need to be very readable, charts and graphics increase interest. Adult education material finds value in creating characters who act as guides or examples through the entire episode of care, i.e. the materials are presented with story-like anecdotes happening with common characters to make the points or show applications of the material.

By design most patient education can be conducted in a group context. By practice it is often not practical to wait for groups to form to begin care.

Skill Building

The essence of the intervention is building a new set of behaviors. That may be:

> Changing diet.
> Changing schedule.
> Increasing or changing activity or physical regimen.
> Changing or creating reliable medication taking
> > routines.
> Changing internal self-talk about disease (or limitations,
> > etc.).

The diagnosis often immediately signals a need for significant changes in a person's life. In essence old habits must be stopped and new ones developed; never an easy proposition. Replacement requires understanding the need, knowing what new behavior you are to do, when you are to perform it and then performing it reliably and often.

The milieu for maximizing change includes:

Present the situation calling for new behavior.

Present the sequence of behaviors in which the behavior to replace occurs.

Present the new behavior to implement.

Personalize the application.

Have participants determine when, where and how this situation is applicable.

Practice the new behavior.

Perform sequence of behaviors in front of peer for feedback and support.

Troubleshoot. Question ease and appropriateness of intervention, vest "buy- in" from participants.

Plan "homework" when new behavior can be utilized.

Live life and practice.

Contact patient and prompt (remind, "nag") support for new behavior.

Debrief and reinforce steps at next meeting.

As with the patient education materials, readability, graphics, common characters, etc. all help with written materials. For improved compliance it is desirable if people leave each meeting with something concretely "in their hands" to remind them of their commitment to new behaviors.

Ideally, all skill building activities can be performed in a group context. Group feedback and public commitments increase veracity of new behaviors.

Prompting

People need support to develop new habits that are life changing. The health educator creates a schedule for support. Calling to check on new habit development. Potentially coming for home visits to help people practice in their real world setting.

Phone calls can work wonders. A kind word, a reminder, joint strategizing to overcome the inertia of change- all can improve outcomes.

Calls are planned and results are documented.

Care Coordination

Helping physicians attend to those aspects of health care which exist outside the practice adds great value and potentially discovers major ways of increasing compliance.

The health educator summarizes all out of practice care the patient's receive. A brief review can identify patterns that have improved or negatively impacted functioning. Other specialist's may have changed medications or given supportive care that impacted behavior; only by seeing these interventions over time can results be identified.

Mutual Support Facilitation

Following assessment and skill building maintenance can be improved significantly by having patient's support each other. The technology around mutual support groups is available. The National Institute for Mental Health has an excellent technical publication on establishing such systems. People learn from each other and provide support that seems to promote growth. Having a group of people a little further along the "learning curve" that can anticipate and provide encouragement for surmounting the trials associated with inserting new behavior into a lifestyle provides a powerful addition to the treatment paradigm. Groups most often have been single disease focused. That does not seem necessary and mixing can add an aspect of generalizability to the situation that seems to help some people.

Groups need to be ongoing. Use of dedicated helpers for people newly in the group (a la "sponsors" or "guides") can improve initial group meeting attendance. Encouragement (or discouragement) of after hours contacts between group members needs to be openly determined. It will happen so it's best to manage it.

Central Support/Account Management

Many practitioners have experienced the phenomenon of inserting a junior clinician in a medical practice to have the clinician leave the practitioners group to go in practice with the physician. To insure your central value to the physician group there must be activities and resources of value that occur on a regular basis tying the physician to keeping a relationship with you. Once a health educator and physician start working together working relationships become automatic. Their exists a need to have support, training, materials updates and performance evaluations central apart from the practice.

Quality assurance functions require sampling the health educators performance and documentation.

Performance updates. Centrally maintaining updates on information, updating patient education, assessment and treatment protocols is a major value to provide.

Regularly scheduled training and potentially providing on site training or one time "clinic" services can go a long way to providing value to the medical practice.

Semi-annual assessments of performance with displays of new materials and troubleshooting of communications will increase direct communications between the physician "client" and the "account manager" at the "home" office.

Documentation

Progress notes must be written for all patient contacts. Because the basis for delivering the service is under the auspices of the physician's practice, documentation fits into the physician's record.

The basis of the services are medical; not psychiatric. Medical records are brief, terse and conform to the problem oriented medical records requirements of the Joint Commission on Accreditation of Healthcare Organizations (JCAHO). Services are "prescribed" by the physician. Insurers and state licensing requirements dictate whether or not the health educator can sign alone or whether all notes must be co-signed or approved by the physician (or contract supervisor).

The reimbursement aspects of service delivery must work for both fee-for-service and capitation billing. In a capitated environment documentation may be unique to the practice, (i.e. payers don't dictate the standards). In a fee-for-service system documentation follows the requirements outlined in the American Medical Association's *International Classification of Disease Ninth Revision (ICD-9) Year 2000*.

Pricing

A simple system for pricing must exist to be attractive to the physician. Most medical groups are not used to value purchasing. They are most comfortable 'buying time", paying a fixed amount for procedures, like they are paid.

In fee-for-service environments having the supplier receive a fixed per cent of revenues collected is a common payment method. Pure fee-for-service payment environments are rare. Mixed capitation and fee-for-service payment is more common (Capitation payments are around one-third of the average physician's income.) Developing a pricing policy that works for both again supports a procedure pricing system.

Generally speaking pricing will peak out around seventy dollars per hour, or alternatively, no more than seventy per cent of all revenues collected. The point in both methods is that the physician's practice must keep a significant amount of revenues generated or they will simply replace your service with one of their own without regard to the additional benefits your services offer.

Personnel and Infrastructure

The requirements for organizing a set of services such as these include the following:

Medical consultation. You will want your protocols and patient education materials reviewed by medical specialists in the areas of focus, e.g. pulmonologist, cardiologist, endocrinologist, etc. The reviews can be of completed work and are not ongoing as much as periodic.

The health educator role can be provided by mental health trained personnel, nurses or educators with training. Experience has utilized a wide diversity of personnel, the issues have more to do with scope of practice, training and supervision. Since it is best to encourage practice within the agreed to materials the functions are best thought of as a technician's activities and in some ways that suggests lesser trained personnel.

Marketing

The utility of such services are quite clear to practicing physicians. The ease with which physicians will organize such a role into their practices depends in large part upon timing. Services demand and payment mix determine a practice's interests in such a provider. Your services must be known and the exchanges (contract performance and price) understood to be desirable. Successful venders must be known in medical trade groups and in local practice areas to be viewed as credible and "worth the chance". Physicians want to see the materials and want to know with some sense of certainty that the financial impacts are real.

There exists a bright future for the application of behavioral technologies in assisting people make personal adjustments to chronic, lifestyle related diseases. The model presented here is but one that will definitely emerge with increasing frequency over time in some form in primary care practices.

Hopefully, this material will stimulate more development and opportunities for improving the lives of others.

REFERENCES

American Medical Association. (1995). *Directory of practice parameters.* Chicago, IL: American Medical Association.

American Medical Association. (1999). *Social and demographic characteristics of physicians in America.* Washington, DC: American Medical Association.

Belar, C. (1995). Collaboration in capitated care: Challenges for psychology. *Professional Psychology: Research and Practice, 26,* 139-146.

Blount, A. (1998). *Integrated primary care: The future of medical and mental health collaboration.* New York: William Warder Norton.

Cummings, N., Cummings, J., & Johnson, J. (1997). *Behavioral health in primary care: A guide to clinical integration.* Madison, CT: Psychosocial Press.

Grandinetti, D. (1999). Midlevel providers: Making their mark in doctor's offices. *Medical Economics, 76*(3), 141-155.

Katon, W., Von Korff, M., Lin, E., Bush, T., & Ormel, J. (1992). Adequacy and duration of antidepressant treatment in primary care. *Medical Care, 30- 67.*

Medstat Group. (1995). *MarketScan database.* Ann Arbor, MI: The Medstat Group.

Padgett, Y. (1997). *Disease management-a special report: Successful strategies and programs for managing chronic diseases under managed care.* Atlanta, GA: National Health Information.

Peek, C. & Heinrick, R. (1995). Building a collaborative health care organization: From idea to innovation to invention. *Family Systems Medicine, 13,* 327-342.

Regier, D., et. al. (1993). The de facto United States mental and addictive disorders service system. *Archives of General Psychiatry, 50,* 85-94.

Rolland, J. (1994). *Families, illness and disability: An integrative treatment model.* New York: Basic Books.

Seaburn, D., Gawinski, B., Gunn, W., & Lorenz, A. (1996). *Models of collaboration: A guide for family therapists practicing with health care professionals.* New York: Basic Books.

Terry, K. (1998, April 27). The disease-management boom: How doctors are dealing with it. *Medical Economics.*

Todd, W. & Nash, D. (1997). *Disease management: A systems approach to improving patient outcomes.* Chicago, IL: American Hospital Publishing.

Woolf, S. (1992). Practice guidelines: A new reality in medicine II: Methods of developing guidelines. *Archives of Internal Medicine, 152*(5), 946-52.

Yurdin, L. (1997). *Primary care assessment of practice needs.* Bellvue, WA: Spectrum Health.

Discussion of Dyer:

Persuasion Criteria in the Business of Disease Management and Behavioral Health

Barbara S. Kohlenberg
Veterans Affairs Medical Center,
and,
The University of Nevada School of Medicine,
Reno, Nevada

Robert Dyer argues that disease management is an important area in medicine, measured both by quality of life, and by direct measures of cost savings. In his paper, he contends that disease management must be marketed, using a business model, to the medical establishment. One point worthy of further elaboration is that though it makes logical sense why there needs to be a serious marketing campaign, at the same time it is surprising. That is, given the increasingly uncontested value in medicine of cost savings and evidence based medical practices, one would think that there would need to be very little "selling", or persuading, indeed. One would want to assume that the data of better clinical outcomes and lower overall financial costs would speak for themselves, but apparently, they do not. In this paper, disease management and Dyer's proposed business model will be discussed. The contingencies involved in persuading medical personnel to implement *any* intervention system coming out of behavioral health will also be considered.

Dyer defines disease management as a systematic series of interventions designed to reduce the suffering experienced by people who have chronic diseases, while also working to maximize the quality of life of these same people. Clinical and economic outcomes are also data of interest when assessing the efficacy of interventions related to disease management. Dyer points out that in the past, behavioral health has been focused on the treatment of "mental health disorders" (anxiety, depression, and substance abuse), and not on providing specific technologies designed exclusively for the management of particular symptoms and lifestyle modifications. He argues that the continued development of behavioral health technologies focused on specific lifestyle behaviors related to specific diseases are going to be an important, and hopefully an increasingly efficacious component of behavioral health in the future.

Dyer then goes on to discuss the specific disease entities of hypertension, diabetes and asthma. He details the huge costs of treating people with these illnesses, and suggests that large portions of these costs are related to the problematic lifestyles of those with the disease. Essentially, the statistics he presents overwhelmingly endorse the cost-savings that could be obtained were behavioral health interventions to be effectively implemented in some of these specific areas of medicine.

A problem inherent in Dyer's analysis is that though disease management programs have great data to support their use, they are not being adopted to the degree one would expect. That is, if the cost savings and improved clinical outcomes generated by behavioral health interventions are believed, and if these cost savings are "the bottom line", then why are these programs not offered pervasively throughout the medical system?

Dyer indicates that disease management programs consistently post from 25-40% medical savings—in addition to significant improvements in the quality of life of the patients who participate. In a survey conducted in 1997 by Spectrum Health (Yurdin, 1997, as cited by Dyer in this volume), one fact that remains both very troubling and challenging and that is that over 70% of primary care physicians surveyed did not offer any lifestyle management services in their practices, though 86% said that they would like to. Based upon this apparent desire of primary care physicians to utilize behavioral health care providers, Dyer then proposes a business model in which behavioral providers contract with medical groups and provide specific interventions focused on specific disease entities.

Dyer's analysis makes logical sense, however it is problematic at several levels. First, there has been many years of empirical work in behavioral health care which has focused on the cost-offset of behavioral health interventions, and a recent meta-analysis puts cost offset at about 20% (Chiles, Lamberg & Hatch, 1999). It seems that these data are really very consistent, and that behavioral health interventions consistently reduce unnecessary medical utilization and costs. It is also known that these costs are more difficult to demonstrate in the last decade given the increasing hold of managed care and overall cost-saving measures (Otto, 1999). Nonetheless, the data from this literature, which focuses mostly on unspecified behavioral health care interventions applied to a wide range of physical medicine conditions, has been very convincing to those of us interested in behavioral health. However, it appears that even the most compelling data may not provide impetus for the implementation of a given intervention.

In medicine, some factions resist or certainly are not embracing what behavioral health interventions have to offer. Fischer (1999) a recent editor of The Journal of Family Practice, notes that while he recommends that physicians remain academically oriented, he resists single disease focused programs that are overly standardized. He states "I worry about attempts to standardize health care, because a good physician is an expert at individualizing care". He also notes that "The therapeutic relationship is your most effective tool, and it cannot be studied with double-blind placebo-controlled clinical trials". These comments certainly illustrate some difficulties with physician acceptance of codified behavioral health care programs.

Poses (1999) argues that physician behavior is resistant to change. He offers as an example, how in the 1980's physicians used empiric antibiotic therapy for patients with pharyngitis more than needed given the underlying prevalence of streptococcal infection. These physicians tended to use the antibiotic because they believed streptococcal infection to be present, though the rate of this infection was in fact overestimated. Interventions designed to improve diagnostic judgements did in fact improve these diagnostic judgements, but had no effect on treatment decisions. This illustrates the point that effective interventions were not relevant in decision making. Poses further argues that physicians tend to make decisions based upon outcome probabilities, rather than using formal decision analysis. They also tend to use the "availability heuristic", in which one uses recollections of cases with similar features to guide decision making, and that the cases usually recalled are those cases that are unusual. This heuristic certainly flies in the face of protocols based upon the average response to treatment.

Physicians are also deluged by tactics from the pharmaceutical companies. Of late, drug manufacturers are marketing directly to the consumer, and consumers are now coming to their doctors and are asking for specific prescriptions. Bell, Wilkes, & Kravitz (1999) found that this "direct to consumer" advertising, which cost 1.8 billion dollars in 1998, is favorably evaluated by consumers. Physicians are now faced with their patients leaving disappointed if they are denied a requested prescription and many may seek the prescription from another provider. So protocols that may be indicated given empirical evidence may lose when the physician has a patient persuading him or her to provide a drug that the TV says is state of the art.

Dyer focuses on the power of behavioral health in the management of diabetes, and presents data that support his contention. However, in a recent paper on diabetes management (Helseth, Susman, Crabtree, & O'Connor (1999), not one physician in the study has a system in place in their office to support patient adherence. No physicians in the study mentioned implementation of any behavioral health strategies that are known to be efficacious.

Similarly, Smyth, Stone, Hurewitz & Kaell (1999) conducted an empirical study in which asthma and rheumatoid arthritis patients had clinically relevant changes in health status when they received an intervention that required them to write about the most stressful experience they had ever experience. Spiegel (1999) comments on the study saying if a medication produced the effects found with the writing exercise, the medication would be in widespread use very quickly. This is because there is an industry that would promote it and that physicians believe they understand the mechanisms of action in a medication while the mechanisms of action of a psychosocial intervention are mysterious. He laments the weakness of data when pitted against the pharmaceutical industry.

While Dyer argues his case from an elegant, data based, perspective, the question still remains: who is to be persuaded and how is this to be achieved? It seems that the culture of medicine is difficult to change once the physician is in practice. Disciplines seem to like to remain intact and they don't necessarily like to refer out. Even in psychology, as evidenced by the debate around prescription privileges, discipline issues do battle with economic contingencies. It may be that the most hope for changing medical practices may be in influencing the educational practices of medical schools. Poses (1999) notes that one effective way to change physician behavior is to give them coursework in statistics and in the principles of reasoning. Perhaps coursework of this sort must accompany or set the stage for the introduction of behavioral health systems to physicians.

In any case, behavioral health care must focuses on how to persuade the medical establishment to use the interventions developed. Product development must be sensitive not only to clinical outcome and cost savings, but must also be user friendly to physicians and must appeal to the culture of medicine. Changing the behavior of the physician and the medical system is as important as developing interventions to change the behavior of the patient seeking health care. Behavioral scientists must learn to produce data that are persuasive to medical systems and these data may be different from what is persuasive to a behavioral scientist.

REFERENCES

Bell, R. A., Wilkes, M. S., & Kravitz, R. L. (1999). Advertisement–induced prescription drug requests: Patients' anticipated reactions to a physician who refuses. *The Journal of Family Practice, 48,* 446-452.

Chiles, J. A., Lambert, M. J., & Hatch, A. L. (1999). The impact of psychological interventions on medical cost offset: A meta-analytic review. *Clinical Psychology: Science and Practice, 6*(2), 204-220.

Dyer, R. (2001). Behavioral technologies in disease management: A new service model for working with physicians. In N. A. Cummings, W. O'Donohue, S. C. Hayes, & V. Follette (Eds.), *Integrated behavioral healthcare: Prospects, issues, and opportunities.* New York: Academic Press.

Fischer, P. (1999). Evidentiary medicine lacks humility. *The Journal of Family Practice, 48*(5), 345-346.

Helseth, L. D., Susman, J. L., Crabtree, B. F., & O'Connor, P. J. (1999). Primary care physicians'perceptions of diabetes management: A balancing act. *The Journal of Family Practice, 48*, 37-42.

Otto, M. W. (1999). Psychological interventions in the age of managed care: A commentary on medical cost offsets. *Clinical Psychology: Science and Practice, 6*(2), 239-241.

Poses, R. M. (1999). One size does not fit all: Questions to answer before intervening to change physician behavior. *Journal of Quality Improvement, 25*(9), 486-494.

Smyth, J. M., Stone, A. A., Hurewitz, A., & Kaell, A. (1999). Effects of writing about stressful experiences on symptom reduction in patients with asthma or rheumatoid arthritis: A randomized trial. *Journal of the American Medical Association, 238*, 1304-1309.

Spiegel, D. (1999). Healing words: Emotional expression and disease outcome. *Journal of the American Medical Association, 238*, 1328-1329.

Yurdin, L. (1997). *Primary care assessment of practice needs.* Bellvue, WA: Spectrum Health.

Accountability for Quality in the Real World: From 30,000 Feet to Ground Level and Back Up

Tom Trabin, Ph.D., M.S.M.
Independent Consulting Practice

The Implications of Industrialization for Quality of Care
From Inflationary Costs to Commodity Pricing
From Benefit Maximization to Cost Containment
From Fragmented Treatment Services to Coordinated Systems of Care
**From Minimal to Extensive Tracking of Organizational Performance
    and Treatment Levels**
From Minimal to Extensive Accountability
    Industry Consolidation and Quality of Care
    Integrated Behavioral Health and Medical Care
Differing Approaches to Maintaining and Enhancing Service Quality
    Differentiating Approaches
    Differentiating Purposes
Organizational Performance Measures and Report Cards

149

Integrated Behavioral Healthcare: Positioning Mental Health Practice with Medical/Surgical Practice

The dawning of the 21st century is a challenging time for behavioral healthcare. If benefit purchasing patterns are indicative, behavioral health-care is perceived as a commodity and its services are being priced accordingly. At no time has it been more important to demonstrate with objective data the value of our services and to differentiate those services to purchasers and consumers on the basis of quality—indeed, it is a necessity for survival. And yet, it is difficult for many to afford the resources to do. Funding and reimbursement cutbacks continue. Recent massive consolidation resulted in downsizing for the larger organizations and in a sense of disempowerment for smaller organizations and individual clinicians. None would argue against the value of quality management initiatives but, as the saying goes, when you're up to your neck in alligators, its difficult to think of how to drain the swamp.

This chapter focuses on the practical and policy challenges of account-ability for quality services in the behavioral healthcare field and industry. The chapter begins with a review of industrialization and recent consolidation developments, and examines their implications for accountability and qual-ity of care. This is followed with a brief overview of differing approaches to quality management and then a more in-depth examination of performance measurement and report cards, including findings from a research study. Next steps are suggested for the behavioral healthcare industry to take for advancing the use of performance measurement for accountability and for enhanced valuation of behavioral healthcare services.

THE IMPLICATIONS OF INDUSTRIALIZATION FOR QUALITY OF CARE

Quality management does not exist in a vacuum; its focus is guided by the context within which it operates. For behavioral healthcare, that context has changed radically in the past fifteen years. Following is a brief review of key changes and the controversial issues regarding quality care they have provoked.

From Inflationary Costs to Commodity Pricing

The economic issues behavioral healthcare confronts at the close of the 20th century are much different than those it faced fifteen years ago. Spiraling inflation of health care expenditures, seemingly out of control, had become a national issue in the 1980s. The adoption of cost containment methods such as those that characterize managed care were just beginning.

Behavioral healthcare was among the more vulnerable targets for cost containment and rate reductions. Managed behavioral healthcare organizations (MBHOs) not only contained costs through effective managed care methods, but also by underbidding each other in a scramble for market share (Cummings, 1998). Employers in both public and private sectors encouraged the bidding war. Over the past fifteen years, behavioral healthcare lost approximately half of its percentage of the health care dollar expended annually (Hay Group, 1999). Few would argue that reductions have removed excess fat only and not cut into the bone of quality care. In fact, many fear that zealous cost containment reduced behavioral healthcare to the economic status of a commodity (Bartlett, 1998).

From Benefit Maximization to Cost Containment

The financial incentives within behavioral healthcare organizations have also changed dramatically. In the 1980s, insuring organizations were much more distinct from provider organizations, and the two types of organizations each had quite different financial incentives.

Insurers did not track or managed treatment patterns closely, and for generating profits they relied primarily upon their investments of health insurance premium revenues in stock and real estate. When their actuaries underestimated treatment utilization and consequent claims to be paid for a given year, insurers would simply raise their premium rates with relative impunity the following year. They had little or no incentive to manage care.

Treatment provider organizations and individual practitioners maximized their own revenues by the type, frequency and duration of treatment they provided. The financial incentive was to generate more expenditures on treatment. Unnecessary psychiatric hospitalizations were the most costly excess in that system.

Increasingly, the line between insurer and treatment provider blurs. Many behavioral healthcare organizations now combine treatment delivery, care management and insurer functions. The conflicting incentives of insurer and provider are brought into much closer alignment. As costs become more contained, public concerns about compromises in quality of care increase, and so correspondingly does the need for credible quality management.

From Fragmented Treatment Services to Coordinated Systems of Care

The fragmented cottage industry of small, separate treatment organizations and individual clinical practices began to disappear in the late 1980s. Many of the same treatment delivery elements of that cottage industry remain, but they are now organized into large systems of care. They share in common, to varying degrees, centralized provider contracting, referrals, and prior authorization of specific treatment plans. These systems create new opportunities for the tracking and coordination of care, and consequently for accountability, that were not possible before.

The industrialization of behavioral healthcare brought tremendous potential for improved treatment coordination. Instead of haphazard selection of a treatment provider, possibly through as crude a method as the yellow pages, consumers now have centralized intake and referral services to call for informed direction to the appropriate level of care and to the clinician with the proper specialty to address the consumer's presenting problem. Since organized care systems incorporate providers at all levels and types of care, care managers are able to continue this guidance throughout the entire course of treatment irrespective of the diversity of therapeutic settings, programs and approaches that may be required. There need be less likelihood of patient care falling through the cracks when in transition from one provider to another.

However, an organized care system can still lead to poor treatment. Highly publicized reports attest to this. Providers may be improperly credentialed who are not well qualified and render inadequate treatment, intake coordinators and care managers may not be properly qualified and consequently demonstrate poor clinical judgment, and the professional culture of the organization may be too weak to resist the financial incentives to under treat. Accountability systems are needed to provide checks and balances so the potential benefits of organized care systems are attained, and the potential for harm is minimal.

From Minimal to Extensive Tracking of Organizational Performance- and Treatment-Level Data

Organized care systems have the capability to track detailed course-of-treatment data across hundreds of thousands of patients in ways that the previous "nonsystem" of the 1980s never could. Their capabilities are further enhanced by the rapid advancement of computer and electronic communication technologies. The potential for increased accountability, improved care, and generation of new knowledge is only beginning to be realized. The more that organized care systems are capable of tracking and reporting on the quality of their services, the more that stakeholders are likely to expect (and insist) they do so.

From Minimal to Extensive Accountability

One of the primary advantages of organized care systems is the heightened degree of accountability. In the 1980s, there was very little accountability possible for the particular course of treatment a patient might undertake across multiple levels of care and providers. Nor was there much accountability for the amount and type of treatment delivered by any single provider. Only the most egregious examples of malpractice were subject to grievance through professional boards, associations, and the courts.

In organized care systems, there are multiple layers of accountability. Regulatory and accrediting organizations set performance standards for both managed care and provider organizations as a prerequisite to bid on behavioral healthcare contracts. They require auditable information to ensure those standards are met. Employers set up reporting and (sometimes a multitude of) other accountability requirements for their managed care vendors. To fulfill those requirements, managed care companies oversee the performance of their provider network and/or staff clinicians by managing care and analyzing data that providers are required to submit. In turn, providers and the consumers they treat may access formal appeal and grievance procedures with managed care companies, and some also have input through satisfaction surveys that the managed care companies are required to disseminate. These and other checks and balances will evolve as multiple stakeholders demand increased accountability for the quality of services provided.

Industry Consolidation and Quality of Care

Most people know from history that industrialization leads to consolidation. For behavioral healthcare this means that companies will integrate vertically (e.g. a hospital develops day treatment programs, acquires outpatient clinics, and develops managed care functions) and horizontally (e.g. several managed care companies merge or acquire each other). The business goals of consolidation in any industry are to obtain greater market share, efficiencies and profitability.

The behavioral healthcare field went through this process at a pace that took most people by surprise. Within little more than a decade, managed care grew from a few companies with a small book of business and little market share to several hundred companies that covered most of the insured population of the United States (Trabin, T. & Freeman, M. A., 1995). Then, in a rapid leap to a next generation of system restructuring, these companies consolidated into a small handful of mega-companies that now cover most of the managed behavioral healthcare business. Three companies alone now cover almost 100 million lives. Will this degree of consolidation be the "right size" for obtaining maximum efficiencies and a high quality of care, or will it prove too unwieldy?

Potential benefits to the field. Industry consolidation has the potential to move the field more easily to consensus on common standards in many areas. For the advancement of quality management, common standards are crucial. Many constituencies, but particularly consumers and purchasers, want such standards for practice guidelines, organizational performance indicators, and treatment outcome measures. Evidence-based practice guidelines, adopted widely, would result in more consistent practice patterns and greater credibility for our field. Widely used organization- and system-level performance indicators would provide consumers and purchasers with comparative data to aid them in selecting their health plan and treatment providers on the basis of quality. Widely used person-level outcome measures would enable scientists and practitioners to improve practice guidelines and further determine what interventions work best with specified conditions.

These goals are likely to be achieved only if the largest companies, as market leaders, make it a high priority. They can involve representatives of different constituencies in advisory capacities to formulate the best standards and insure a broad consensus. If they decide to take this high road, they might also use their consolidated bargaining power to obtain increased contract prices for funding of more substantial quality initiatives.

To advance further in quality and efficiency of services, the behavioral healthcare field also needs common standards for electronic communication and computer-based patient records. The few largest companies with most resources may decide it is in their best interests to invest in the purchase and customization *or Web-based outsourcing of standardized* practice management, outcomes measurement and electronic communication software that can subsequently be used by their provider network at low cost. This would greatly ease if not end the frustrating demands placed upon providers to use differing forms from each of a dozen or more manage care companies with which they contract. Industry wide cooperation in meeting common data requirements may then become a reality, at an affordable cost. As a result, industry wide quality management initiatives based on data could take a giant leap forward.

Potential harm to the field. A more negative scenario is also, of course, quite possible and fraught with danger. The expense from some of the recent acquisitions and mergers was extremely costly, resulting in substantially increased debt. For those companies that are publicly traded, it also resulted in plummeting valuation of their stock. The pressures upon them are intense to actualize the efficiencies of consolidation quickly, reduce debt and enhance profitability. Their short-term tactics to accomplish these challenges include employee layoffs, consolidation of operating systems across newly acquired companies, rationalizing provider networks, and adopting a conservative approach to investments in new quality initiatives and information system components to support those initiatives. Financial pressures are also prompting delegation of some responsibilities and related costs onto network provider organizations, many of whom are financially vulnerable and unable to bear the burden. These are not the best of times to ask companies to invest in new quality initiatives for their own improvement, let alone for the greater but less direct benefit of the field.

The managed care focus on reduction of direct costs is resulting in further cuts in reimbursement rates for providers. Rate reductions during the past ten years already drove many skilled mental health professionals and provider organizations out of the market. What result will the new reductions have? We know from research that the therapeutic skill and other specific characteristics of the clinician were vital components of what resulted in treatment effectiveness. Even the most ingenious quality management initiatives will be limited in effectiveness if many of the best and brightest clinicians leave the field.

Another potential threat to quality in the restructured behavioral healthcare industry will come from the large bureaucracies created within the newly consolidated managed care giants. An essential aspect of bureaucracies is to develop and base decisions upon an extensive set of rules. At their best they provide informed guidelines for decision support. At their worst, they provide a set of decision rules that employees apply rigidly across situations for which those rules may at times be inappropriate. In contrast, the nature of behavioral healthcare treatment is highly personal and individualized. To the extent that managed care becomes bureaucratized and devoid of human and professional discussion, there is increased danger that some care management decisions will be unintentionally but inevitably misguided with harmful results.

Centralization versus decentralization and quality management. An important set of strategic decisions for each of the large consolidated managed care companies is to determine which functions are best maintained centrally for efficiency and quality control, and which are best decentralized. Their decisions have vital implications for how to most effectively and efficiently manage the quality of their services. This section will address a few of the functions that have the most bearing on quality management.

Although organized care systems may delegate service functions to multiple organizations across many sites, they remain ultimately accountable for the overall quality of their services. These systems usually centralize the design and production of their forms, which provide the structure for how data is collected. They also centralize the selection of performance and outcome measures to be used, and the practice guidelines to be disseminated and tracked for adherence. It is usually at the local provider and managed care sites that the data is actually collected and then transmitted electronically or by mail to a centralized site where it is aggregated and analyzed at the system level. Increasingly, organized care systems rely upon information system specialists to structure the data from multiple sources into data warehouses for easier analysis. Innovations in database technology now make possible these warehouses capable of analyzing large amounts of aggregated, restructured data.

Managed care practices vary widely with regards to how centralized they make the care management functions. Large national companies with provider-contracted networks will provide some triage and referral from their headquarters office to sites nationwide, but will also have regional offices that perform those functions for employer contracts that require a regional presence. These same companies tend to manage ongoing care through prior authorization from their national or regional offices if they reimburse their providers on a fee-for-service basis. If they pay providers on a case rate or capitation basis, they tend to delegate at least some if not most of the care management functions to the contracting provider organizations. Those managed care companies with staff models tend to use care management methods at the local site. To the extent that care management functions are delegated to a local provider organization, the delegating managed care company must find ways to manage quality and collect quality-related data from a distance.

Delegated accountability along provider distribution channels. Network model managed behavioral healthcare companies are increasingly delegating at least some care management functions—and related reporting accountability—to their contracting provider organizations (Bobbitt, B., Marques, C. & Trout, D., 1998). One of the results is a complex layering system that, at its most extreme, can involve prospective patients in describing their presenting problems to several complete strangers over the telephone. A not unlikely scenario is:

1. The prospective patient calls the managed behavioral healthcare organization (MBHO) and speak to an intake coordinator who refers the prospective patient to the regional independent practice association (IPA) or "mega-group."
2. The prospective patient then calls the regional IPA or mega-group and speak to an intake coordinator who refers the prospective patient to the local group practice in his/her geographic area.
3. The prospective patient then calls the local group practice and speak to an intake coordinator who refers the prospective patient to an appropriate provider.
4. The prospective patient then calls the provider to set up an appointment.

The obvious problems with this worst case scenario are its consumer unfriendliness, time wastefulness, and excessive use of administrative resources. Also, at each step in the channeling of those services, part of the premium dollar is taken and is no longer available for direct patient care. It goes something like this:

1. Purchaser contracts with a large HMO or insurance company which keeps part of the premium dollar.
2. Subcontracts to a carveout MBHO which keeps part of the premium dollar.
3. Subcontracts or pays fee-for-service to regional IPAs or mega groups which keep part of the premium dollar or reimbursement for services.

4. Subcontract or pay fee-for-service to local group practices which keep part of the premium dollar or reimbursement for services.
5. Reimburse clinicians at low rates (e.g. $30-$40 per billable hour for non-M.D.s plus overhead expenses) to provide highly professional clinical services.

Every industry post-consolidation has the challenge of designing effective and efficient distribution channels for its goods and services. Because the nature of treatment services are so personalized in the behavior healthcare industry, the distribution channeling of those services from a nationwide, centralized operation is particularly challenging. The layering described above may seem unnecessarily convoluted, consumer-unfriendly, time-consuming, and resource-intensive. Certainly there is room for improvement or, in business terms, need for rationalization of services.

While recommendations for how this rationalization of services can best be accomplished are beyond the scope of this chapter, the brief discussion above of the trends and problems is relevant as part of the context for quality management. With multiple layering of responsibilities for care among distinctly separate organizations, the overall system of care's task of demonstrating accountability for quality of services has become enormously complex and expensive.

Integrated Behavioral Health and Medical Care

Another vital trend in the restructuring of behavioral healthcare services is the reintegration of those services with medical care. Other chapters in this book focus exclusively and extensively upon this trend as it pertains to both primary and specialty medical care, so it will not be necessary to go into depth here. Suffice it to say that the medical cost offsets that integration can provide are not only beneficial financially, but also represent measurable reductions in human suffering that can be considered part of quality management.

There are unique challenges to quality management arising from the integration of behavioral healthcare and medical care. First, and most often discussed, is the practical challenge of measurement. In truly integrated systems, such as Health Maintenance Organizations (HMOs) that do not contract out specialty services, all service data is available. However, in carve-out managed behavioral healthcare, the task of obtaining pharmaceutical and medical data from other companies to analyze with the behavioral health services is daunting (Coke, J., 1996). Contracts with purchasers and between health plans must be written to encourage this data-sharing, and difficult legal issues of confidentiality and data privacy must be addressed. NCQA's Health Plan and Employer Data Information Set (HEDIS) 2000 features a new antidepressant medication measure that will prompt working through some of these challenges (Coltin, K. and Beck, A., 1999).

Another set of challenges to quality management from integration relate to the longstanding trend in many medically-dominated organizations to under value and inadequately fund behavioral health services. If integration is truly at the level of organizationally restructured care management and service delivery, then these dangers must be anticipated and addressed. Carve out managed behavioral healthcare grew so successfully during the past decade partly in response to public demand for a richer behavioral health benefit than was offered by HMOs. For various reasons, particularly the bidding wars for market share, the differences in benefits offered by carve-outs are not as pronounced as they once were. However, it may be argued that the reduced benefit is a problem to be corrected, not a reason to end carveouts. For the purposes of this chapter on quality management, the point is that benefits too meagerly funded limit the potential for quality services, and necessitate stringent reporting requirements on quality as a check and balance against doing harm.

Differing Approaches to Maintaining and Enhancing Service Quality and Accountability

Among the most powerful and underrated motivators guiding behavior within organizations are corporate culture and values. These factors are set by and communicated from top management—the chief executive officer and senior management. Some providers—individual practitioners, provider organizations and professional associations—maintain that the proper values and professional training should obviate the need for them to be overseen by managed care. Some managed care executives maintain, in similar fashion, that the proper corporate culture and values should obviate the need for them to be overseen by accrediting and regulatory organizations. Both sets of detractors express the belief that corporate culture and values are better differentiators and predictors of ethical and quality service than are objective measures.

Many of the organizational leaders whose opinions are paraphrased above are astutely insightful regarding the limitations of our current objective measures. Some are also reluctant about and reactive to these changes in our behavioral healthcare system. Their arguments do not wholly satisfy the public need for checks and balances to potential excesses arising from the varying financial incentives within our healthcare system. For those public concerns to be addressed systemically, accrediting and regulatory agencies with independent auditing capabilities seem to be needed. These agencies must stipulate clear requirements that can be met through documentation and/or performance data. Some of the larger purchasing organizations and coalitions also possess and use these capabilities, but they are too few and inconsistent to totally replace the functions of regulatory and accrediting organizations.

Differentiating Approaches

Books have been written that articulate systematic approaches to quality management within organizations, a summary of which is beyond the scope of this chapter. This section very briefly reviews the major types of approaches, contrasting some of them for purposes of clarity, and focusing on a few examples of their current applications in behavioral healthcare.

Quality assurance and continuous quality improvement. The traditional quality assurance approach focuses upon identification of problems and their amelioration. In contrast, continuous quality improvement approaches encourage ongoing collection of data from multiple sources to identify opportunities for improvement, irrespective of whether egregious problems are identified. During the past decade, the latter approach became extremely popular with American industry in response to global competition. Elements of quality improvement are now incorporated into the accreditation standards of both the National Committee for Quality Assurance (NCQA, 1997) and the Joint Commission for Accreditation of Health Care Organizations (JCAHO, 1997).

Accreditation, performance measurement and report cards. Accreditation standards tended, until recently, to focus primarily on the documentation of organizational structures and processes. Accrediting organizations such as NCQA and JCAHO are beginning to add performance measurement to their set of requirements, so that data-based results are monitored. The performance measures they have initially developed tend to analyze elements of process (e.g. access, utilization) but the intention is to move more to outcomes. A few organizations, such as NCQA, have taken performance measurement to a new level with "report cards". These report cards compare the performance of similar types of organizations on standardized measures and are intended to guide purchasers and consumers in making selection decisions based on quality. They will be described in more depth in a succeeding section of this chapter.

External accountability and internal quality improvement. Quality assurance and related methods have been driven primarily by external requirements from regulatory and accrediting organizations. The relatively recent enthusiasm with continuous quality improvement methods have added an internal focus. Ironically, it is because of the externally imposed requirements to have an internal quality improvement program that has broadened the adoption of this approach.

Outcomes measurement, outcomes research, and outcomes management. Outcomes measurement is increasingly used in behavioral healthcare organizations. The methodology is more similar to program evaluation than outcomes research, since there is usually no experimental design, the results are used only for purposes of meeting the organization's accountability requirements and quality improvement goals, and the results are consequentially not generalizable to a broader population. The outcome measures are brief but tend to have at least some psychometric research behind them to address reliability and validity concerns.

Outcomes management was most prominently introduced and articulated by Paul Ellwood (Ellwood, 1988) to describe the ongoing collection, analysis and use of outcome data within organizations as a basis for efforts to improve clinical processes. To be effective, the data must include details of treatment protocols as well as outcomes. The organizational culture must be committed to the value of outcome data for quality improvement. This is a sophisticated quality management approach that is still rare in behavioral healthcare organizations.

Consumer satisfaction and dissatisfaction. Consumer satisfaction surveys remain the most common form of patient self-report data collected routinely by behavioral healthcare organizations for use in quality management. Some organizations erroneously present the results of these surveys as information on treatment outcomes, but the research literature is clear that satisfaction is a different factor than outcomes (Lunnon, K. M., & Ogles, B. M.).

Consumer advocacy groups, particularly in the public sector, have criticized most satisfaction surveys as designed to pull for high levels of satisfaction. They have suggested other item wording to also pull for dissatisfaction and for other important factors (Ganju, V., 1998). Their perspective was incorporated into at least one consumer survey instrument that is now widely used in the public sector (MHSIP Task Force on a Consumer-Oriented Mental Health Report Card, 1996).

Differentiating Purposes

Behavioral healthcare organizations vary widely in the degree to which they employ quality management methods, and the methods they select. Their selection decisions are based partly on their organizational culture and values, partly on the basic standards set by regulatory and accrediting agencies as a required floor for competing, and partly on what the market might reward as competitive advantage.

Most behavioral healthcare organizations undertake quality management for the primary purpose of meeting requirements dictated by organizations external to them. These include purchasers and payers with whom they have contracts, regulatory agencies, and accrediting organizations. A recent study indicated, for most organizations, that even internal quality improvement efforts are focused primarily upon requirements set by these external organizations (Kramer, T., Trabin, T. et.al., 1997). These economically tight times clearly result in an organizational focus on survival, not high-minded idealism.

Nevertheless, there are a few organizations which go well beyond what is required. Some may do so out of an entrepreneurial spirit, hoping it will bring them competitive advantage and new business. A few others do so because they think that the use of data to continuously improve patient care is simply the right thing to do, and therefore necessary. Some wonderful examples of this have been described elsewhere in the literature, where outpatient clinics and group practices have used linkages between assessment, practice guidelines, and outcome measurement to guide their treatment planning and continuously improve their clinical processes (Person, J., 1999; Wade, W., 1999).

The need for more sophisticated forms of quality management is greater when viewed from the perspective of the entire behavioral healthcare system. A predominant public perception of behavioral healthcare services is that they are significantly less valuable than medical interventions, cannot be differentiated on the basis of quality, and therefore can be priced as a commodity service. It is vital that we counter that perception convincingly to resolve the financial crisis our field has entered. To do so effectively, we need quality management methods we can implement successfully on a broad nationwide level—particularly practice guidelines, organizational performance measures, and treatment outcome measures (including medical cost offset). Without the support of strong data, talk about quality has little impact.

Of the varying types of quality management, the following sections of the chapter will focus primarily on those used for accountability at organizational and system-of-care levels. In particular, we will review those that are performance measurement-oriented and have the potential for broad impact across the entire behavioral healthcare field. No less important, practice guidelines will be addressed by another author in a different chapter of this book.

Organizational Performance Measures and Report Cards

Evaluation of the quality of behavioral healthcare services for accreditation purposes traditionally focused on structure and process measures. The audits used to assure compliance with quality assurance and accreditation requirements centered on assuring proper credentialing of clinicians, proper documentation of an appeals processes, and other structural and process features of quality assurance. These requirements provide a necessary infrastructure to support quality service, but they fail to provide a basis from which purchasers and consumers can compare the outcomes and value of different organizations when selecting services.

In contrast, performance measures use data to focus upon results *that can be compared across multiple organizations.* As an example of how accreditation standards for organizational processes translate into performance measures, consider this example within the performance domain of access to care:

> Accreditation Standard: Patients receiving routine outpatient psychotherapy obtain timely appointments.
>
> Performance Indicator: The percent of patients receiving routine outpatient psychotherapy who express satisfaction with the timeliness of their appointments.
>
> Performance Measure: The percent of patients receiving outpatient psychotherapy who endorse "usually" or "always" to the item "In the last 12 months, how often did you get an appointment for counseling or treatment as soon as you wanted" on the Experience Of Care and Health Outcomes survey.

The results of an organization's performance measures can be compared against an internal baseline and with other organizations for benchmarking purposes. The comparisons can also be incorporated into organizational performance "report cards". The performance data, particularly when benchmarked, can be used for accountability, quality improvement, better informing consumer choice, system and program planning and management, meeting contract requirements with purchasers and payers, monitoring system change, and (with proper design) contributing to the scientific understanding of services and outcomes (Evaluation Center@HSRI, 1998).

An increasing number of stakeholder groups advocate for behavioral healthcare organizations to be held accountable for their service performance by submitting standardized data that can be used to compare them against each other. The performance domains of greatest interest to these stakeholders are access to care, utilization, appropriateness of care provided, and clinical and functional outcomes achieved by patients. Consumer satisfaction with various aspects of services is typically interwoven into these domains, although some regard satisfaction as a distinct domain of it own.

Report cards that encourage accountability through comparative data on organizations are a new phenomenon for behavioral healthcare. They are only possible because of the dual development of organized care systems with the capability of tracking many aspects of the care, and technologies that enable organizations to store large amounts of data in flexibly structured ways for rapid processing and analysis. The organizations which commonly submit data for use in these report cards range from general medical health plans with behavioral health components (such as HMOs), specialty managed behavioral healthcare organizations, and large integrated delivery systems. These organized systems of care are the primary entities controlling health care services in the United States, including access to treatment and the type and amount of treatment delivered for a substantial portion of this country's population.

The Art and Science of Performance Measure Development

Because of the expense and high stakes to participating organizations, those who develop performance measures included in report cards must do so carefully in a manner that is likely to produce both clinically and financially useful results. Attention is given to identifying the most useful indicators to purchasers and consumers, and the best ways to measure them. NCQA has developed the most elaborate and clearly articulated criteria, along with the most systematic methods for implementing them in measurement selection (NCQA, 1997). The criteria they consider include:

> Relevance: meaningfulness to key stakeholder groups, clinical importance for treatment, financial importance, cost effectiveness, strategic importance,

controllability (within the organization's power to impact results), variance among systems (make a difference for comparability), and potential for performance improvement;

Scientific soundness: clinical evidence that the behaviors to be measured make a difference, reproducibility, validity, accuracy, necessity and feasibility of case-mix adjustment/risk adjustment, and comparability of data sources;

Feasibility: precision of specifications, reasonableness of costs, allowance for confidentiality and data privacy constraints, logistically feasible, and auditable.

Considerations in Report Card Implementation

The data collection and reporting required to produce valid report cards are expensive undertakings for the submitting organizations as well as for the report card vendor. Data collection can cost an average-sized health plan or delivery system of a similar size over a million dollars annually. To meet data reporting requirements, a participating organization must have a well-developed information system infrastructure, expert staff dedicated to data collection and analyses, and effective coordination of efforts with contracting providers.

In addition to the costliness of data collection, there are substantial business risks to the participating organizations in sharing publicly the comparative results. If an organization's performance is low, it must move quickly to correct its deficiencies, or risk losing business. Furthermore, the money invested in quality measurement could instead be used to reduce premiums, add customer service features, or expand marketing efforts. Some organizations may regard spending money on comparative performance measurement as potentially undermining other important aspects of their business mission.

Current Report Card Initiatives

There are *at least* three major behavioral healthcare report card initiatives that are both ongoing and national in scope, and several other initiatives that are closely related:

PERMS. The American Managed Behavioral Healthcare Association (AMBHA) developed approximately twenty performance indicators to provide comparative information on access, quality, appropriateness, and satisfaction, with regards to their services. AMBHA represents specialty managed behavioral healthcare companies. Its member organizations, in aggregate, provide mental health and substance abuse treatment coverage for approximately 100 million people. With such a large client base, the collection of data is an extensive and expensive undertaking.

AMBHA's performance indicators are organized into a report card called *Performance Measurement for Managed Behavioral Healthcare Programs (PERMS)* in 1995 (AMBHA, 1995). AMBHA's approach is pragmatic, focusing primarily on measures that require administrative data collected routinely. AMBHA completed the pilot phase of data collection and analysis for PERMS 1.0 in 1996, and learned which technical and administrative areas required attention in order for the next phase to be implemented successfully. At the time of this book's publication, they are likely to have completed data collection, analysis and reporting for PERMS 2.0.

HEDIS. The National Committee for Quality Assurance (NCQA) is the predominant accrediting agency for managed care organizations. Compliance with their accreditation and performance standards is becoming a prerequisite for managed care companies to bid on many contracts. Consequently, the impact of NCQA standards is substantial. In addition to their accreditation procedures, which focus primarily on process standards, NCQA has developed a report card called the *Health Employer Data Information Set (HEDIS)* to measure the results of actual performance (NCQA, 1997). Many of AMBHA's PERMS measures were considered for inclusion into HEDIS, and several were incorporated. HEDIS is revised annually, with new measures added. The proportion of measures devoted to behavioral healthcare is small but growing.

MHSIP consumer–oriented mental health report card. The Mental Health Statistics Improvement Program (MHSIP) *Consumer-Oriented Mental Health Report Card* (MHSIP Task Force on a Consumer-Oriented Mental Health Report Card, 1996) focuses particularly on managed care for publicly-funded programs. Its development was funded through the federal Center for Mental Health Services (CMHS), and is intended as a performance evaluation framework for states to adopt as they transition their mental health and substance abuse services into managed care. The content focuses on consumer perceptions of care and their outcomes more than other report cards, and it relies less on routinely collected administrative data. CMHS has awarded grants to most states to implement aspects of the report card, and has incorporated those aspects into their quality improvement programs.

Related initiatives. In addition to the above-mentioned three report cards, several related initiatives are underway that are worth mentioning:

> Several state mental health agencies have developed report cards of their own, including Indiana, Iowa, Massachusetts and Texas.
>
> The Joint Commission for Accreditation of Health Care Organizations (JCAHO) plans to require performance measurement reporting for the behavioral healthcare organizations it accredits. Separately, it also began an initiative called ORYX, which requires that organizations contract with an outcomes software vendor to collect and analyze treatment outcome data.
>
> The Council for Accreditation of Rehabilitation Facilities (CARF) convened two annual summits of leaders in performance measurement to advise them on best indicators and measures, and have developed a set they recommend organizations use which seek accreditation from them.
>
> The National Association of State Mental Health Program Directors (NASMHPD) developed a framework and listing of most commonly used measures across state mental health departments.
>
> The Institute for Behavioral Healthcare conducted the first series of empirical studies with performance measures in behavioral healthcare. The studies investigated the degree to which different measures were used, perceptions of the relative feasibility and cost of implementing the measures, perceptions of the relative value of the information provided by the measures, and benchmarkable standards set for each measure. Some of the key findings of the studies are summarized in a later section of this chapter.

Providing an Empirical Base for Report Card Development

In 1995, the Institute for Behavioral Healthcare's National Leadership Council (NLC) began a series of performance indicator research projects to provide an empirical base that would accelerate the advancement and quality of report cards. The NLC included more than three hundred leading organizations in the behavioral healthcare industry that, together, accounted for most of the managed behavioral healthcare coverage and organized treatment delivery in the United States. Their studies were designed with the guidance of interdisciplinary task forces representing organizations from key sectors of the field, such as managed care organizations, community mental health centers, integrated delivery systems and specialty behavioral health facilities, and behavioral group practices. Each was conducted collaboratively with technical support provided by the research staff at the Institute for Behavioral Healthcare, the University of Cincinnati Department of Psychiatry, and University Managed Care, Inc.

The first study was conducted in 1995-96. A task force of experts representing different segments of the behavioral healthcare industry first conducted a careful review of major report card initiatives in the field to identify key performance domains and associated performance measures. A pilot study of NLC organizations was conducted to obtain further information about performance domains evaluated routinely in naturalistic settings. Five major performance domains were identified (access, clinical appropriateness, quality of care, outcomes, and prevention), along with the indicators thought to be most widely used within each domain. NLC organizations were surveyed to determine which of 69 indicators they were actually using, and how meaningful, valid, and feasible they considered each indicator to be. The results were published in 1996 (Kramer, T., Trabin, T., et.al., 1996) and presented at national conferences.

The NLC decided a useful next step in studying performance indicators would be to target the indicators identified in the first study as the most widely used within each domain, and analyze organizations' actual experiences with measuring them. It was thought that the empirical results derived from the study could serve as an important adjunct to expert opinion for organizations seeking to identify the performance indicators that are most pragmatic and value-added to measure and use.

Methods

A task force of members representing behavioral group practices, managed care organizations, community mental health centers, and integrated delivery systems was convened to establish the research objectives, design the survey, and develop the data collection methodology. A draft of the survey instrument was circulated to NLC representatives from approximately thirty organizations, and their feedback was incorporated into the final version.

Survey instrument. Twenty-eight performance indicators identified in the first study as most commonly used were selected for this study's more in-depth analysis. The survey included demographic questions regarding the responding organizations, questions regarding their experience with implementing each performance indicator, and questions regarding the benchmarking standards they set for themselves with each indicator. A complete description of the survey can be found in Table 2. A few of the questions asked regarding each of the indicators were:

> The estimated level of staff time required for tracking the
>   indicator.
> The estimated level of cost to track the indicator.
> The estimated value of tracking the indicator for purposes
>   of quality improvement.
> The estimated value of tracking the indicator for external
>   reporting purposes.
> What performance standards the organization set for
>   itself with regards to the indicator.

Participants. All NLC members were surveyed; 106 responded, resulting in a return rate of 40%. The total number of respondents included 15 (14.2%) managed care organizations (MCOs), 17 (16.0%) behavioral group practices (BGPs), 54 (50.9%) community mental health centers/social and rehabilitation service agencies (CMHCs), 16 (15.1%) integrated delivery systems/specialty behavioral health facilities (IDS/SBFs), and 4 (3.8%) who identified themselves as belonging to an "other" category. They ranged widely in number of sites, clinicians, and covered lives.

Procedure. The Institute for Behavioral Healthcare mailed surveys to all members of the NLC with instructions for completing it within a specified period of time. All surveys were coded so that anonymity of the respondents could be maintained. Data entry and analyses were subsequently performed by the authors of this report at the University of Cincinnati and at the Institute for Behavioral Healthcare.

Response options for four of the questions were structured so that their results could be compared with correlation statistics. The four questions addressed in this way were: 1) estimated staff time to track each indicator, 2) overall costs to track each indicator, 3) estimated value of each indicator for internal quality improvement, and 4) estimated value of each indicator for external reporting. In addition to the summary, these results are reported in more detail in Table 1. A composite "cost-effectiveness" score for each indicator was also derived and is listed in Table 2 with a brief summary.

Results

Highlights of the study are excerpted from the original publication and are shown in the Results and Conclusions sections below:

Estimated staff time and costs required for tracking indicators. There was a .97 correlation between the amount of staff time required to track each indicator, and the overall costliness of tracking. This suggests that management regards the cost of staff time as the primary contributor to the cost of tracking these indicators, and regards the more substantial cost of an information system infrastructure as a fixed and essential cost of doing business.

The indicators rated by the combined industry segments as requiring the most staff time and highest overall costs to monitor were primarily process indicators. They are typically found in accreditation standards, in contrast to outcome and performance indicators usually found in report cards. They are:

> Percent of inpatient cases audited for medical necessity.
> Percent of inpatient cases reviewed for adequate documentation.
> Percent of medical records audited for quality.
> Written plan for monitoring quality of care.
> Percent of inpatient cases reviewed with the medical director for medical necessity.
> Percent of providers recredentialed annually.

The other indicators rated as staff time-intensive and costly to monitor were related to the measurement of clinical outcomes. Because of their costliness to administer, they typically are not required in most report cards at this time. They are:

> Percent of patients having reduced symptoms after treatment.
> Percent of patients having improved functioning after treatment.

The six indicators rated by the combined industry segments as requiring the least staff time and as least costly to track all reflect the domain of Access. They are performance indicators commonly found in major report cards and in purchaser reporting requirements:

> Average length of stay in a partial program.
> Average length of stay in an intensive outpatient program.
> Inpatient days per thousand (enrolled members).
> Waiting time for scheduling routine office visits.

Telephone call abandonment rate.
Average length of stay in an Inpatient program.

EstimatedValue of Indicator for Internal Quality Improvement and for external reporting. There was a strong, statistically significant (.85) correlation between the perceived value of information provided by each indicator for internal quality improvement and for external reporting purposes. This indicates a strong convergence between what organizations find useful to improve their internal processes, and what they need to report to external agencies.

The indicators rated by the combined industry segments as most valuable for either quality improvement or external reporting were all performance and outcome-oriented measures, typically found in report cards. None were process indicators, more typically found in accreditation standards and quality assurance audit procedures. These particular performance and outcome-oriented indicators are best categorized in domains that reflect Access to Care, Quality of Care, and Outcomes of Care. They are:

Acute inpatient days/1,000 (enrolled members).
Outpatient visits/1,000 (enrolled members).
Percent of patients reporting overall satisfaction with quality of care.
Percent of patients with adverse outcomes.
Average length of stay in an inpatient hospital program.
Percent of patients having improved functioning following treatment.
Percent of patients readmitted after a specified period of time.

The indicators rated by the combined industry segments as providing the least value for internal quality improvement and for external reporting purposes were the two indicators within the Prevention domain. This may reflect the fact that payers have failed to establish strong incentives for

	Staff Time	Cost	Quality Improvement
Cost	0.97		
Quality Improvement	0.02	-0.03	
External Reporting	-0.17	-0.18	0.85

Table 1

Correlations among staff time, cost, internal quality improvement, and external reporting.

behavioral health promotion, prevention and demand management programs at the current time. These "low valued" indicators are:

Dissemination of information on behavioral health and prevention issues.

Psychoeducational prevention groups in place.

Other indicators rated as among the least valuable for both quality improvement and external reporting are:

Percent of inpatient cases reviewed for adequate documentation.

Average length of stay in a partial hospital program.

Interrelationships between Indicators. The previous two sections review ratings for the indicators with respect to the four dimensions of Staff Time, Cost, Internal Quality Improvement, and External Reporting. These four dimensions were rated on a scale that can be considered linear and continuous, thereby permitting a correlational analysis. Table 1 summarizes the findings:

As was mentioned in the preceding two sections and indicated in the table, there is a highly significant correlation between staff time and overall costs involved in tracking the indicators, and a similarly high correlation between the perceived value of the indicators for quality improvement and for external reporting purposes.

The most interesting findings in the table are the lack of significant positive correlations between the resources required to track these indicators and their perceived value. In fact, three of the four correlations are negative, although none significantly so. These findings have important implications for the industry which will be discussed in the concluding section of this report.

Cost effectiveness of indicators. A composite "cost-effectiveness index" was derived by adding the rank order numbers for each of the indicators evaluated in this study on the four items as follows:

1. Staff time for tracking the indicator (least time= 28, most time = 1)
2. Costs to track the indicator (least costly = 28, most costly =1)
3). Value for internal quality improvement (most valued = 28, least valued = 1)
4. Value for external reporting (most valued = 28, least valued = 1)
5. Value for external reporting (most valued = 28, least valued = 1)

Indicator (Rank ordered from most to least cost-effective)	Cost-Effectiveness Score
1. Acute inpatient days/1000	104
2. Acute inpatient average length of stay	95
3. Outpatient visits/1000	94
4. Intensive outpatient average length of stay	86
5. Percent of patients readmitted after specified period	82
6. Percent of patients reporting overall satisfaction with quality of care	80
7. Telephone response time by answering phone calls	77
8. Telephone call abandonment rate	76
9. Waiting time for scheduling routine office visits	75
10. Outpatient average number of sessions	74
11. Waiting time for scheduling emergent visits	72
12. Percent of patients satisfied with access to care	71
13. Partial hospitalization average length of stay	64
14. Percent of patients having improved functioning after treatment	60
15. Percent of patients with adverse outcomes	57
16. Percent of claims paid within specific period	53
17. Percent of inpatient cases reviewed for adequate documentation	51
18. Percent of cases following written guidelines for High-Risk procedures	50
19. Percent of patients having reduced symptoms of treatment	47
20. Percent of patients whose quality of life improved after treatment	40
21. Written plan for monitoring quality of care	36
22. Percent of inpatient cases reviewed with medical director for medical necessity	35
23. Written criteria available to determine medical necessity for each level of care	35
24. Percent of providers recredentialed	33
25. Psychoeducational prevention groups in place	33
26. Dissemination of information on behavioral health and prevention issues	31
27. Percent of medical records audited for quality	26
28. Inpatient cases audited for medical necessity	25

Table 2

Cost-Effectiveness ranking of indicators in descending value.

Table 2 shows the relative cost-effectiveness of each indicator rank-ordered from most to least cost-effective. The more cost-effective indicators were primarily in the Access domain, and cover waiting time and utilization information. It is interesting to note that a patient satisfaction indicator (overall quality of care) and an outcome indicator (number of hospital readmissions) also ranked as among the most cost-effective. Traditional documentation-oriented quality assurance indicators and prevention services ranked among the least cost-effective.

Standards established for indicators. There was surprising concurrence across industry segments regarding standards for most of the indicators. In addition, detailed results for each indicator, broken down separately by industry sector, were displayed with graphs and charts in over a hundred pages of appendices. An executive from a managed care plan can look up what managed care companies reported their benchmarking standards to be for a given indicator, and the executive director of a community mental health center can look up what community mental health centers reported as their standards for the same indicator.

Study conclusions. Perhaps the most significant finding of this study is that organizations were able to make clear distinctions between more and less cost-effective performance indicators. At a time when many behavioral health-care organizations are experiencing downward price pressures and declining profit margins, the recommendation or requirement to increase performance measurement can place a troublesome burden on organizations who are struggling to remain viable in the marketplace. In this context, ratings of the comparative cost-effectiveness of different performance indicators offer valuable information to guide the efforts of those who develop report card indicators and accreditation requirements. It is important that the indicators and requirements they select are ones that maximize the likelihood of quality improvement at the least cost.

Clear patterns were apparent in respondents' ratings of the relative cost-effectiveness of performance indicators. Access (e.g.,. wait time) and utilization (average length of stay, days/1000) measures dominated the list of the most cost-effective indicators. An outcomes measure (inpatient readmission rates) and a measure of consumer satisfaction (with overall quality of care) were also among the top ten. The latter two indicators were regarded as more costly to measure, but were also clearly regarded as providing very valuable information.

Among the lowest on the list of cost-effectiveness ratings were traditional documentation review-oriented quality assurance indicators. This finding clearly suggests the importance of re-evaluating the appropriateness of traditional accreditation standards. Also among the least cost-effective indicators were those related to education and prevention services. While preventive services were clearly worthwhile, the findings from this survey indicate that providers and managed care payers were not motivated to invest in prevention. Purchasers of behavioral healthcare services have yet to recognize the need to create strong incentives for developing behavioral health promotion, prevention, and risk management services.

This study confirmed the growing power of purchasers to drive the quality and accountability agenda. Respondents to the survey reported a strong relationship between the types of performance data they were required to report to external audiences (e.g., commercial and public purchasers, health plan payers, accrediting agencies and regulators), and the types of performance data they most use for their organizations' internal quality improvement efforts. As purchasers increase and refine their awareness of the types of performance data they can request from managed care and provider organizations, they will be in a better position to truly influence the behavioral healthcare market towards greater quality and accountability through the application of value-based purchasing methods.

The study revealed a surprisingly high level of agreement among organizations, even across different segments of the behavioral healthcare industry, with regards to appropriate standards for some of the most commonly used performance indicators. It is doubtful that this would have been the case ten or more years ago. As purchasers form purchasing coalitions, and as provider and managed care industries consolidate, consensus on standards increases. This creates a basis for hope that our field can develop common measures and data collection methods, common standards from which to benchmark, and the capability to provide comparative data across similar types of organizations for selection decisions. This is essential if the behavioral healthcare field is to substantiate the value of their services to purchasers and consumers in a manner sufficiently compelling to circumvent the trend towards turning professional services into a commodity. Comparable and objective data are required to make this shift so that purchasers and consumers can be assured of receiving accessible, appropriate and high quality care.

Challenges for Report Card Implementation

What does the future hold for report cards? To be effective, they must address several major challenges.

Most organizations find it expensive to meet the performance measurement and reporting requirements of even one purchaser or accrediting organization, let alone several. This dilemma is exacerbated when organizations must also meet the different reporting requirements of multiple external payers. Eventually there will need to be considerable overlap if not actual consolidation among report cards.

An initial and highly significant effort to accomplish this consolidation is conducted by the American College of Mental Health Administrators, which began in 1996 to convene Summit meetings and task forces of leaders in performance measurement and accreditation standards to develop a consensus on the most important performance indicators for widespread use across all mental health services. They published a report of their conclusions in 1998, after which they took the next step of convening a group of the major accrediting organizations to obtain consensus on a reduced set of indicators.

Since the accrediting organizations have tremendous influence on behavioral health organizations, this first-time collaborative effort is regarded as significant. After more than two years of meetings and intensive work, this group released a document with their conclusions in February, 2001.

Another significant consensus initiative for common performance measures was initiated by a group of leading performance measurement experts within the substance abuse treatment field. Named the Washington Circle Group, they developed eight performance measures recommended for adoption by those organizations and systems of care that assess and treat adult substance abusers. They released a report detailing their measures in autumn of 2000. The measures are being considered for adoption by NCQA and other major national organizations.

In autumn of 1999, the federal government's Substance Abuse and Mental Health Services Administration (SAMHSA) launched the most broad-based initiative yet to consolidate performance measurement efforts for the behavioral health field. For its first year, the initiative held many working meetings with public and private sector organizations that developed major performance measurement report cards for the behavioral healthcare field. Representatives participated from the major accrediting organizations, ACMHA and the Washington Circle Group mentioned previously, along with provider and managed care trade associations, consumer groups, and government agencies. Consensus was reached on approximately 20 indicators for adult mental health services and 7 indicators proposed by the Washington Circle Group for adult substance abuse treatment. These indicators, along with others that address substance abuse treatment prevention, were presented for consideration at a national Consensus Forum on Performance Measurement for Mental Health and Substance Abuse in March, 2001 at the Carter Center. Leaders of this initiative hope the Forum will further galvanize this initiative, help it evolve from standardized indicators to standardized measures, and also promote the same for behavioral health services serving children and their families.

Many of the indicators identified by both the ACMHA and the SAMHSA initiatives are measured most effectively through consumer surveys. Currently, no standard survey instrument exists that is widely used throughout both public and private sectors of the behavioral healthcare field. However, at the time of this writing one such measure still under development has considerable momentum towards widespread adoption. The Experience of Care and Health Outcomes (ECHO) is an attempt to integrate the best elements of the MHSIP Consumer Survey and the Consumer Assessment of Behavioral Health Services (CABHS). It is, at the time of this writing, being piloted for inclusion in NCQA's HEDIS and as a requirement for NCQA accreditation.

Several other accrediting and regulatory organizations are regarding it with great interest. If it succeeds, it will provide the field with a standardized measurement instrument able to provide comparisons between and benchmarks for organizations along key performance indicators valued by the entire field.

Information system standards are also needed. These should address common data elements, software interoperability, electronic communication, and information exchange with protections for data privacy and confidentiality (Axelson, A., Geraty, R., Hill, E., 1995; NCQA, 1997).

Of these standard-setting needs to be addressed, data privacy and confidentiality are paramount. Computerization exacerbates the public perception already present of data privacy infringements due to managed care. With increased use of the Internet for transmission of health care information, the challenges of securing data privacy increase. Technological locks and keys are plentiful, such as firewalls, data encryption and biometric passwords. More important are organizational policies, procedures, values and staff training to respect and secure the privacy and confidentiality of patient data. Without these, sophisticated technological security devices will be for naught. Organizational policies will be somewhat guided by new federal regulations developed and released by the Department of Health and Human Services in late 2000 through the Health Insurance Portability and Accountability Act. These regulations set standards for how health care information should be recorded and exchanged, with particular attention to coding sets and to data privacy and security. However, organizations will still be responsible for creating the internal culture to respect and strictly abide by those regulations.

Another important standard-setting initiative is Decision Support 2000+ (DS2000+), sponsored by SAMHSA's Center for Mental Health Services. This 5-year project, in mid-course at the time of this writing, is focused on defining behavioral health-specific data standards for enrollment, encounters, treatment guidelines, system guidelines, consumer outcomes, organizational and system performance, and other elements. DS2000+ is intended to advance the national data infrastructure for behavioral health so that accountability for quality services can be enhanced through organizational comparability and benchmarking, and so that new knowledge may be generated for the field.

In order to be comparable, data submitted from multiple organizations must first be collected through the same methodology and reported using identical formats. Adjustments for severity of illness and demographic characteristics of the study population may also be required in order for meaningful comparisons to be made. Without this attention to methodological issues, we will be comparing apples and bananas. Report card developers must address disparities in interpretation of the measures and in measurement capabilities among organizations by providing clear, highly specific instructions to them on the measurement methods required to collect performance data.

It is a monumental and extremely expensive task to monitor with audits the data collection process across multiple organizations for compliance with prespecified and standardized methodologies. Yet these safeguards, or something similar, must be put in place to give credibility to the report cards in which so many will have a stake.

To be widely used it is necessary for the complex information contained in report cards to be presented in a format that is easily accessed and understood. Computer technology can enable users to access the comparative information they need easily and efficiently through online services. Most users will only want data on a few variables comparing the performance of a limited number of prespecified organizations. Research is needed to determine the type and format of information that consumers and purchasers of behavioral health services will find most user-friendly.

Even with all these conditions, report card sponsoring organizations must still provide considerable education to potential users on how they can obtain and use the information they need. In this way, report cards have the potential to substantiate the value of behavioral healthcare services and to provide a framework for value-based selection and purchasing decisions by purchasers and consumers.

SUMMARY AND CONCLUSIONS

In this chapter, we reviewed the dramatic changes in how the behavioral healthcare field is structured, from cottage industry to industrialization and consolidation. We critiqued the potentials those changes create for both benefit and harm. Building checks and balances into the system through accountability for quality of care can work to maximize the benefits of industrialization and minimize the likelihood of harm.

We reviewed many approaches to accountability for quality, including quality assurance and quality improvement. We also reviewed many methods, including performance and outcome measurement, medical cost-offset studies, and practice guidelines. The primary method focused upon was performance measurement, because of its accountability function for large organizations and entire systems of care. We have passed the time where expressions of good intention and professionalism sufficed to assure quality in behavioral healthcare. The time of accountable data requirements has arrived. Measurement shortcomings notwithstanding, its value for the field and industry is undeniable.

Advances in outcome and performance measurement and innovative approaches to quality improvement have slowed somewhat in behavioral healthcare. Commodity pricing policies and industry consolidation have been discouraging, and have caused the industry to catch its breath and wonder about strategy and direction. During such times, the will required to continue expensive outcome and performance measurement and other quality-focused activities is substantial. The expense can seem unsupportable. Nevertheless, it is especially during such a time that we must continue our efforts to demonstrate convincingly that our services are not commodities. They can be differentiated by various dimensions of quality, value-priced accordingly, and monitored through data to ensure that value is maintained.

REFERENCES

Abt Associates. (2000). Decision support 2000+. Rockville, MD: Center for Mental Health services, Substance Abuse and Mental Health Services Administation.

American College of Mental Health Administration. (1997). *Preserving quality and value in the managed care equation.* Pittsburgh, PA: The American College of Mental Health Administration.

American College of Mental Health Administration. (2001). A proposed consensus set of indicators for behavioral healthcare. Pittsburg, PA: American College of Mental Health Administration.

American Managed Behavioral Healthcare Association. (1995). *Performance measures for managed behavioral healthcare programs.* Washington, DC: American Managed Behavioral Healthcare Association.

Axelson, A., Geraty, R., & Hill, E. (1995). Dialogue—Can we agree on common forms, language and standards for electronic data communication? *Behavioral Healthcare Tomorrow, 4*(1), 42- 49.

Bartlett, J., Cohn, C., & Mirin, S. (1998). Can quality survive continued downward price pressures? *Behavioral Healthcare Tomorrow, 7*(2), 49-53.

Bobbitt, B. L., Marques, C. C., & Trout, D. L. (1998). Managed behavioral health care: Current status, recent trends, and the role of psychology. *Clinical Psychology: Science and Practice, 3*(1), 53- 66.

Coke, J. (1996). Integrating behavioral and medical/surgical data. *Behavioral Healthcare Tomorrow, 5*(5), 73-76.

Coltin, K. and Beck, A. (1999). The new antidepressant medication measure for HEDIS 2000. *Behavioral Healthcare Tomorrow, 8*(3), 40, 41 & 47.

Cummings, N. (1998). Spectacular accomplishments and disappointing mistakes: The first decade of managed behavioral care. *Behavioral Healthcare Tomorrow, 7* (4), 61-63.

Ellwood, P. M. (1988). Outcomes management: A technology of patient experience. *New England Journal of Medicine, 318*, 1549.

Ganju, V. (1998). From consumer satisfaction to consumer perception of care. *Behavioral Healthcare Tomorrow,* 7(4), 17-18

Hay Group. (1999). *Health care plan design and cost trends, 1988-1998.* Washington, DC: National Association of Psychiatric Health Systems and the Association of Behavioral Group Practices.

Human Services Research Institute. (1998). *Toolkit on performance measurement using the MHSIP consumer-oriented report* Cambridge, MA: Human Services Research Institute.

Joint Commission on Accreditation of Health Care Organizations. (1997). *Comprehensive accreditation manual for managed behavioral health care.* Oakbrook Terrace, IL: Joint Commission on Accreditation of Health Care Organizations.

Joint Commission on Accreditation of Health Care Organizations. (1997). *ORYX: The next evolution in healthcare.* Oakbrook Terrace, IL: Joint Commission on Accreditation of Health Care Organizations.

Hoosier Assurance Plan (1996). *Provider profile report card.* Indianapolis, IN: Family and Social Services Administration.

Kramer, T., Trabin, T., Daniels, A., Theriot, R., Freeman, M.A., & Williams, C.(1997). *Performance indicator measurement in behavioral healthcare: Data capture methods, cost-effectiveness, and emerging standards.* Portola Valley: Institute for Behavioral Healthcare.

Kramer, T., Trabin, T., Daniels, A., Mahesh, N., Freeman, M.A., Bernstein, S. & Dangerfield, D. (1996). *Performance indicators in behavioral healthcare: Measures of access, appropriateness, quality, outcomes, and prevention.* Portola Valley, CA: Institute for Behavioral Healthcare.

Lunnon, K. M. & Ogles, B. M. (1997). *Satisfaction ratings: Meaningful or meaningless?* Behavioral Healthcare Tomorrow, 6 (4), 49-51.

Mental Health Statistics Improvement Program Task Force on a Consumer-Oriented Mental Health Report Card (1996). *The MHSIP consumer-oriented mental health report card.* Rockville, MD: Center for Mental Health Services.

National Association of State Mental Health Program Directors President's Task Force on Performance Indicators Technical Workgroup (1998). *Performance measures for mental health systems.* Washington, D.C.: National Association of State Mental Health Program Directors.

National Committee for Quality Assurance. (1997). *1997 Standards for accreditation of managed behavioral healthcare organizations.* Washington, DC: National Committee for Quality Assurance.

National Committee for Quality Assurance. (1997). *Health plan employer data and information set* (Vols. 1 and 2). Washington, DC: National Committee for Quality Assurance.

National Committee for Quality Assurance. (1997). *Health plan employer data and information set, volume IV.* Washington, DC: National Committee for Quality Assurance.

Persons, J. (1999). Showcase studies: How to integrate practice guidelines and outcomes measurement into an outpatient group practice. *Behavioral Healthcare Tomorrow, 8* (3), 45-47.

The Washington Circle Group (2000). *Improving performance measurement for alcohol and other drug services.* Rockville, MD: Center for Substance Abuse Treatment, SAMHSA.

Trabin, T. (1998). Industry consolidation and quality of care: Ambivalent partners? *Behavioral Healthcare Tomorrow, 7* (3), 8, 39.

Trabin, T. & Freeman, M. A. (1995). *Managed behavioral healthcare: History, models, strategic challenges, and future course.* Tiburon, CA: CentraLink Publications.

Wade, W. (1999). Showcase studies: How to integrate practice guidelines and outcomes measurement into a community mental health center. *Behavioral Healthcare Tomorrow, 8* (3), 42-45.

Discussion of Trabin:

The Best and Worst of Times for Behavioral Mental Health Practice

S. R. Thorp

J. Gregg

R. Niccolls

W. T. O'Donohue

University of Nevada, Reno

Trabin presents an informative account of the recent and dynamic history of the healthcare industry. His thesis is that behavioral healthcare is in a financial crisis (losing about half its allotment of health care funds since the mid-1980s), and needs to demonstrate its worth to organized managed care, treatment providers, and consumers. He proposes that behavioral healthcare services are not commodities because they can be differentiated in terms of quality and cost-effectiveness. He argues that these services can enhance their value by taking advantage of performance measurement.

The context for this proposal must be emphasized. Trabin repeatedly comments about the pressure for managed care companies to increase profit, decrease the debt incurred by consolidation, and increase efficiency. Reimbursement rate reductions have driven many provider organizations and mental health professionals out of the market, and consumers have increasingly voiced concern about decreasing access or quality of services. However, Trabin points out that this may be the best of times for behavioral healthcare in that opportunity abounds for improvement of the industry.

Due to the consolidation of hundreds of managed care companies into a relatively small number of "mega-companies" with centralized quality management resources, companies can now track literally hundreds of thousands of patients during their treatment. These data can be stored, analyzed, and communicated quickly thanks to the rapid advancement of information technologies. This combination of data resources and practical data management set the stage to potentially improve treatment coordination, enhance patient care, and generate new healthcare knowledge.

Trabin puts out a call for standardization. He states that purchasers and consumers who seek access to appropriate and effective care require compa-

Integrated Behavioral Healthcare: Positioning Mental Health Practice with Medical/Surgical Practice

rable and objective data across managed care systems. To this end, Trabin would like to see practice guidelines, performance indicators, outcome measures, software, information systems, data collection methodology and reporting formats, policies, procedures, and staff trainings conform to universal standards. Certainly, if the methods of data collection, storage, and reporting are universal within an organization it will reduce the cost of data management. Yet, why would managed care companies be motivated to conform in the other domains?

Trabin properly devotes much of his argument to the incentives that spurred insurers, treatment providers, and consumers toward the current state of affairs in managed care. However, he allots little space to the factors that will motivate change from this point. He said that the largest companies might *decide* to take the "high road" by pursuing standardization and by investing time and money to insure a "broad consensus" and "substantial quality initiatives" (p. 158). Again, why would they do this? More generally, what influences the decision-making of managed care companies?

Much as treatment providers are governed by managed care, the decisions of managed care companies are shaped by the contingencies put in place by the regulatory and accrediting organizations. Internal review and quality management practices are dependent on these external agencies. Since regulatory and accrediting agencies can influence managed care, influence should be exerted on *these* agencies to help produce change at the level of organized healthcare (and therefore the provision of quality treatment). These agencies can influence the industry through report cards and audits to maintain the credibility of the report cards. More importantly, these reports hold weight for managed care organizations because their results dictate financial incentives (or constraints).

A last point involves the targets of studies trying to establish an empirical base to improve the quality and dissemination of report cards. The study described in this chapter, conducted by the Institute for Behavioral Healthcare's National Leadership Council, presents an extensive and interesting approach. The researchers chose to begin the study by reviewing report card initiatives and surveying existing behavioral healthcare organizations. In developing a survey instrument, the most commonly used performance indicators were consistently chosen for inclusion. Although this is a reasonable starting place, it necessarily limits the choices of respondents and therefore the results of the study. This is a problem especially because, as stated previously, internal review is influenced by external review procedures. In other words, as was evidenced in the resulting correlations shown in Table 1, the respondents were essentially rating survey items on two dimensions: (1) staff time/costs and (2) value for quality improvement/external reporting.

These results are confounded because the respondents are familiar with the existing values of the external reporting agencies and the existing methods for measuring and calculating staff time/costs. In a sense, then, the survey is asking, "What parts of the status quo do you think are most relevant and practical?"

This bias might help to explain the "low valued" indicators for prevention (for which there were only two items included out of twenty-eight), because as Trabin notes there are not currently sufficient perceived incentives to promote prevention programs. It is quite possible that an empirical analysis of prevention programs would demonstrate financial benefits for HMOs (through fewer claims to be paid each year, for example) while maintaining pragmatic approaches to treatment and assessment.

Another point that is missed by the study involves the ability to manipulate the factors that are considered worthwhile and the effects of this manipulation. For example, can we change the number of acute inpatient days per year? If so, what would the long-term consequences be? It is certainly feasible that decreased inpatient days would lead to a greater utilization of outpatient services, increased use of medications, or increases in the number of individuals who need care but go without. The analysis of change and its effects is an area that seems well suited to the strengths of behavioral healthcare management.

Again, managed care organizations are under pressure to consolidate, reduce debt, and increase profit. It is unlikely that these organizations will invest enormous amounts of time, effort, and money in quality management services that may or may not benefit them. Although the quality assurance process will be costly to managed care organizations, they will not disappear. As Trabin indicates, the time is ripe for a science of healthcare utilization and outcome. It would be a shame if we confused the goals of efficient, affordable, effective healthcare with that which is easy and profitable.

8

Managed Care: Cost and Effectiveness

Ian A. Shaffer, M.D.
Ian A. Shaffer and Associates, LLC,
Reston, Virginia

Integrated Behavioral Healthcare: Positioning Mental Health Practice with Medical/Surgical Practice

INTRODUCTION

Managed behavioral health care has brought about some fundamental changes in the way behavioral health care is delivered. Most of the prominent managed behavioral health care companies, several of whom who have now been merged into the two large behavioral health care companies, were formed in the early 1980's. This chapter will review some of the history and practices of managed behavioral health care. We will also explore the cost impact of this changing health care system and some measures of its effectiveness. While there has been much rhetoric suggesting that managed behavioral health care has negatively impacted the quality of treatment, there is little evidence to support that. There is a great deal evidence however to support the fact that treatment is much more focused and targeted with providers being asked to specifically state the nature of the problem they are treating, the treatment plan, the goals of that treatment plan, the methods they will use to determine how successful they are in meeting the goals, as well as acknowledging progress along the way.

Training for most behavioral health care clinicians in the 1960's and 1970's and in some degree even to this day, focused on meeting the individuals and working through issues that arose in therapy. Therapies tended to be non-directive and issues evolved over time. Managed behavioral health care has brought a fundamental change in that area, requiring that providers specifically determine through comprehensive assessments, the nature of the difficulties in the plan. Moreover, with an expanding base of knowledge regarding the problems and treatments that work for those specific problems, managed care is no longer accepting of providers treating individuals according to the philosophy upon which they were trained.

Pre-Managed Care Costs

In order to understand some of the costs prior to managed care; one must understand the nature of the benefit plans that were available. Benefits for behavioral health care were almost exclusively for inpatient treatment and outpatient treatment only. The concept of covering alternative levels of care did not exist. In this model, there were extremely high costs and lengths of stay in the inpatient area with limited utilization of outpatient treatment. This was very clearly incented by the nature of the insurance benefit plan. Inpatient care was covered often at a minimum of 80% and in some cases at 100% of cost.

Further, it was not uncommon for hospitals at that time to waive the 20% co-pay, particularly given the fact that patients stayed in the hospital for an extended period of time. Thus, individuals experienced no personal costs to an extended inpatient stay for themselves or a member of their family. On the other hand, there was limited outpatient coverage. Frequently, the coverage was approximately 50% of an outpatient's psychotherapy session. However, there was also a limit on the amount of reimbursement, so in some cases for example, one could see a benefit that reimbursed at 50% up to a session cost of $50. Given that in early 1980's, psychotherapy costs were in excess of $100 per session, a patient could easily be facing an out of pocket expense of $100 per each outpatient psychotherapy session. Thus, when people were having difficulties, it was financially easier to go into the hospital and experience no out of pocket costs, than to enter outpatient psychotherapy where they could face costs of $100 per week or more.

With the incenting of hospitalization and the rapid proliferation of proprietary hospitals, employers began to experience large annual increases in their costs. It was not uncommon for employers to experience 15-20% annual increases in the cost of their behavioral health care. Not only were employers experiencing actual dollar increases on an annual basis, but also behavioral health care was climbing in terms of the percentage of their health care dollars expended on behavioral health care. When some of these employers began to study their costs, they found that the behavioral health care dollar represented in excess of 10% of the entire medical costs, while these funds were being consumed by less than 5% of their population.

Emergence of Managed Care

One of the initial methods of containing costs was to limit behavioral health care benefits. This began prior to the formation of managed behavioral health care companies and occurred as employers had difficulty determining how to contain these rising costs, that were experienced by many as out of control.

As managed care grew on the scene; they began to focus on managing utilization. This meant that clinicians were required to pre-authorize all inpatient care and maintain continuing authorization throughout the treatment process. This method of concurrent review became increasingly popular after many plans had utilized a retrospective review process. This retrospective review process is extremely difficult for providers and consumers of care. Providers have delivered care and expect to reimbursed. Consumers have obtained care believing that their health care benefits would assist them in managing the costs. With retrospective review, consumers would face the possibility that an insurer would deny payment, and they would then be left expected to pay for services that have already been delivered. In the prospective model, consumers could then decide whether they wanted to pay for services out of pocket and would also have some information as to why services were not being reimbursed. Over the fifteen years of evolution of managed behavioral health care, plans have become much more sophisticated in providing specific information to consumers when authorization for benefit is being denied.

Managed behavioral health care is delivered in several models. Health plans, such as Kaiser and Group Health Cooperative of Puget Sound, have their own internal behavioral health departments that generally manage care through a staff model or a network model, but within their overall health plan. On the other hand, many employers chose to utilize a managed behavioral health care carve out company. In this model, the employer or health plan carves out its benefits for mental illness and substance abuse treatment to an entity that specializes in managing this component of health care. The carve out companies have all developed a network of individual clinicians in most major disciplines, as well as contracts with facilities and programs. Care may be delivered through this network or from outside this network, recognizing that there is a differential in benefits to the consumer for utilizing the network versus non-network coverage. The carve out company provides clinical care management, where treatment is reviewed and authorization of benefit is made. In a significant number of cases, the carve out companies will also process claims for services and will directly reimburse the providers or forward the payment information to the check processor.

There are a number of models within managed behavioral health care. Large self-insured companies contract with these managed behavioral health care carve out companies to provide administrative services. In this model, the client company is at risk for their own health care costs. The managed care organization provides the network, the care management and claims processing. The carve out company is reimbursed on a per employee per month basis with performance guarantees most frequently in the areas of access to providers, responsiveness to beneficiary telephone calls and requests, and claims processing. It is important to realize in this model, a decrease in actual health care dollars spent is a direct benefit to the self-insured company.

In a second model, the managed behavioral health care company accepts the risk for health care costs. In this scenario, all of the services provided under the administrative services model are present. Performance guarantees also remain present usually for the same key areas noted above. The key difference here is that the client company, who engages an MBHO in this method, has fixed their costs, and the MBHO must manage the risk as part of the overall contract. In this model, companies are reimbursed on a per member per month basis.

Another component of managed behavioral health care today is the employee assistance programs. Early in managed behavioral health care, employee assistance was separate and there was significant tension between EAPs and MBHOs. While some of this tension continues, it is important to realize that many of these programs have worked hard to develop an interface and understand the components that each bring to the care of individuals. Employee assistance programs can take a variety of forms. They can be a telephonic service that refers individuals to treatment, after providing telephonic counseling on one hand, to those that may provide as many as eight sessions with an EAP counselor on the other. A number of companies have made these EAP programs the front end of their behavioral health care program. This can be done through their own internal EAP or in some cases by purchasing an integrated behavioral health care program from an MBHO. In this model, the MBHO provides the EAP services as well as the full managed behavioral health care program. Generally consumers access the EAP for initial assessment and treatment. In a number of cases, issues can be resolved within the EAP and individuals do not need to access their behavioral health care benefit.

Costs and Managed Care

As mentioned earlier, self-insured companies were frequently experiencing 15-20% annual increases in their behavioral health benefit costs prior to managed care. Many of these companies experienced cost decreases of 25-40% in the first year of implementing a managed behavioral health care program. There are a number of components impacting the overall decreasing costs. With the precertification process for inpatient care, as well as the encouragement of alternatives to inpatient care, there was a decreased likelihood that individuals would enter acute care facilities. Moreover, when individuals did enter the hospital, there was a decrease length of stay. Over the past ten years, there has been a steady decline in the average length of stay in acute care hospitals. At the same time that the length of stay was decreasing, MBHOs contracted with facilities to provide acute inpatient care. These contracts frequently extracted 40-50% cost decreases and were developed on a full per diem basis. Thus, all services provided by the hospital, were covered by a single per diem rate. This significant decrease in unit cost further decreased the total dollars spent. Finally, MBHOs developed fee schedules for outpatient clinicians that developed some certainty in the overall unit costs for outpatient care and this too impacted the overall costs. Figure 1 demonstrates that inpatient costs dropped from 50% of the overall mental health costs in 1988 in one study, to 22% of the costs in 1995. It is important to understand that this represents a dramatic decrease in funds utilized for inpatient care. In 1988, that 50% of a dollar not only represented a higher percentage, but it also represented a higher unit cost. Thus, the actual dollar decrease is greater than the differential, between the 50% and the 22% as the overall dollars spent in 1995 on inpatient care was significantly less than those paid in 1988.

It is also important to note, in one study, that costs between 1976 and 1982 increased on average 6.1% per year for inpatient care. Between 1982 and 1990, there was a 20 decrease in the inpatient community hospital days. In 1990, when you begin to look at this, combining the decreased utilization and the decreased unit costs, the overall cost was about 20 billion dollars less than would have been expected with the absence of these changes.

There was an impact on costs on the outpatient side as well. Within disciplines, these were initially reduced 10-15%. At the same time, however, there was increased use of masters prepared therapists. With this change in discipline mix, companies experienced 20-30% decrease in costs because of the fee differentials between the various disciplines. This was combined with a decrease in the number of outpatient visits per thousand lives. Several companies studied, experienced a 25-35% decrease in visits per thousand lives. A significant component of that was the fact that the number of visits per episode of treatment was decreased. It is important to realize this because data, later in this chapter will point out, that while costs were decreasing, the number of people accessing care was increasing.

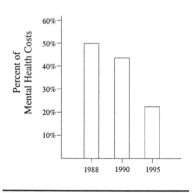

Figure 1

A 1995 study on inpatient costs.

The employee assistance program also had an impact. As mentioned, many of these programs encouraged individuals to seek initial assessment and treatment through their EAP program. This has been shown to decrease cost in behavioral health care programs by as much as 25%.

One of the most significant contributions of managed care to the field of behavioral health care delivery has been the encouragement and reimbursement of alternative levels of care. This not only includes traditional residential treatment, but also the use of partial hospitalization programs for acute care, day treatment centers fort the long term mentally ill, and structured outpatient programs for substance abuse, eating disorders and other behavioral problems. The presence of these alternatives has contributed to the decrease in inpatient care. Depending on the severity of an individual's condition, some were in a position to be directly admitted to a partial hospitalization program and not enter an inpatient acute care facility. Moreover, once stabilized in an acute care facility, patients could then be transitioned to less intensive levels of care to continue their treatment. At a time when only inpatient and outpatient care existed, there was a need for a much higher level of clinical improvement because of the significantly less intense treatment when comparing inpatient and outpatient care. However, those individuals who now could actively participate in an alternative level of care, could return home to the support of family and friends, while attending an intense program of treatment. In reviewing several clients, we noticed that the appropriate use of alternatives could lead to a decrease cost per inpatient episode of treatment between 20-50%.

Figure 2 points the return on investment that several employers have experienced through the use of managed behavioral health care programs. This data has been derived form self-insured companies who study the return on investment they receive for the costs of their administrative services program. This example demonstrates that this client company experienced a savings of $3 in their behavioral health care program, for every dollar spent with us. As you can see, by year four, they were experiencing a $9 return on each dollar spent on the program. In our global competitive economy, where many of these self-insured companies are very concerned about their overall costs, this is a very powerful statement. It is important to understand at the same time, that many of these firms feel very strongly about their individual employees and dependents of their employees receiving the care they need. They are not interested in denying access to care as a means of saving money. They are however, interested in ensuring that the overall health care dollar is utilized in a meaningful way.

The presence of the cost containment that has taken place in managed behavioral health care,

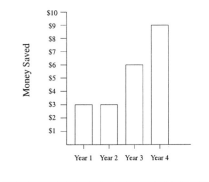

Figure 2

Client return on investment over a four year period.

has opened the door for a discussion on benefit parity. In 1996, the federal government passed a mental health parity act. This act requires that employers not discriminate on annual and lifetime dollar maximums between their general health care benefit and their behavioral health care benefit. At the same time however, there is no requirement that there be parity if the benefit is described in terms of hospital days and outpatient visits. Finally, if employers experience an increase in health care costs of greater than 1% that can be directly attributed to mental health care parity, they can apply for and receive an exemption from the parity act. Clients have responded in mixed ways, with some changing their annual lifetime maximums to meet the general health care dollars, while others by changing their benefits from dollars to days and visits. Clearly the discussions regarding the behavioral health care parity, could never have taken place when the costs of the treatment of mental illness were escalating out of control. In the presence of the cost predictability described above, employers are willing to engage in the discussion. At the same time, there is significant amount of concern in the employer community, as they are still unclear as to whether this benefit will be manageable in a parity environment.

A SAMHSA report on the impact of parity, notes that the cost increases with parity in managed care are less than 1%. Moreover, the author notes that implementing parity and a managed care program can frequently lead to savings in excess of 20% of current costs. In summary, managed care has clearly demonstrated its ability to reduce and stabilize costs. In the face of these treatment and cost reductions, providers have proposed that the overall quality of care has diminished. Unfortunately, little data to demonstrate quality of treatment or the outcomes of treatment was collected prior to managed care. As a result, it is difficult for us to make comparisons to what occurred previously. In the next section, we will begin to discuss some measures of the effectiveness of managed care and its impact on treatment.

Effectiveness in Managed Care

In this section, we are going to look at some of the impact that has been measured in managed care programs. While there is an ongoing debate as to the impact of managed care on overall treatment, it is clear that there is no debate about the fact that managed care has dramatically increased the accountability of providers in delivering care. It is important to recognize that this accountability extends beyond the providers, to the managers of care. Their client companies to ensure and that services meet timeliness standards monitor MBHOs. With this increased accountability, providers have felt the intrusion of being questioned as to the nature of their decisions. While providers have suggested that this intrusion is impacting quality of care, it is clear that this oversight has required providers to be much more definitive in what they are treating and what the goals of treatment are. Finally, if a disease management program is involved, there is an increasing awareness of accountability developing on the part of consumers of care. It is important that consumers learn about decisions being made with regard to their treatment and actively participate. Along with this, there is an increasing recognition that our health care system must move away from an acute illness to a wellness system. This will necessitate an involvement of consumers in these wellness programs. Weight loss programs and exercise programs are two examples of the type of wellness programs being offered. Along with this, active participation in one's treatment and adherence with agreed upon treatment goals and activities is important.

In considering the effectiveness of a managed care program, there are a number of domains that will be addressed. We have already clearly addressed the effectiveness of managed care in containing cost. At its initial inception, managed care evolved as a result of costs that had escalated out of control. Thus, it was clear that one of the early goals of managed care was to contain costs. We have seen earlier in this chapter that this has been successfully accomplished. The next goal is to focus on issues of effectiveness as it relates to consumer of care rather than the payer of care.

In addressing these issues, we will look at five domains. These will include access to care, the impact on unexplained treatment variability, clinical outcomes, functional improvement, and consumer satisfaction. People will argue that one or another of these domains is more important. For example, clinicians will often focus more on clinical outcomes as the measure of effectiveness in care. However, consumers in advocacy groups, point to the importance of consumers being satisfied with the treatment that they receive and that this treatment will lead to an overall improvement in their ability to function in their world. They point out that improvement of the clinical situation, while important, is not an end unto itself and that we must pay attention to the overall impact of treatment on the life of the consumer.

I. Access

Access to behavioral health care prior to managed care came in many forms. One company studied its employees and dependents referral patterns and found that the majority of decisions as to whom they would go to for treatment came from studying the yellow pages. Also, as hospitals proliferated in the 1980's, they developed toll free help lines that individuals could access. These lines were often marketed as a place where people could seek referrals for whatever care they needed. Unfortunately, many of these were used to encourage hospital admissions. In many cases, consumers were not aware that the facilities were on the other side of the

Year	Penetration Rate
1995 (Pre-capitation)	10%
1996 (Post-capitation)	14%
1997 (Post-capitation)	11.5%

Table 1

Penetration rates in a medical population.

country. Some of these hospitals went so far as to provide airline tickets and taxi services in order to get consumers to come. With the arrival of managed care, access included the presence of clinical referral lines that individuals could call. These referral lines, manned by clinicians, would discuss the individuals needs and make referrals as appropriate. A key component of these referral lines was the ability to ensure that those with urgent and emergency needs were seen promptly.

Other ways in which patients received access to care included referrals from their employee assistance professionals, directly accessing providers from recommendations from friends or family, or the referral by a primary care physician. While these types of referral had taken place prior to the presence of managed care the emergence of managed care lead to a questioning of each particular referral as to its appropriateness. As a result, some referral patterns, such as specific facility referrals by employee assistance professionals, was changed. The overall goal, on the part of all concerned was to provide the consumer with a prompt and appropriate referral.

Penetration rates in behavioral health care were not well known. It is has been suggested by some that the overall penetration rates were 2-4% prior to managed care. Studies by some of the clients in a commercial population suggest that these penetration rates are now between 6 and 9%. Another critical factor in understanding access, was the impact of the implementation of a managed care program by a self-insured company. As mentioned earlier in this chapter, the companies experienced a 25-40% decrease in costs. At the same time, during that first year, they generally experienced a 15% or greater increase in the number of people accessing care.

Table 1 demonstrates the penetration in a Medicaid population in the State of Colorado. You will note, as there is continuation in the treatment program, that there has been an increase in the number of people accessing care over three years. Table 2 also notes the length of time it takes to obtain appointments. Access to care must not only represent the presence of an adequate network, but also the ability to get an appointment as rapidly as

possible. This data demonstrates
that with the ongoing management
of the Colorado program, there has
been a significant drop in the number of days required to obtain appointments.

	Average Days Needed to Obtain Outpatient Appointments
Pre-capitation	
(Pre-September 1995)	7.5
Post-capitation	
June 1996	3.5
December 1996	2.0
December 1997	3.2

Table 2

Average days to obtain outpatient appointments.

While many clinicians will
point to the fact that the presence of
a benefit package and an adequate
network will not necessarily get you
care because of the need for certification. It is clear that absent this
access, care cannot take place. Another aspect of this access is the fact
that individuals in increasing numbers continue to come for treatment,
suggesting along with the satisfaction data, that they are pleased with the
treatment they are receiving.

II. Treatment Variability

One of the concerns that client companies have expressed with respect to
behavioral health care, is the marked variability in treatment. From a benefit
manager's perspective, they see many people with similar illnesses being
treated in dramatically different ways. This is compounded by the fact that
they do not receive any adequate explanation for the variability. This has the
result of raising questions from those benefit managers as to the specificity and
value of treatment.

The National Committee for Quality Assurance (NCQA) and MBHOs
recognize the importance of minimizing treatment variability. As a result,
those organizations seeking NCQA accreditation will need to develop and
maintain clinical practice guidelines. This actually follows an initiative on the
part of a number of companies, to develop treatment guidelines as a way to
address treatment variability. It is important to recognize that practice guidelines do not represent a cookbook approach, which directs a provider to follow
a very specific treatment protocol, for every patient. An effective treatment
guideline will delineate the types of treatment known to be effective for an
illness. To the extent possible, first and subsequent choice therapies will be
explained. A provider is not required to do everything within a treatment
guideline. However, if a provider is to vary significantly from that guideline,
that provider should be able to justify his or her treatment decisions. For

example, if a patient is profoundly depressed, and their level of concentration is such that they may not be able to participate in psychotherapy, medication should be considered. If medication is not utilized, then the provider should have a reasonable rationale to explain that. A guideline should not mandate the use of such treatment, but must mandate that every element of a treatment guideline be considered and effective decisions made based on the guidelines and the individual under treatment's current clinical condition. The overall impact of treatment variability clearly requires further study.

III. Clinical Implications

Managed care has brought about a series of clinical considerations. First and foremost, managed care has put upon the providers a demand for individualized treatment plans. As has been stated in the past, there is no magic to once a week psychotherapy. Patients may need to be seen more frequently and less frequently, depending on their clinical condition. The key component is the importance of making sure that each treatment plan is focused specifically on the problems the individual consumer is experiencing.

Another important aspect is the need for continuity of care. The Health Plan Employer Data Information Set (HEDIS) report of NCQA asked that MBHOs measure the percentage of patients who are seen following hospitalization. Given the level of acuity that individuals requiring hospitalization have, combined with the fact that inpatient treatment is utilized for stabilization, makes it clear that follow up is critical. By measuring this, health plans are able to put into place a continuous quality improvement process to increase the number of people seen.

Table 3 demonstrates the implications and importance of treatment follow up. A 1993 SAMHSA National Advisory Mental Health Council Report points to a significant increase in relapse rate in Schizophrenia, Bipolar Disorder and Major Depressive Disorder when follow up care does not take place. Table 4 points out some of the experience that we have had in the Colorado Health Partnership, in developing follow up for adolescents in treatment. This table clearly demonstrates the fact that in this managed care program; there has been a significant increase in adolescent follow up. While some would argue that the follow up measures by themselves do not demonstrate the overall effectiveness of treatment, it is clear that in the absence of follow up, no treatment can take place. It is again, important to recognize that managed care has brought an increased awareness of this data and need for us all to monitor our effectiveness in this area.

	Relapse Rate without Treatment	Relapse Rate without Treatment
Schizophrenia	80%	25%
Bipolar Disorder	81%	34%
Major Depression	85%	18%

Table 3

  Implications of follow-up. From SAMHSA National Advisory Mental Health Council, 1993.

Managed care is also raising a need for increased emphasis on the coordination between primary care physicians and other health care providers. It has been reported that up to 60-70% of visits to primary care physicians are by individuals for whom there is no diagnosable biologic disorder. The importance of coordination of care in assisting primary care providers and addressing these behavioral health care issues, can lead to significant improvements as well as medical cost offsets. Moreover, the coordination of care between primary care and behavioral health care clinicians can assist in avoiding iatrogenic illnesses that might potentially occur as a result of an inadvertent conflict in therapy.

Another measurement that is receiving a great deal of attention is readmission rates. Here again, prior to managed care, the data is unclear as to the hospital readmission rate in many commercial self-insured accounts. Managed care organizations use this data to study the drivers of readmission rates, in an attempt to diminish those rates and improve overall clinical status for individuals. In tracking some of the commercial data, we find that readmission rates frequently range from 5-15%. Table 5, shows thirty day readmission rates in the Colorado Medicaid population. Here, the readmission rates are all below 10%. It is important to point out that while there is not a great deal of data on readmission rates that has been published, anecdotal data has suggested that readmission rates in an unmanaged Medicaid population can exceed 25-30%. The current monitoring suggested by the table presented indicates an awareness on the part of managed care to continue to monitor this data actively and be as effective as possible in diminishing readmission.

These clinical issues have raised some significant questions. The key question, that remains to be answered, is does managed care lead to different clinical results? The data suggested here would indicate that the likelihood of people's improvement is dramatically improved as a result of increased access and attention to follow up and readmission rates. Providers on the other hand, would suggest that quality has been negatively impacted by the virtue of the fact that patients are receiving shorter treatments focused at functional deficits. Managed care's perspective is that these improvements in process would put patients into a situation that increases the likelihood of

Time Span	Stage	Percent of Patients Receiving Recommended Mental Health Care	Total Number of Patients
1995 - 1996	Baseline	58%	n = 248
1996 - 1997	Year 1	86%	n = 127
1997 (6 months)	Year 2 (in progress)	92%	n = 84

Time Span	Stage	Percent of Patients Receiving General Health Follow-up	Total Number of Patients
1995 - 1996	Baseline	93%	n = 248
1996 - 1997	Year 1	100%	n = 127
1997 (6 months)	Year 2 (in progress)	100%	n = 84

Table 4

Development of follow-up for adolescants.

positive results. One of the arguments that is presented about these measures is that they do not directly measure the clinical impact of the treatment. While this point is well taken, and points to the fact that more study is needed, the process measures represent an excellent proxy that demonstrates the clinical improvements brought about by managed care.

IV. Functional Improvements

The area of functional improvement is one that has not been focused on a great deal by clinicians. For the most part, prior to managed care, clinicians focused on the signs and symptoms that were presented to them and utilized psychotherapy in response. Consumers point out that the elimination of clinical issues is only a part of what is important. Ultimately for improvement to be meaningful there must be an overall improvement in the individual's functional status.

The first area of functional status that must be focused on is that an individual's self care. Activities of daily living are frequently attended to when patients are in inpatient or residential treatment centers. However, it is important that providers pay attention to an individual's ability to maintain activities of daily living and what their living arrangements are as part of their overall treatment. If these areas can have a significant impact on the outcome of treatment, it is important that the provider address some of these during the treatment process. An example here is one of those receiving treatment for substance abuse that might be planning to return to a home where active substance abuse is continuing. The likelihood of avoiding relapse is small and these issues must be addressed in treatment. Consumers also point out that an individual's self-confidence is tied to their improvement. Thus a provider must work to encourage an individual to move forward in their life to the best of their ability. Finally, there needs to be attention the financial status of the individual. Devising a treatment plan or goal that is not consistent with an individual's financial situation is doomed to failure. Even if the clini-

Year / Quarter	Readmission Rate
1996 - Quarter 3	9%
1997 - Quarter 1	6%
1997 - Quarter 2	7%
1997 - Quarter 3	5.6%
1997 - Quarter 4	5%
1998 - Quarter 1	5.3%

Note: Readmission reports as high as 80% in the 1980's

Table 5

Readmission rates in a medical population.

cian is successful in removing the clinical syndrome, the presence of these real life concerns can undermine that progress and lead to prompt relapse.

The second area that becomes important is that of relationships. These relationships need to be looked at in terms of the home, interpersonal social situations, and work situations. These areas again, can have a dramatic impact on the long-term outcome of the removal of any clinical syndrome. Providers, while focusing on the clinical syndrome, must also focus on the impact of these relationships in order to provide external support that can minimize future difficulties. A supportive family and work situation can go a long way in assisting in recovery. On the other side, relationships that are problematic can undermine progress. In a study at ValueOptions we learned that the risk of suicide can be dramatically increased by a negative change in an individual's relationships and that a number of serious suicide attempts have followed these changes.

An area receiving increasing attention is that of the educational, vocational component of an individual's life. Employers are particularly interested in issues involving absenteeism or situations where individuals are at work, but are functioning far below their capability. An additional component of this is the increasing awareness of the impact of disability on an employer's overall benefit costs and ability to maintain function in their work. Employers are moving forward with disability management, working to combine the presence of disability within a treatment plan that is sufficiently intense to assist the individual in returning to work as soon as possible, and also has built within it, the return to work plan.

In devising treatment plans, clinicians are being asked now to focus on the individual in the context of their work situation. For example, in devising the treatment plan, patients are now being asked to be aware of the type of work situation the individual is in. Individuals who work in safety sensitive positions or whose jobs are in jeopardy require specific attention within the treatment plan, to addressing these concerns.

The data to date is largely anecdotal. There is an effort in education by managed care organizations to help providers understand the importance of workplace issues and to address them within the treatment plan. While the overall impact has yet to be studied, and more specificity in this area is required, it is clear from the anecdotal evidence that long-term outcomes for consumers are significantly increased when these key components of an individuals life are taken into account.

There are a variety of types of measurements that are beginning to take place. Employers are increasingly measuring, with more specificity, the impact of absenteeism and disability. Also, they are looking to understand more about the impact of job performance for those who are in attendance at work.

Another type of measurement that can take place is that of the physical area. As suggested in work by Nicholas Cummings, targeted focused treatment, addressing specific clinical disorders and stress can have a significant impact on overall health care costs. At the same time, it has a significant impact on individual's overall functioning.

V. Consumer Satisfaction

Consumer surveys done within many MBHOs reveal over 80% satisfaction by the consumer. Consumers are asked to rate the referral practice when they have used the MBHO's referral line, their interaction with the MBHO's staff, both clinical and customer service, the provider from whom they received treatment and their overall treatment. They are also often asked whether they feel the treatment has resulted in positive change for them. Consistently, the numbers come back above 80% satisfaction. This immediately raises the question of reconciling that data to the managed care backlash and complaints that are often presented by the lay press. It is important to recognize that as hard as we try, there is always the potential for problems to occur within treatment. This took place prior to managed care, and in fact, the concerns about providers care and the malpractice suits pre-managed care, in many states, lead to malpractice insurance crisis in the 1970's. Since often these issues related to single cases by individual clinicians, one would not see lay press articles of this nature. However, one does see articles that talk about overall rates of treatment that become questionable. For example, a recent article in the Washington Post, pointed to the fact that the Cesarean section rate within the Mid-Atlantic geographic region was significantly higher than in other areas of the country. It is generally in this fashion, that one will see questions about provider's care.

Managed care on the other hand, is a larger entity and often viewed as a concept, rather than a group of individuals, clinicians and administrators who are advocating on behalf of consumers. Moreover, there are many different types of managed care but they all tend to get lumped together in spite of their differences some of which were noted earlier in this chapter. When one looks at the number of cases treated by managed care organizations, it is unfortunately inevitable, that some problems will occur. The three largest managed behavioral health care companies, manage in excess of 100 million people, using over 60,000 network providers, with a penetration rate of a conservative 6%. It is important to see that over 6 million individuals will be in treatment each year. Most of those cases go very well and require no intervention from the managed care organization. Others go well with some intervention on behalf of the beneficiary by the managed care organization, and a few unfortunately, do not go well. The lay press would have us believe that this is a function of managed care, and ignore the fact that from the time of the Flexnor Report in the early 1900's, there have always been situations where cases did not go as well as one would have hoped for a variety of reasons. Since managed care presents a fundamental change in the way health care is delivered, it has become the entity upon which to focus wrath. An example of this is an unfortunate case in North Carolina where a young man successfully committed suicide. The individual had care not certified at one point by his managed care organization. Over a number of years, this same case has been used as evidence for problems within managed care. While that one case was being brought up over and over again, managed care continued to involve itself with successful treatment of over 6 million people per year.

In that context, one can clearly understand why satisfaction rates remain high for the large bulk of consumers. One very important factor in managed care is their desire for continuous quality improvement. Managed care continually oversees itself, auditing its decisions and reviewing its clinical guidelines. Thus, one of the most prominent aspects of managed care's effectiveness, has been to raise awareness of the need to measure what we are doing, holding ourselves all accountable, and working in a continuous quality improvement environment.

IMPACT OF MANAGED CARE

Managed care has had an impact in three areas: the client company, the consumer, and the provider. From the perspective of the client company, there has been a decrease in their overall costs for behavioral health care services. Moreover, there has been a development of some cost predictability, which has lead to a willingness to enhance benefits. Many self-insured companies were willing to enhance their benefits when they moved from an indemnity program to a managed behavioral health care program. Moreover, while there is much anxiety about the concept of parity, more of these companies are willing to consider parity because of the efforts of managed care in containing costs and helping further clinical understanding. Finally, there is a beginning to clinical predictability in treatment of a company's beneficiaries.

The consumer now has increased access. They can not only seek care, as they did in the past, but they can now utilize the resources of the clinical departments of MBHOs to find appropriate treatment providers. Along with this, they have experienced a decrease out of pocket expense for treatment. As has been pointed out in the Rand study on the utilization of medical services, there is a significant decrease in the use of services as copayments increase. The increased access and decreased out of pocket expenses have come with some change. While access has increased to care, the number of clinicians that one can access has decreased through the development of provider networks. However, these networks are sufficiently large to allow consumer choice, even though that choice is not to everyone. Many plans however, have impacted that by allowing open choice through a point of service plan, with increased copayments for choosing outside the network. If one looks at the increasing numbers of individuals receiving care through managed health care, one can see that although there continues to be a great deal of anxiety and concern about managed care, individual employees and their dependents are interested in managing their own health care costs and are willing to enter managed care programs to do so. The negative component of all of this change has been the fact that the health care system has become more complex for consumers to navigate. Managed health care programs must spend more time helping consumers more fully understand the nature of these programs and how they can function within them.

The most significant change, as a result of managed care, has taken place from the perspective of the provider. The provider is now being asked to justify treatment plans to the consumer and to a manager. When these treatment plans demonstrate significant variability from standards, that variability is being asked to be justified. Many providers in the past based their treatment on where they were trained. Now they are being asked to be much more specific and select treatment based on consumer clinical condition, the other factors that impact potential improvement, and the knowledge of the disorder and treatments that are effective. Providers understandably, resent this intrusion and see managed care as responsible. It is important to note that managed care was in response in escalating costs and treatment variability and the necessity of treatment justification becomes a vehicle to assist companies in becoming more comfortable with the health care dollars they are spending. The providers are also experiencing an increase their administrative work. The justification of treatment plans will take place either through telephonic certification reviews, outpatient treatment reports or electronic interactions. This new record keeping endeavor adds time to the provider's workload. Further, the provider is being asked to maintain an appropriate clinical record and share appropriate clinical information with other health care providers for that consumer.

With all of this, one of the most important aspects is that there has been a significant decrease in provider income. The reduction in income comes from both a decrease in units of service provided and a decrease in the unit cost. Managed care has required providers to treat individuals in a focused manner and utilize multiple levels of care as appropriate. This has led to shorter lengths of stay at higher levels of care and shorter episodes of treatment overall. Some would argue that these reductions have negatively impacted quality of care. Data to support that statement is lacking. In fact, the tendency by some to question the overall value of treatment has led payers to push reimbursement rates down. This push from employers and others leads to rate reductions which when combined with a decrease in units of service leads to the income decreases.

This combination of an increased need for treatment justification, an increased administrative workload, and a decrease in income, has lead to a strenuous pushback by providers on managed care. It is important for all of us to realize that managed care is only a means to an end. That end involves being better able to define the nature and quality of treatment and in doing so, reduce the variability and thereby improve results and contain the costs. It behooves the providers to begin to find ways to work with managed care, to assist the providers in dealing with some of these clear concerns that are being presented to them.

SUMMARY

This chapter has reviewed some of the history of the development of managed care and the types of programs available. It has also looked a data regarding costs before and after managed care. Prior to managed care, companies experienced large, steady increases in the costs of behavioral health care. They responded initially by limiting benefits and ultimately by developing management programs. With the inception of managed care, an increased number of people accessed treatment, while the overall costs for the company client went down.

Along with the focus on cost, there has been an increased focus on the accountability of treatment provided to consumers. Providers are asked to be aware of treatment guidelines and to explain variability from the guidelines. This is a very important issue. Managed care organizations do not propose to dictate and prescribe treatment. They will however, ask for justification of variability in treatment or justification when current treatment is not effective and the treatment plan is not being changed. Managed care has begun to develop data on various aspects of clinical care such as access, follow up and readmission. This data collection must continue to expand beyond traditional scientific research.

While the scientific research is important and must continue, it is equally important for us to learn what happens when treatment occurs in the general population, under the care of a general clinician. Our study of this information provides us the opportunity to develop methods to improve care provided by practicing clinicians, by dealing in measures that are important for clinical outcomes and meaningful to the consumer.

REFERENCES

Cummings, N. A. (1997). Behavioral health in primary care: Dollars and sense. In Cummings, N. A., Cummings, J. L., & Johnson, J. N. (Eds.), *Behavioral health in primary care: A guide for clinical integration*. Madison: CT, Psychosocial Press.

Manning, W., Wells, K., & Buchanan, J. (1989). Effects of mental health insurance: Evidence from the health insurance experiment. Santa Monica, CA:RAND.

National Committee for Quality Assurance. 1998 MBHO Surveyor Guidelines: For the Accreditation of Managed Behavioral Healthcare Organizations.

Schwartz, W. B. & Mendelson, D. N. (1982). Why managed care cannot contain hospital costs – without rationing. *Health Affairs Summer 1992*, 100-107.

Discussion of Shaffer:

Effectiveness and Cost in Managed Care

Ole J. Thienhaus, M.D.
University of Nevada School of Medicine,
Las Vegas and Reno

Managed care is not a monolithic concept. Rather, the term encompasses a continuum of organizational structures for the financing and delivery of health care services. The various structures are most appropriately operationalized according to the distribution of financial risk among the payers (insurers, employers etc.), providers and facilitators (hospitals, brokers, clinics etc.) that are involved in the health care delivery system. At one end of the continuum there are managed care organizations providing administrative support, such as utilization review, to traditional insurers. At the other end, there are organizations that have taken on the full risk of a capitated insurance product. In either case, the advent of managed care has profoundly impacted the US health care market. And, some say, no segment in that market has been affected more than the community of mental health care professionals.

Managed care has greatly promoted the principles of evidence-based medicine in the area of mental or behavioral health. Historically, patients who came to see a mental health clinician could expect to receive treatment according to the chosen provider's expertise, not according to the needs dictated by their clinical condition. The managed-care-driven emphasis on outcomes has changed that. Providers have to justify their recommended treatment vis-à-vis those who pay for it, and, if the treatment does not work, they must expect to change it.

The vilification of managed care due to anecdotally reported adverse results is uncalled for. What counts are aggregate outcomes. And in this area, the introduction of managed care has, indeed, most probably increased access to mental health services and reduced their cost to those who ultimately pay for it, namely the consumers. This observation has added powerful ammunition in the debate about "parity" for mental health. With adequate resource

Integrated Behavioral Healthcare: Positioning Mental Health Practice with Medical/Surgical Practice

utilization management, it is argued, putting mental health services on a par with medical or surgical benefits will not substantially add to the actuarial risk of health insurers. Therefore, premiums would not dramatically increase. The managed care industry appears to be emerging as an ally of the National Association of the Mentally Ill (NAMI).

If managed care is so good, why do mental health clinicians cry foul? Why are all the major professional organizations — the American Psychological Association, the American Psychiatric Association, the National Association of Social Workers — so unanimously and vociferously opposed? A number of answers may be proposed to answer that question.

For one, there is a profound communicative gap between traditional clinicians on one side and managed care organizations on the other. This gap is based on fundamentally different frames of reference. The clinician is, and must be, responsive to his or her client's needs. The clinician must retain a highly individualized perspective in order to function as his or her patient's advocate.

By contrast, managed care organizations deal in populations. The manager of a managed care organization seeks improvements in value for the insured population at large—even if the occasional individual care recipient is unhappy with his or her benefits. This has, of course, always been the insurance industry's perspective. But traditional indemnity insurance stayed out of the doctor-patient relationship. By contrast, the utilization managers of managed care organizations dare to intrude.

But there are also more substantive issues involved. Managed care is obviously not a panacea to solve the challenge of simultaneously optimizing quality of care, access to health care and health care cost containment. Since managed care started its meteoric rise in the late 1980s, more Americans have joined the ranks of the uninsured whose number is now estimated at 43 million. The initial flattening of cost increases has begun to disappear. For 1999, at least seven percent increase in national health care expenditures is forecast, almost three times the expected rate of consumer price index increases.

The recent health care cost increases are, to be sure, partly due to cumbersome government regulations and intrusive micromanagement. The ever-increasing role of costly technology in our response to health care needs also plays an important role. But there is also a disturbing trend toward anti-competitive consolidation on the vendors' side of the managed care market. The number of managed care organizations is decreasing, the average size of managed care organizations, in terms of insured lives and in terms of capitalization, is increasing, and in some geographic areas, the market-sustaining phenomenon of competition has largely disappeared. Monopolies invariably engender price increases to consumers.

Related to this consolidation, there is a growing preponderance of for-profit players in the market. Such organizations may be good at cost-cutting. But the greater efficiency, which translates into income-squeezes on providers (facilities as well as professionals), means reductions in "medical loss ratios." This term defines the percentage of gross income used to pay for care as opposed to the portion that is returned to the managed care organization's shareholders. In other words, part of the greater cost effectiveness takes on the form of a shift of income from providers to shareholders.

The intrusion of profit motives is nothing new to health care: After all, independent, licensed providers have, over many years, sought to maximize their individual incomes from patient care activities. However, the introduction of the profit motive on a corporate scale into the health care market does change the health care market's dynamics. Shareholders have, ultimately, no professional accountability to sick people looking for help. And the actual professional providers cannot forget that in their respective professional codes of ethics the services they provide can never be reduced to a commodity.

In the area of care for the chronically mentally ill, the success of managed care to replace traditional models of behavioral health care is arguably mixed. The conceptual model of mental illness in managed care is an episode-of-illness concept. This model can be expected to work best for patients with adjustment disorders or situational stress problems. It is more difficult to apply to patients who suffer from schizophrenia or dementing conditions. The implosion of Tennessee's TennCare experiment, when applied to the chronically mentally ill Medicaid beneficiaries of that state, may not be typical. But it certainly should be reason for caution in predicting success of transferring managed care results in the private sector to public health problems.

Certain principles of managed care are likely to endure. These include the healthy emphasis on accountability and the measurement of outcomes as a function of cost: The concept of value — long appreciated in other areas of the consumer market — has finally been brought to behavioral health care, thanks to the managed care revolution.

Other aspects are likely to wash out. We are undoubtedly beginning to see the end of initial cost-savings due to eliminating certain ineffective practice types. But regulatory limitations and monopolistic tendencies are exerting their countervailing influences, and costs are beginning to rise again. The administrative cost ("overhead"), associated with a proprietary and fragmented payer system, is not being addressed by the managed care concept as it now exists. In the long run it seems illusory to attach hopes for realizing true market efficiencies to a product that by necessity can never meet economists' specification for a commodity in a market operating under the conditions of perfect competition.

Practice Guidelines and the Industrialization of Behavioral Healthcare Delivery

Steven C. Hayes
Jennifer Gregg
University of Nevada, Reno

Integrated Behavioral Healthcare: Positioning Mental Health Practice with Medical/Surgical Practice

INTRODUCTION

We have three major purposes in this chapter. First, we want to convince the readers that practice guidelines are not an arbitrary development in the field. Our logic, in outline form, will be that managed behavioral care marks the transition of this economic sector to full scale industrialization. Practice guidelines are a necessary component of an industrialized behavioral health care delivery system because they help ward off threats to successful industrialization. Second, we want to convince the readers that practice guidelines, done properly, hold out great hope for consumers, managers, payors, and providers alike, but only if they are properly done, with participation of all the major stakeholders. We will describe the Practice Guidelines Coalition process as a good example of what needs to be done. Finally, we will discuss where practice guidelines fit within an integrated system of evidence-based care.

The Non-Arbitrary Nature of Practice Guidelines

The Industrialization of Healthcare Delivery

There are not many times when you can see the future, but there is an exception when the speed of change is so fast that the present and the future are the same thing. You know you are in one of those times when you can say the same sentence in the present or the future tense and makes equal sense either way. The personal computer provides an example. At one point early in the development of personal computers you could say "personal computers will be big" or "personal computer are big" and it was just as sensible either way. People who fully realized what that meant easily made successful investments by betting on the future they could already see. Biotechnology or the internet provide other recent example. The same applies, we would argue, to clinical practice guidelines.

In a span of less than a decade managed care has risen from a minor player to be the dominant force in private and public healthcare delivery (Frank, McGuire, Notman, & Woodward, 1996). The essence of managed care is not its form—there are many competing forms and new varieties are emerging every few months—but its nature. Managed care represents the industrialization of healthcare delivery (Cummings & Hayes, 1996).

Industrialization involves the systematized production of goods or services in large-scale enterprises that are responsive to the enterprise-wide bottom line. There are thus three defining characteristics of industrialization: large size, constant systematization, and the overall enterprise as the ultimate economic unit. These three characteristics put the productivity of an individual into the context of the productivity of an entire enterprise. The economic unit of interest goes beyond the worker, the family, the cottage, or the manor, to that of the firm. Technical efficiency and productivity generally rises during industrialization because tasks can become more systematized, worker skill and training can be better fitted to the tasks, mechanization and technical aids can amplify the skills and output of individuals, and efficiencies in the entire system are refined through innovation and competition.

If anyone doubts that industrialization is the process that is impacting healthcare delivery, consider this: the mental health needs of over 90 millions Americans are today controlled by *two firms*: Magellan and Value Options. In the year 2000 each of these firms expects to add one to eight million more consumers to their systems. There can be little doubt that we are already in an era where the delivery of behavioral health services resides in large-scale enterprises that are systematized to provide these services in a fashion designed to produce a positive, enterprise-wide bottom line. By definition, this means that healthcare delivery is industrializing.

Opponents of managed care, and there are many, need to distinguish specific forms of industrialization from the process itself. Specific managed care arrangements can and will change. Some will die out over time. But no one should think that this means that industrialization per se will be reversed. Never in human history has a major economic sector industrialized and then deindustrialized. It is unlikely to happen in healthcare delivery.

The reasons for industrialization are many, but the single biggest factor was the excess costs incurred by fee for service healthcare deliver. In fee for service healthcare, insurance was an industry, but healthcare delivery was not. Providers essentially ran their own "mom and pop" businesses. Healthcare delivery was very much like the small family farms so common in the first half of this century, prior to the era of the industrialization of agriculture

(Drum, 1995). Third party payers became increasingly subject to any escalation in costs that occurred. Cost escalation was relatively unconstrained since the contingencies operating in this system did not encourage efficiency or effectiveness. If patients stayed in therapy as long as provider felt it was necessary, providers would benefit since third party payers would usually reimburse for this amount without information on the need for treatment or its outcome. Providers learned to work the system. There was a rapid proliferation of private psychiatric hospitals and addiction treatment centers (Cummings, 1995; Trabin & Freeman, 1995). The number of behavioral healthcare training programs also increased.

Indemnity based health insurance companies faced with escalating costs were forced to maintain their profits by charging higher and higher premiums to businesses and individuals purchasing their policies. Costs for behavioral healthcare began skyrocketing. For example, during a five year period, from 1987 to 1992, the average yearly premium for mental health and substance abuse paid by employers increased from $163 per employee to $318, an increase of nearly 100% (Shoor, 1993; Strosahl, 1994). Both government payers (e.g., Medicare and Medicaid) as well as business and industry were unable to absorb any further increases in costs.

The industrialization of healthcare delivery has occurred so rapidly because large scale managed care enterprises were readily able to reduce cost while maintaining reasonable quality, primarily by driving down both unreasonable utilization and the fees charged by facilities and providers. Value Behavioral Health, for example, could reduce costs 40% while *increasing* access by 25% during first year after they took over an indemnity-based behavioral healthcare system simply by eliminating coverage for those who had been seeing a psychotherapist for years without clear justification, cutting therapists who tended to see the patients for years, and demand somewhat lower payment of clinicians (Shaffer, this volume).

These changes gave better overall value to payers and consumers. As time has gone on, however, the reduction in reimbursements has had serious consequences for some providers, who are working harder for less, and there is a broad perception that quality of care is beginning to suffer. In just a few years it seems that we have wrung out about all that we can using cost containment mechanisms. The rise of public support for legislation and regulation shows that MCOs are now cutting into the bone. Yet competition has reduced profit margins to a sliver.

With costs down, the next major area of improvement has to be value. In theory an emphasis on value can cut costs by reducing per incident costs and especially by reducing further demand for services through effective and efficient services. As the industry consolidates, this begins to make good economic sense, since consumers stay with given firms for longer and longer periods.

Stages in Industrialization

Industrialization tends to go through four stages, and these stages are being followed quite closely in the industrialization of healthcare deliver systems (Hayes, Barlow, & Nelson-Gray, 1999).

1. In the early stages of industrialization, *vendors proliferate and consumers are confused.*
2. In the confusion, *poor quality products succeed but then die out as the overall quality of products increases.*
3. As products become better understood, *vendors and product lines are consolidated and external review increases.*
4. Finally, in a mature marketplace, *known firms offer known commodities of known quality, cost, and value in a stable external review environment.*

You can see these stages in a recent example: personal computers. In stage one, hundreds of software and hardware firms competed, each one claiming that their systems or programs were better. Customers were confused. Consumers had a hard time knowing if an 8 bit operating system was better than 16 bit, if Apple's system was better than IBM's; or if DOS was better than TRS-80. In stage two, computers began to get better and better. Some firms (e.g., Leading Edge) undercut the market with cheap clones but they later began to fail under the weight of returns, poor service, and the poor reputation these bred. In stage three, consolidation occurred. We went from dozens of popular word processors, to one giant and two also rans. Half a dozen computer makers survived with significant market share. Litigation and legislation began to be focused on the industry. People began to resent the hegemony of MicroSoft. We are now entering stage four. Variability in features, quality, and cost, occur within a known range and provide choice to the consumer who may, for example, choose slightly less sophisticated technology in exchange for a lower price. Changes in external review continue however (e.g., the anti-trust suit against MicroSoft) which indicates that the marketplace is not yet fully mature.

The health care delivery industry is proceeding through this same developmental sequence and has recently reached stage three. Vendors did indeed proliferate chaotically and consumers were terribly confused. Even three years ago a Louis Harris poll showed that a majority of US citizens did not know that "managed care" meant or what a "health maintenance organization" was (Gannett News Service, 1996). Quality was uneven and some vendors succeeded by cutting needed services (Manderscheid & Henderson, 1996). The industry has seen a tremendous degree of consolidation and a major increase in external review as any glance at the newspaper will show. Litigation, accreditation, legislation, and regulation are now an inherent part of the landscape of managed care. The healthcare delivery industry is trying to find ways to increase quality and efficiency through means other than mere cost reduction.

The Enemies of Industrialization

There are four big enemies of success in this stage. *Consumer confusion and fear* is one enemy. Fearful consumers are slow to buy and quick to complain. Confused consumers will make poor buying decisions that do not reflect the real value of competing products or services, and thus maintain inefficiencies in the system.

The second enemy is an *unpredictable context that too rapidly alters the playing field for competition*. This slows industrialization because investors become uncertain and because business errors are more likely. Challenging contexts per se are not necessarily bad because they tend to weed out strong and weak players. But unpredictability is another matter.

A third enemy is the *failure to demonstrate increased value*. Value is a measure of the quality and convenience of an item per unit of cost. Industrialization tends to occur when value leaps forward as a result of large scale, systematized enterprises, by reducing cost, or by increasing quality and convenience, or both. The personal computer industry, for example, has produced more and more powerful computers, for less and less. Value thus shot up. Mechanized production of shoes showed a different pattern. Quality did not necessarily increase over the shoes made by a good craftsperson, but the cost of shoes plummeted, and value rose. If value is not demonstrated, however, the main support for industrialization is removed.

A final barrier is *unexplained product variability*. Unexplained variability leads to an inability to improve quality and efficiency. Suppose a manufacturer is making a car and there is a poorly designed part. If the part varies too much in ways unknown to the maker (e.g., through manufacturing tolerances that are too large) the part might be fine in one car and a problem in others. If the part was made with good tolerances its bad design would be much more easily detected. Any industrial entity must know what it is producing and selling, and unexplained variability interferes with that knowledge.

Enemies of Behavioral Healthcare Industrialization

Each of these four enemies of industrialization currently exists in the behavioral healthcare delivery sector. Consumer confusion and fear is exacerbated by the consumers perception of a loss of control. This is due in part to the complexity and rapidity of the changes in healthcare delivery. Plans themselves are confusing and difficult to understand. This perception is also due in part to an actual reduction in the range of plans offered by employers as they increasingly direct employees into lower cost options.

The context underlying managed care is relatively unpredictable due to rapidly evolving business and political events. Legislation such as the patients' bill of rights, lawsuits, or entirely new business models adopted by competitors provide a constant threat of rapid change. Ironically, however, some of these threats to predictability (e.g., suits over coverage practices) will increase the predictability of the business context in the long term because they will weed out excesses that the public does not support. That has been the experience in other sectors of the economy going through external market regulation and litigation.

There is indeed a widespread belief that the healthcare industry has failed to produce or to demonstrate value. Outcomes are unclear and consumers are increasingly beginning to believe the managed care reduces cost at the expense of quality.

Finally there is huge unexplained product variability in behavioral healthcare delivery. An enormous range of treatments exist for any disorder, and clinicians factors (e.g., theoretical orientation), not patient factors, seem to dominate as the source of variability in treatment decisions.

Thus, behavioral healthcare delivery faces every one of the major threats to successful industrialization. The industry has a built in bias toward any steps that will help solve these problems.

THE ROLE OF PRACTICE GUIDELINES IN REDUCING BARRIERS TO INDUSTRIALIZATION

Clinical practice guidelines are statements of the best available evidence in specific practice domains for the purpose of advising practitioners in their professional work. Unlike standards of practice, guidelines encourage but do not require that practitioners be guided by this evidence. Guidelines serve as summaries, reminders, prompts, and suggestions, not requirements.

Clinical practice guidelines have long existed in physical medicine, but their advent in behavioral healthcare is recent. Most of the activity in the area dates back only into the early 1990's. Some examples of developments in this area include the development of a depression guideline by the Agency for Health Care Policy Research (published in 1994), the recommendation in support of clinical practice guidelines from the Second Summit of Applied Psychological Organizations (1992), the formation of the Task Force for Empirically Validated Treatment by Division 12 (Clinical Psychology) of the American Psychological Association(1995), the convening of a Conference on Scientific Standards of Psychological Practice (1994), the publication of the first practice guidelines from the American Psychiatric Association (1992), the formation of the Practice Guidelines Coalition (1996), or the requirement that at least two behavioral health practice guidelines be implemented in accredited behavioral healthcare organizations by the National Committee for Quality Assurance (1998).. It is fair to say that at the present time clinical practice guidelines are only beginning to hit behavioral health in a meaningful way.

Despite their recency, it seems that that clinical practice guidelines are bound to develop in managed care organizations for a simple reason: In each of the four areas that can slow industrialization, clinical practice guidelines are at least potentially helpful. It is for that reason that practice guidelines are a non-arbitrary aspect of the current healthcare scene. Unless industrialization per se stops in the healthcare delivery sector, the growth of practice guidelines will continue.

Consumer confusion and fear may be reduced by practice guidelines because in principle they can provide a quality floor and a more known product. If payers and consumers know that a system follows empirically-based practice guidelines, it is less likely that untested methods will be used before methods known to be successful are tried. If delivering these methods requires certain kinds of training or a certain number of sessions, payers and consumers know that it is more likely that such resources will be made available. Practice guidelines can reduce clinicians' fear by providing more protection again arbitrary and capricious reimbursement decisions.

Contextual unpredictability may be reduced by practice guidelines for several reasons. Systems may be less subject to political battering if a credible practice guideline is being followed since it provides a kind of empirical shield against unwarranted criticisms and attacks. Practice guidelines can reduce contextual unpredictability by reducing and channeling the pressure of regulation, legislation, accreditation, and litigation. If practice guidelines were broadly implemented, they would help level the playing field and prevent competitors from succeeding by reducing the quality of care in areas covered by guidelines.

The production and demonstration of value can be increased by practice guidelines because evidence of compliance with practice guideline provides evidence of quality of care. Further, if the guidelines produce better, faster, more long lasting desirable clinical outcomes, then they may produce cost savings through a reduction of the demand for services. At the system level, guidelines could provide a principled basis for the construction of mental health benefits as helping to direct the pre-certification and utilization review process on a case by case basis. Evidence-based practice guidelines could provide clinicians access to scientifically valid decision support tools that would help identify the procedures most likely to be effective. Finally, guidelines may help companies better allocate professional resources by providing a better match between the existing skills of clinicians and the types of core procedures recommended in guidelines. Costly doctoral professionals, for example, may be better suited to supervising a empirically supported protocol than in delivering most of the services themselves.

Probably the biggest issue for clinical practice guidelines, however, is whether they can reduce unexplained variability in treatment. In principle this seems likely, since following a practice guideline, by definition, should produce less variability than following nothing. It is not yet known, however, whether this theoretical expectation will be upheld. In all likelihood the answer will be complex, since probably some guidelines in some areas and in some formats will produce better outcomes than others. Focusing on a reduction in variability leads to the conclusion that penetration, not perfection, is most important. Even a highly flawed guideline, it widely read and followed, sets the stage for system improvement since these flaws can be detected and corrected. Among other things, this means that guideline acceptability to stakeholders is paramount, since resistance by any major sector will tend to reduce penetration and recycling and improvement.

Practice guidelines so directly help with the major problems faced by industrial healthcare delivery systems that they *will* be developed. And, in fact, every large managed care firm is involved with guideline implementation. Many have been involved directly in developing them. But the guidelines being developed are not ideal.

Political Problems in Current Clinical Practice Guidelines

Probably the biggest source of clinical practice guidelines right now is the industry itself. Unfortunately, those developed inside the industry tend to be proprietary and thus are not open to scrutiny and orderly change. They are often not based on the best available evidence, especially those developed by inhouse staff. Industry guidelines also tend to overemphasize cost-reduction over quality outcomes and each firm has their own, which leads to a nightmare for clinicians working with several firms.

Those developed by specific disciplines or guilds tend not to have broad penetration, in part because they lead to professional in-fighting inside managed care firms as, say, social workers resist being directed by psychiatry guidelines. Guild guidelines tend also to be narrowly focused, and are biased by the values, goals, and roles of the specific guild or discipline. This is not a problem if they are applied only within specific disciplines, but even here guidelines not yet widely enough adopted that disciplines can reach their members.

Those developed by the government or private foundations tend to be dominated by professionals and scientists seeking comprehensive statements, and as a result they are long, complex, and clinician unfriendly. These guidelines are at a much level higher than that of the typical clinician, who often is a masters level provider with fairly general training in mental health treatments. Such guidelines tend to offer far too many recommendations to be practical, instead of focusing on the few clinical procedures that empirically are associated with good outcomes. They are also characterized by expensive and lengthy development cycles, taking a million dollars or more over a multiyear period. They have often been biased by political and professional in-fighting. Thus, almost all of the guidelines efforts now underway – industry, guild, and governmental – have problems.

There are other challenges faced by guidelines regardless of where they are developed. Many clinicians fear that these documents will be used as standards that specify cookbook-fashion what professionals must do. Properly implemented, guidelines provide a guide, but it is *expected* that often they may not fit. When they do not, the clinician need not follow them, but the clinicians may be asked whether the guide was considered. In essence, guidelines target *unexplained* variability, not absolute variability. The fear is nevertheless quite real.

And there are many other barriers to overcome. Our most popular diagnostic system is notoriously weak, especially in its treatment utility. We have a very large weakness in specification of technology. A related problem is that we often describe procedures in a way that makes theoretical orientation a major barrier and source of conflict. There is a major divide between psychosocial and biobehavioral approaches. And consumers will have to be given choice or guidelines will never be accepted. Most guidelines also have not meaningfully integrated consumer and clinician views about treatment acceptability and burden of receiving or delivering given services into recommended actions.

Problems in the Science Base for Clinical Practice Guidelines

The final group of problems is in our scientific culture. Guidelines are not purely scientific documents. They are meant to provide clinical guidance. They are not the place for scientific tomes and endless equivocation, and for guidelines purposes scientists need to learn to speak with a clear voice. Yet we have very few one-handed scientists: almost always scientists say "on the one hand this and on the other hand that." That tendency is not helpful in guideline development.

An even more serious problem lies in the scientific literature itself. Our outcome research is also far too dominated by efficacy research. We have hardly begun to develop appropriate methods for effectiveness research and to implement them regularly. For that reason, data on clinician acceptability, client acceptability, and system applicability, among others, is usually not available. Evidence-based practice guidelines in the current environment usually will not include some of the kinds of data that may most predict whether the actual implementation of the guideline will lead to positive change.

Our current models of treatment development and dissemination are based on the FDA model of drug development. In this three-stage approach, pilot work is done by the pharmaceutical company, testing specific drugs with specific medical conditions. If the data are promising, large scale efficacy testing is then conducted, often with federal dollars. Dissemination research follows, especially to look for side effects, and continues following FDA approval as the delivery system itself continues to monitor impact and safety factors. Practice guidelines would be one form of "stage three" dissemination. The problems in transporting this model to mental health are considerable but the federal government forced the issue in the late 1970's and early 1980's as it began to fund only specific treatments for specific disorders. At the insistence of the leadership of the National Institute of Mental Health, federal funding was reorganized and proposals, reviews, and funding went through sections that were organized in terms of particular diagnostic categories. Researchers were required to specify their interventions in a technologically precise manner. It is relatively easy to meet this requirement in pharmacotherapy, because it is easy to specify a pharmacological treatment, but psychosocial interventions are another matter. Treatment manuals and extensive adherence and competence measures became a virtual requirement for funding in the psychosocial area.

Compared to the state of the literature in the 1960's and 1970's, these changes have been positive in the main, at least as considered from a scientific point of view. It is now possible to conduct treatment outcome research in a fairly well controlled and replicable manner. This in turn has allowed us to begin to sort out to the most effective approaches for particular kinds of problems.

As more and more bells and whistles have been added to the typical clinical research study, the FDA model of treatment development has had the undesirable effect of increasing the distance between some aspects of the health care delivery system and our existing data. Let me give some examples.

Cost of Training

There is nothing in the current research system that demands that treatment technologies be simple to train. Researchers generally refuse to consider the cost of training as a significant component of their research program. One can understand the rationale. After all, the researcher is first attempting to determine whether a particular approach is effective. It seems almost unfair to treat the extraordinary means that researchers might use to make sure that therapists are well trained as a kind of "cost." Efficacy is the first requirement of the FDA model—in this approach we can always get to cost in stage three dissemination research

But the health care delivery system does not have this luxury. Use of a technology in their systems is inherently a matter of dissemination, and that immediately involves cost considerations. Dissemination research, furthermore, is both largely absent and often ill conceived when it does occur. Researchers think of dissemination research as proof of the transportability and generality of impact of specific technologies—clinical efficacy writ large. Health care administrators think instead of fit within their systems. Imagine the dismay of a clinical researcher who might realize that a favorite technology might have to be fundamentally altered to fit a system. By the rules of the FDA model, the whole process of treatment testing would then have to begin all over.

Broad Versus Narrow Focus

The FDA model calls for specific treatments for specific problems. If these "problems" were functional entities that might make a lot of sense, but practically everyone knows that syndromes are no such thing. Yet researchers can only secure funding if they claim that their treatment technologies apply to specific syndromes. Researchers become "experts" in these same narrow areas. They write books about them; they given workshops on them. They sit on review panels that are organized by these topographical entities.

The health care delivery system views it differently. Clinics cannot afford to have "experts" in every syndrome and empirically supported technology. They need broad approaches that are known to be effective, saving specific training for fairly costly disorders (e.g., borderline personality disorder; panic disorder). But to make the claim that an approach is broadly applicable is to fly in the face of both academic contingencies and the process of federal funding. And without federal funding, clinical outcome research is now basically impossible, since the FDA model has made it enormously expensive.

Technique Proliferation and Fractionation

Researchers need to make a name for themselves in particular areas in order to advance in the academy and to develop reputations that contribute to their success in obtaining research grant funds. One of the best ways to do this is to develop particular treatments that are "all your own". This has led to a proliferation of manuals, the full impact of which we are only now beginning to feel. There are literally dozens of cognitive behavior therapy manuals now available covering almost every conceivable syndrome. Many of these manuals are quite similar and yet they go under different specific names. Each has their own particular training methods, adherence measures, competence measures and the like. New researchers are scrambling to get on the train. Unless something changes, the dozens of CBT manuals will be the hundreds in a short time.

Clinician Acceptability

Clinician acceptability is one of the most fundamental areas where there is a disconnect between your usual research methods and the health care industry. In the typical research study therapists are selected for their willingness to be trained in the methods of interest. If a clinician has a problem with the underlying model in a particular technology, that person would be unlikely to be selected to be trained. Yet that very person—or other like persons—may need to be trained in the health care system as particular technologies are disseminated. Behavior therapy carries a particular burden in this regard because a behavioral model often flies in the face of the deeply held beliefs of some clinicians.

Adherence and Competence

Adherence and competence measures, while of great use in a research setting, are not necessarily directly applicable to the delivery system as we have developed them. They are just too costly, intrusive, and complex. Yet health care delivery systems must know what treatment is being delivered in order to improve their product. Researchers have to help provide simple means of assessing whether given treatment technologies are being implemented and properly used, but that need is not yet on the radar screen. As a result, in the current phase of development in the delivery system, clinicians merely need to learn to use the right words without necessarily changing what they do in actual practice. For example, an astounding number of clinicians claim to be "cognitive behavioral therapists" despite the fact that many have had no training in this approach and are not favorably disposed to it. A recent case in which psychoanalysts were using the term "relapse prevention" to describe their usual psychodynamic approach to addiction is an example.

How to Combine Technologies

Everything we know about clinical practice in physical medicine or behavioral health suggests that clinicians will modify and combine treatment technologies when they use them. However much the researcher might wish it were otherwise, it simply is not realistic to expect that this will not happen. The recent Phen-Fen case provides an interesting example both of the pervasiveness of this approach and of its problems. In this case, two medications that each worked separately and were approved for use in weight reduction turned out to have serious health side effects when combined.

The lessons from this case are twofold. First, combinations will be used. Second, they need to be examined empirically. In the behavioral health area, unlike the Phen-Fen case, toxic combinations would problem go on indefinitely because our means for detecting problems are so limited. There may not be as many obvious examples of combinations that could be detrimental in behavioral health, but the possibility must be explored.

Practice Guidelines and Effectiveness Research: Finding a Solution to the Scientific Problem

Our current approach to effectiveness is a technique-oriented version. In this approach, the central goal of effectiveness research is the unambiguous statement of the relation between use of a technique or approach and clinical impact in the context of existing healthcare delivery systems. In this kind of effectiveness research, we try to learn whether clinicians can be trained to use a given technique properly, and if so whether it will it will be effective and cost-effective on defined populations in real world settings. This is a straightforward extension of efficacy research that seemingly takes advantage of all that we have learned to do there (e.g., defining technique and populations). The problem is that precious few systems and clinicians will play along. Few systems will demand that clinicians follow a given protocol with certain cases, and certainly not with non-volunteer clinicians. Few system administrators will want to face the political heat that would be needed to implement such a plan. Thus, perversely, the noisy real world context seemingly makes controlled effectiveness research impossible, even though the whole point is to examine work in that context empirically. That is the basis on which some have claimed that correlational research or even simply post-hoc surveys are the only alternative available (Seligman, 1995).

As this issue applies to practice guidelines, if we do not change our models of effectiveness research we will not get the real world data we would like to have as input to guidelines, nor will we have the ability to evaluate these guidelines in effectiveness research. There is another approach to effectiveness research, however (Strosahl, Hayes, Bergan, & Romano, 1998). This approach seems to fit the empirical needs in the area of guidelines rather well. In the "Manipulated Training Method" client outcomes are assessed in a large group of clinicians (say, pre-post measures on all clients starting treatment for a month or two by every clinician in the group), and then these clinicians are randomly assigned to training and no training conditions. If there is a reason to do so, there can also be comparison training or control training conditions, much as in efficacy research. Client referral continues as before (a key point), and outcomes are then assessed in the clients of subgroups of clinicians post-training, including clinical impact and system impact (e.g., cost-effectiveness). This method can be focused on specific populations (e.g., conduct it with clinicians in an anxiety disorders clinic, or prescreen clients and focus only of those with a given problem), but it can also be conducted with the kinds of general clinical populations many clinicians deal with daily. Ideally (for scientific reasons), some measures should be taken of what the clinicians actually do in treatment, but in principle even this is not necessary. After all, if clients get better faster after training we know that *something* important changed in the clinician's behavior as a result of training. In practical terms, that is all we may absolutely need to know. Adherence and competence do apply to the *trainers* behaviors, however.

In our article (Strosahl et al., 1998), which was recently published in *Behavior Therapy*, we gave an actual example of this effectiveness research method. It did not have all of the bells and whistles of the method in the abstract, but it had most of them and the results were interesting. Eighteen clinicians participated—mostly master's level with an average of 5.2 years experience—from the Group Health Cooperative of Puget Sound (a large regional HMO). Eight were trained in ACT, while 10 were not. All of their new clients were assessed for a month, pre-treatment and five months later (N=59). Training consisted of a 2-day workshop, a 3-day intensive clinical training, distribution of a detailed treatment manual, and 12 monthly 3-hour group supervision sessions. We told clinicians to use ACT methods only when they seemed appropriate (specific guidance was given about the things that might indicate usefulness of an ACT approach) and to feel free to combine ACT techniques with other methods. After one year of training, their new clients were once again assessed for a month, pre-treatment and five months later (N=67).

After training, ACT trained therapists were far more likely to be finished with therapy at five months in the eyes of the client, and were more likely to agree with the client's assessment in that regard. Medication referrals were reduced significantly, and client ratings of the degree to which they could cope with the problem that brought them in were significantly enhanced. In short, clients got better faster, cheaper, and better following training.

This approach is relevant in two ways. First, it shows something of what should be done in the evaluation of practice guidelines. It is not enough to write them. They also have to be implemented, and done so in a way that will make a difference. Ultimately, that difference must reside in clinical outcome or the whole purpose of guidelines is unmet. The methods currently available for dissemination research, however, are a poor fit to the needs of the heath care delivery system. Manipulated training studies provide a much better fit and one that could enhance the evaluation of clinical practice guidelines.

Second, if similar results were available in several areas, guideline development itself would be greatly enhanced, since the task then would be to describe the methods that had been shown to improve clinical outcomes when implemented in specified training programs. Clinical improvement from being guided by the literature would not merely be hoped for, but instead would be expected, since dissemination impact would already be known.

PRACTICE GUIDELINES DEVELOPMENT

The Bottom Up Approach: Simplify, Simplify, Simplify

When guidelines are thought of in industrial development terms, the perfection of initial guidelines is far less important than their penetration. Imagine that a fairly weak set of guidelines is developed, widely used, and is evaluated. The places where the guidelines are helpful or useless would quickly be known. This very information could feed into guideline improvement when the guidelines themselves were revised. Over time the guidelines should do a better job and the quality of the system itself will improve as a result. Now compare this situation to one in which a near perfect set of guidelines is developed and not widely used. The adequacy of the guidelines will not be known, and problems in implementation will have no impact on future draft of the guidelines. Even if future scientific progress leads to guideline modification, no positive long term effects can occur until the guidelines penetrate. Thus, while guideline quality is important, guideline penetration is much more so. Guidelines are themselves a quality improvement process that will be spread out over decades.

This has comforting implications. Empirical clinicians do not need to wait forever to get perfect data (especially in the area of clinical effectiveness or utility) since guidelines themselves will help produce the needed data. It also means that two things are paramount: a) the acceptability of guidelines to clinicians, systems, and consumers, and b) the ability to recycle and improve guidelines over time.

We know only a little about how to improve acceptability, but it seems logical that the guidelines have to be simple, short, clinician friendly, and sensitive to client preferences and needs. In order to step around guild infighting they should be multi-disciplinary, but yet not interfere with more

focused discipline-oriented guidelines that specific disciplines are developing. That suggests that guidelines should focus on core clinical processes that
everyone agrees upon. They have to be practical for systems to use, concrete,
and be readily available. To avoid political in-fighting they should be based
on a broad consensus about the best available evidence.

To a degree, acceptability and quality may conflict in practice guidelines.
Guidelines of the sort just described focus on the floor, not the ceiling, and for
that reason the improvements in outcome they are likely to produce will be
incremental. Conversely, detailed guidelines that suggest a change in practice
for most clinicians may have a greater likelihood of changing clinical outcomes (if they are high quality) but a much lower change of being accepted.
Managed care systems with a great deal of control over clinician behavior
might think of "top down" guidelines for that reason, but in the vast majority
of clinical settings a more "bottom up" approach seems indicated.

Frequent recycling carries other implications: guidelines have to be fast
and inexpensive. A guideline that cannot be developed in six month and that
costs much more than $100,000 is one you cannot revise every two years.
Anything revised less frequently is old news. This precludes the gigantic
tomes some guidelines efforts have produced. Recycling also suggests the
value of a bottom up approach. Top down guidelines will almost certainly cost
more to develop, maintain, and implement, than bottom up guidelines because the former is more detailed and intrusive. Bottom up guidelines aims for
evolutionary not revolutionary change. Their simplicity makes them less
expensive to develop and easier to implement.

Producing Clinical Guidelines

Who will produce evidence-based clinical practice guidelines and how?
The most logical immediate answer is the government, but history has shown
that government cannot do it. A federal agency designed to do just that (the
Agency for Health Care policy Research) self-destructed in the attempt when
back surgeons disagreed vehemently with a back pain guideline issued by
AHCPR and took their objections to Congress. This was an object lesson for
federal bureaucrats, and there is little chance that other federal agencies will
now travel that same path.

Specific managed care companies have a hard time getting enough access
to enough expertise, getting buy-in by diverse constituencies and stakeholders, and producing guidelines that are not biased by the economic motives of
the company. Specific disciplines and guilds tend to produce guidelines that
are just too narrow to be adopted by other disciplines.

Research scientists have a hard time being practical and succinct, and their literature review processes tend to be too broad and unfocused to be efficient. Consumer and advocacy groups tend to overemphasis the views of members and leaders, even if the literature does not agree with these biases. Furthermore almost every development process currently available is either too inefficient, too narrow, too expensive, too top heavy, too closed, or too lengthy. All of these problems increase as the number of guidelines increases. We simply do not yet know how to develop guidelines in a way that will work at full build out.

THE PRACTICE GUIDELINE COALITION EXPERIENCE

The Practice Guidelines Coalition (PGC) experience provides a possible approach to guideline development that might help move the field in a positive direction. PGC is a developing organization launched by two national meetings called the *National Planning Summit on Scientifically-Based Behavioral Health Practice Guidelines.* The meetings, held in Orlando in November 1996 and Minneapolis in June 1997, gathered together over fifty representatives from managed care associations, other behavioral health care provider groups, behavioral science associations, professional groups, consumer groups, and the government. A list of organizations that participated in the National Planning Summits is shown in Table 1.

The representatives met to consider how best to work together to promote better behavioral health care delivery through evidence-based practice guidelines. The meetings were sponsored by the Association for Advancement of Behavior Therapy (AABT) and the American Association of Applied and Preventive Psychology (AAAPP), and were funded by grants from the Office of Behavioral and Social Sciences Research at the National Institutes of Health and by the Substance Abuse and Mental Health Services Administration. The meetings identified the central mission of a possible coalition, laid out the core interests of the various constituencies, and resulted in a unanimous decision to launch a development process that could lead to a membership based Practice Guidelines Coalition.

Initially, attendees at the November meeting had a hard time being comfortable with each other. The atmosphere was respectful, but the tensions were palpable. One professionally oriented representative, for example, introduced herself by saying that she welcomed the opportunity to work together to fight managed care. The managed care representatives wondered aloud if the scientists were ivory tower eggheads and the professionals were

Academy of Psychological Clinical Science
Agency for Health Care Policy Research
American College of Mental Health Administration
American Academy for Child and Adolescent Psychiatry
American Association for Marriage and Family Therapy
American Association of Applied and Preventive Psychology
American Managed Behavioral Health Association
American Psychiatric Association
American Psychological Association
American Psychological Society
American Society of Addiction Medicine
Association for Advancement of Behavior Therapy
Association for Ambulatory Behavioral Health
Association for Behavior Analysis
Association of Child and Adolescent Psychiatric Nurses
Center for Mental Health Services
CHAMPUS
Consortium for Clinical Excellence
Council of Behavioral Group Practices
Department of Defense
National Council on Quality Assurance
Division 12 (Clinical) of the American Psychological Association
Division 17 (Counseling) of the American Psychological Association
Division 33 (MRDD) of the American Psychological Association
Expert Consensus Consortium
Gerontological Society of America
Institute for Behavioral Health Care
International Society of Psychiatric Consulting Liaison Nurses
Mental Health Programs
NAMI
National Association of Psychiatric Health Care Systems
National Association of Social Workers
National Council of Community Behavioral Health Care
National Institute on Drug Abuse
OBSSR Committee on Use of Behavioral Procedures
Office of Behavioral and Social Sciences Research, National Institutes of Health
Park Nicollet Guideline Project
Society for a Science of Clinical Psychology
Society for Behavioral Medicine
Society for Education and Research in Psychiatric Nursing
Society for Social Work and Research
Substance Abuse and Mental Health Services Administration
The Health Maintenance Organization Group
Veteran's Administration

Table 1

Groups with Representatives Participating in the National Planning
Summit Process (Either Meeting)

mere protectors of the guild. The hard core scientists sat back, arms folded, taking a skeptical eye on every statement.

But then something quite remarkable began to happen. First, the group began to listen. David Barlow gave a brilliant talk on the history of efforts to link science to practice. Clarissa C. Marques, then of the American Managed Behavioral Health Association (AMBHA), captured the attention of the group as she talked about how the industry was trying to link quality care to an empirical base.

Next, then the group began to talk to each other. A series of break out discussions put all the barriers the group would have to face on the table, along with the possible benefits of cooperation. The participants began to take each other more seriously. They began to let go of the cardboard cutout views they had of each other.

The group began to identify what they needed, and then what they needed of each other, and in so doing, they began to identify possible benefits of cooperation. For example, the flip chart that the group generated in the first meeting about the kinds of guidelines needed from an interdisciplinary group such as the one that was assembled said the following (edited only for reader understanding):

> Target high need areas.
> We need ultra-brief guidelines in some settings.
> Should identify consensus.
> Should be based on overlap between existing guidelines.
> Should include guidelines in clincal problem areas (e.g., suicide; compliance), not just syndromes.
> Some guidelines may need to be expansive, others not.
> Multidisciplinary guidelines should not interfere with disciplinary guidelines.
> Need both minatory and hortatory guidelines.
> Guidelines should be reverse engineered from outcomes.
> Should have goal of increase functionality and quality of life, bot just symptom reduction.
> Should mesh with best available evidence.
> Should be user friendly.
> Must have significant input from practice base (field developed and tested).
> Should have criteria for entry and exit.
> Should have adherence tools.
> Should have indications for pharmacology.
> Should be revised continuously.

Connected to entire system (primary care, etc.).

Should address treatment failure options.

Should foster empowerment and self-help.

Should include psychoeducational and self-management.

Should include indicators for consultation.

Should be oriented toward community.

Should have validation program linked to it.

Should start with high priorities, such as (in adults) anxiety, depression, substance abuse; (in children) ADHD; (in adolescents) Substance abuse or eating disorders.

Should include prevention, v-codes, growth issues.

Dependent variables (processes, outcomes and measurements of them) should be attached to guidelines.

Ethically, clinicians should inform patients of guidelines-driven treatment plans and of the evidence for it.

Guidelines that actually meet all of these requirements simply do not exist, and the group realized this immediately as the list was generated. As the groups began to discuss their hopes and fears, representative from opposing groups began to see the issue is a new way. It is useful to examine the hopes and fears of each group. What follows is that list, brainstormed at the first meeting, and formally presented at the second, broken down by stakeholder. Behavioral health systems and managers emphasized the following points:

Clinical practice guidelines developed via cooperation between the industry and key scientific, professional, and consumer associations is a very attractive product

The development of clinical practice guidelines should involve the active participation of a variety of industry constituencies (AMBHA, THMOG, IBH, CentraLink, Council of Group Practices, Association of State Directors of Mental Health, Veteran's Administration, etc.).

When target areas are identified, clinical practice guidelines have to be developed quickly (within 3-6 months) and renewed regularly to keep pace with developments in the industry.

Practically useful clinical practice guidelines have to be simple and focus on the "critical few" core clinical processes.

Clinical practice guidelines need to focus on processes and procedures, not on the discipline of the provider.

Clinical practice guidelines must avoid any appearance of proprietary, discipline, profession, guild or self-serving interests.

Clinical practice guidelines should focus on the evidence and avoid any attempt to dictate health care policy per se at the industry level.

Professional associations and guild had a quite different list:

Clinical practice guidelines must be not be academic tomes, but products designed to help practitioners make decisions in the context of daily clinical practice.

Clinical practice guidelines must be user friendly in how they present core clinical concepts.

Clinical practice guidelines cannot become a "straight jacket" that supplants individual clinical decision making and the development of new and creative clinical approaches.

Clinical practice guidelines are the most applicable when they focus on the broad context of clinical assessment and decision making and leave the details of clinical implementation up to the practitioner.

Clinical practice guidelines cannot appear to reflect specific guild or association interests.

Clinical practice guidelines cannot favor any particular type of treatment (i.e., drugs versus psychotherapy, long term versus short term psychotherapy), unless there is a clear and agreed upon evidence basis for such a recommendation.

Scientific associations had a different set of concerns:

Scientifically based clinical practice guidelines must be grounded in a systematic and careful method of assessing and interpreting the existing research base.

Clinical practice guidelines should focus on effective assessment, treatment, and prevention processes and procedures, not on disciplinary interests.

Clinical practice guidelines should incorporate recommendations about how to assess clinical functional outcomes and over what time frames.

Clinical practice guidelines must be based in a coherent mechanism for describing the "strength" of a clinical practice recommendation, based upon the available evidence.

Clinical practice guidelines can include expert opinion, when the clinical topic is critical and the evidence is either scant or inconclusive, but these recommendations must be clearly distinguished from those based on scientific evidence and steps should be taken to subject such recommendations to empirical test as soon as possible.

Clinical practice guidelines should have a self correcting function that is tied to research in the field.

Clinical practice guidelines should be updated periodically based upon changes in the evidence base or in expert opinion.

Consumer and advocacy groups had other concerns:

Clinical practice guidelines need to be built to attend to the best interests of the client and his or her immediate family members.

Consumers of behavioral health services must be a significant source of information about preferred outcomes of those services.

Clinical practice guidelines should not make treatment recommendations that place undue hardship on significant others as a part of treatment.

Clinical practice guidelines should not make recommendations that in effect deny a client access to care, even if there is no effective treatment available.

Clinical practice guidelines should state clear parameters for appropriate assessment of clinical and functional outcomes and recommend procedures for assessing those outcomes.

Federal and foundation entities added a few additional points:

Clinical practice guidelines must be built through a consensus process that includes all of the major constituencies in the behavioral health industry.

Clinical practice guidelines must be developed in a cost efficient way that includes the option of incorporating existing practice guidelines.

Clinical practice guidelines must help with the process of dissemination of science regarding effective behavioral health procedures.

Clinical practice guidelines should exist in some type of national center or clearinghouse, whose main goal is to coordinate development, refinement and dissemination.

Clinical practice guidelines should be developed by the behavioral health constituencies, not by governmental agencies per se.

What can be seen from these lists is that the concerns of stakeholders are legitimate and understandable. Furthermore, these imply enormous linkage between stakeholders. For example, the behavioral healthcare managers want cooperative, evidence-based guidelines, but they also want them to be developed in a cycle that takes no more than six months. The latter figure stunned the scientists in the room, who wanted evidence-based guidelines as well, but were not sure if such a short development cycle was possible. Between each pair of stakeholders there was a bi-directional set of interests, worries, needs, and a prod to change. To consider another example, the consumers wanted evidence-based care where possible, but wanted more attention to functionality, which was a bit of a challenge to the more purely syndromal thinking of many research scientists, practitioners, or funders.

By the end of the meetings, there was genuine enthusiasm for the idea that a bridge needed to be built between the industry, science, and the professions, with the active involvement of consumers, government, and other interested stakeholders. The PGC was born.

The central mission of the Practice Guidelines Coalition is the development of a multi-disciplinary, multi-organizational partnership that is dedicated to better behavioral health care through the dissemination and implementation of non-proprietary clinical practice guidelines for behavioral health providers that are based on a broad consensus about the best available evidence. Participants generally agreed that credible non-proprietary practice guidelines are best fostered through a broad, consensus building process based on a working partnership among all the key constituencies in behavioral health, avoiding any hint of disciplinary, professional, corporate, or guild bias. It was broadly agreed among the participants that the Practice Guidelines Coalition will be open to all major organizations relevant to behavioral health care who wish to foster the goals of the Coalition. The Coalition intends to develop clinical practice guidelines that are brief, evidence-based, readily understandable by practitioners, focused on core clinical processes and measurable outcomes, nationally disseminated, multi-disciplinary, and available in the public domain. The coalition is attempting to construct processes of review and development that are empirically sound, efficient, open, and participatory.

These PGC processes of guideline development are worth describing. The PGC guideline panel itself consists of eight members:

First, there are two respected scientists who are not strongly identified with a treatment or assessment model in the area of the guideline. They function more like "jurors" as in the NIH consensus conference model. Their role is to sort through the evidentiary summaries, articles and narrative summaries and organize their response to the core clinical and assessment questions, along with a statement of scientific confidence in each recommendation. Normally, one of these scientists will be non medically trained; the other will be medically trained. These scientists will expected to seek counsel from their colleagues in the event critical data is missing from the evidence reviews or when the evidence is hard to sort out and more expertise may be required.

Second, there are two behavioral health practitioners from different disciplines, whose role is to review and incorporate statements of expert opinion/best practice innovation into the guideline, to provide the panel with perspective about the likely practice impacts of scientific recommendations, to review their ease of application during a normal behavioral health service, and to review the user friendly attributes of the guideline format. These representatives do not represent an association point of view, but rather the practitioner point of view. Up to this time, each PGC panel has had one doctoral and one master's level practitioner.

Third, there are two behavioral health industry representatives, one public sector and one private sector, whose role is to address the implementation aspects of the guideline as it is being developed. This may involve questions around comparative costs of two treatments with equal efficacy, feedback when recommendations are becoming too esoteric or specialized to be feasible in a typical delivery system, etc. In their industry representation role, these individuals should interact with industry members in the Coalition to assure that all viewpoints are being considered.

Finally, there are two consumer advocates, one being a direct recipient of care and one representing the larger advocacy community such as significant others impacted by a behavioral health condition and the demands of treatment. These consumer advocates keep the panel focused on consumer and family needs and preferences, they help construct meaningful consumer information that would be attached to the guideline, and they look at feasibility in terms of personal cost, retention in treatment, burden of care placed on the family and so forth..

There are five possible sources of data input into the scientific review process:

> 1. The most published and most cited authors in the area over the last ten years (out of both PsychLit/MedLine) are asked to nominate what they consider to be the three most important articles in the area
> 2. The top 25 highest citation impact articles over the last ten years in this area from the Science Citation Index and the Social Science Citation Index.
> 3. Limited numbers of raw articles submitted from participant organizations as representing important findings (limit of five)
> 4. Evidence tables, conclusions, and supporting articles from participant organizations. Existing guidelines may be part of this form of evidentiary material, provided that they are based on identifiable evidence tables and scientific review.
> 5. Articles suggested by the panels themselves.

Several articles are weeded out that come in through this process, namely, purely theoretical articles that do not review existing literature, animal studies without clear links to human concerns, and articles not focused primarily on the content area. If need be, the scientific subcommittee further weeds out articles on the basis of relevance or quality to limit the input to no more than approximately 50 articles. The goal of this process is to filter out relatively unimportant articles from ever being considered rather than doing a more comprehensive literature search and then using quality ratings as the filter.

These articles are examined by a scientific sub-committee, that is advisory to the scientists on the main panel. The scientific subcommittee is composed of 4-5 experts in the particular area Each must have excellent credentials, and must represent a range of constituencies and competencies. The scientific subcommittee essentially combines the scientific input into evidence tables and conclusions, for use by the main panel.

Each member of the subcommittee reviews 10-20 articles, and completes an evidence evaluation form for each. The key section of the evidence evaluation form is the "Conclusions and impact" section. In this section the subcommittee scientists are asked to examine the list of questions being considered by the guideline panel, and to list conclusions that they draw from the article that speak to the guidelines questions. The subcommittee members try to state conclusions in terms of core clinical procedures and processes, where possible, and avoid phrasing statements in terms of discipline or orientation.

The guidelines questions addressed include the following:

What is the best established and most appropriate method of assessment for this condition? Are there assessment methods that should not be used?

Are there any age, sex, racial, ethnic, religious, economic, disability, social/familial or work setting factors that might mitigate how this problem presents or might influence treatment selection, likelihood of response or retention in treatment? Are there functional outcomes in any of these areas that should be measured?

What treatments have been shown to be effective with this problem? What core interventions in this treatment are most associated with positive clinical response? Is there evidence regarding the acceptability of recommended treatments with providers? What is the probability of positive treatment response based upon a review of "completers" data? Are there treatments with more variable or poorer outcomes that should not be employed? If there is more than one effective treatment, is there a significant cost differential between the two? Is this cost differential mitigated by other factors, for example, reduced relapse rates?

What are the consumer acceptance data like with the recommended treatment (s)? Are there differential drop out rates that might effect the population effectiveness of the treatments? What information should consumers receive regarding the risks and benefits of this treatment? Are there potential side effects that might affect treatment acceptability?

What is the estimated time frame for positive clinical response? What assessment procedure is recommended for measuring clinical response and when should it be used? What should be done if a patient is not responding as expected to the treatment? When should an alternative treatment be added or substituted for the existing treatment?

What are the most commonly occurring co-morbid conditions? How do they influence treatment selection and prognosis? Are there functionally distinct subgroups within this problem area, either diagnostically or in terms of underlying etiological or maintaining processes? Are there differential treatment considerations related to subgroups?

Is this a recurring problem that is subject to relapse? What is the relapse rate in patients who have responded to the preferred treatment(s)? What methods should be employed to prevent relapse?

Is there evidence that primary prevention or health promotion interventions can forestall the appearance and/or progression of this condition? If so, what are the core components of such effective interventions?

The main panel then works through this same list of questions, this time benefiting from the give and take from the different stakeholders they represent, and from the different data they bring to the table. The goal is to whittle down the input to the core clinical issues involved. The resulting product (and an associated consumer guideline) is shared among a broad range of constituent groups for input.

AN EXAMPLE OF THE RESULTS OF THE PGC PROCESS

Two demonstration guidelines projects, in panic disorder and the management of chronic back pain, have been conducted by PGC. The panic process is instructive and will be described here.

From the nominations submitted by participating organizations, the eight-member main panel was formed. The panel was composed of:
Two scientists, for whom panic disorder was not their main area of research: G. Terrence Wilson, PhD, a psychologist from Rutgers University and Gail Stuart, RN, PhD, from the Medical University of South Carolina;

Two industry representatives: Gary Mihalik, MD, MBA from the private sector (Greenspring of Illinois) and Wendy Wade, PhD from the public sector (South Central Community Mental Health Center in Bloomington, Indiana);

Two consumers: Cyma Siegel, RN, a consumer herself and founder, editor, and publisher of the National Panic/Anxiety Disorder Newsletter , and Jerilyn Ross, MSW, President of the Anxiety Disorders Association of America; and

Two clinicians: Cheryl Al-Mateen, A Virginia psychiatrist, and Deborah Jackson, MA, a counselor in the Washington DC area.

The next step involved in the development of the panic disorder guideline was the selection of the scientific subcommittee. Again relying on the recommendations of participating organizations and associations, a six-member scientific subcommittee was formed. This subcommittee consisted of the two scientists nominated to the main panic disorder panel, as well as Michele T. Laraia, PhD, RN, CS, Medical University of South Carolina, W. Stewart Agras, M.D., Department of Psychiatry, Stanford University, William Sanderson, Ph.D., Albert Einstein College of Medicine, and Kathy Shear, M.D., Department of Psychiatry, University of Pittsburg. The articles gathered in the data collection process were then distributed to these subcommittee members, such that each articles was independently reviewed by at least two of the panel members. The committee members then met for a one-day meeting in New York City, where they created a cohesive document of the state of the science, that was then passed on the main panel. The main panel met a short while later, and in just under two days, came to consensus.

By focusing only on the relatively black and white areas that are clearly known and are agreed to through a multi-discipinary process emphasizing consensus and clear evidence, a remarkably brief and clinician-friendly guideline resulted. The draft guideline is shown in Table 2. In small type format the primary document can fit on both sides of a legal sized sheet of paper. The guideline lays out a working definition of panic disorder, issues relating to the assessment of panic disorder, as well as recommendations for psychosocial and pharmacological treatment, and the selection between, and combination of, the two types of treatment. Additionally, the guideline addresses issues of comorbidity, prevention, typical length of treatment. To be of use when there is not enough time even to read four bulleted pages, individual emboldened words in the guideline provide a quick overview. This overview version can be read in about a minute.

The guideline also has two appendices: a medication appendix delineating various pharmacotherapy types and dosages, and an appendix expanding on the psychosocial components laid out in the guideline. A consumer guideline was also developed, containing similar information as the main

WHAT IS PANIC DISORDER?

Recurrent, unexpected panic attacks—a discrete period of intense fear or discomfort, in which **four** (or more) of the following **symptoms develop abruptly and peak within 10 minutes**:

>Palpitations, pounding heart, or accelerated heart rate
>Sweating
>Trembling or shaking
>Sensations of shortness of breath or smothering
>Feeling of choking
>Chest pain or discomfort
>Nausea or abdominal distress
>Feeling dizzy, unsteady, light-headed, or faint
>Derealization (feelings of unreality) or depersonalization (being detached from oneself)
>Fear of losing control or going crazy
>Fear of dying
>Paresthesias (numbness or tingling sensations)
>Chills or hot flushes

1 month or more of **persistent concern** about having another attack **or**

>**Worry about** the implications or **consequences** of panic (e.g., fear of loss or control, going crazy, or social humiliation).

or

>A significant behavioral change related to the attacks (e.g., **agoraphobic avoidance** of panic producing situations).

What Should be Ruled Out?

>Direct physiological effects of a substance (e.g., Caffeine Intoxication).
>General medical conditions that can cause panic-like symptoms.
>Not better accounted for by another mental disorder (e.g., PTSD).

Figure 1

Draft PGC Panic Disorder Guideline.

Basic Facts About Panic Disorder:
> Tends to be **chronic**
> **Co-Morbidity is common**. Usually at least one other
> > disorder is present, including:
> > > Depression
> > > Substance abuse
> > > Other anxiety disorders
> > > Personality disorders

Associated with notable suffering, disability, and **functional impairment** (e.g., social withdrawal, employment or school difficulties).

Lifetime prevalence rates (With or Without Agoraphobia) between 1.5% and 3.5%. One-year prevalence rates between 1% and 2%.

> **Age:**
> > Occurs across the age range. **Children may be as responsive** to treatment as adults.
> > In the **elderly panic can be complicated** by the normal aging process, medical co-morbidities, and concomitant pharmacological therapies, and thus may be misdiagnosed or left untreated.

> **Gender:**
> > More **prevalent in women**, particularly panic with extensive agoraphobia.
> > Symptom severity worsens during the **menstrual cycle** and may improve during pregnancy in some women.

> **Racial differences:**
> > Seems associated with hypertension and with sleep paralysis in African Americans.

> **Belief systems:**
> > Incidence and prevalence seems **consistent across ethnic/ racial** groups.
> > Presentation and interpretation of symptoms is affected by ethnic, racial, religious, and family belief systems.

What Goes Into Effective Clinical Assessment?

> Consider using a **screening questionnaire** instrument for detection.

Figure 1 (continued)
> Draft PGC Panic Disorder Guideline.

Conduct a **thorough clinical interview** assessing history
and current symptoms—consider using a structured
clinical interview to guide you.

Assess initially and on an on-going basis for:

Number and severity of panic attacks
Severity of anticipatory anxiety
Severity of agoraphobic symptoms
Suicidal ideation and attempts
Panic attacks
Missed work/school
Underachievement at work or school
Self-care
Routine social behavior
Quality of life

Assess for co-morbid conditions initially and on an on-going basis
(particularly depression, substance abuse, agoraphobia, other anxiety disorders, and caffeine use). To **rule out medical conditions** that mimic panic,
consider medical history with appropriate laboratory tests.

What Assessments Are Not Helpful?

The **MMPI, projective tests, and neuropsychological
testing** have not been shown to be particularly useful
in diagnosing panic disorder or measuring response
to treatment.
There is **no medical test** that diagnoses panic disorder.

What Treatments Are Helpful?

Effective Psychosocial Treatment
The strongest evidence supports the effectiveness of a psychosocial
interventions that include the following (see Appendix I):

Psychoeducation about the symptoms, the disorder, and
the specific role of fear of bodily sensations.
Exposure to the interoceptive reactions that comprise
and cue panic attacks.

Figure 1 (continued)

Draft PGC Panic Disorder Guideline.

Cognitive restructuring to change maladaptive thought processes.

Training in proper breathing, to avoid hyperventilation, breath holding, shallow breathing, and other common breath problems occasioned by anxiety

In vivo **exposure to phobic situations.**

Effective Pharmacological Treatment

The strongest evidence supports the effectiveness of **SSRIs, TCAs, MAOIs, and high potency benzodiazepines** (see Appendix II). There is comparable efficacy among these medications. The effectiveness of maintenance medication to prevent relapse has not been firmly established.

How Do Effective Treatments Compare?

The clear majority of patients show a **positive response to either** psychosocial or pharmacological treatment.

Both are **equally effective in acute phase** (12 weeks) treatment.

Effective **psychosocial treatment has greater durability** than pharmacotherapy.

In studies comparing effective psychosocial treatment to a single form of effective pharmacological treatment (imipramine), **dropout rates for pharmacotherapy are higher.**

Are Combining These Two Forms of Treatment Best?

The data show that **combining benzodiazepines** with effective psychosocial treatment **reduces treatment efficacy** when compared to psychosocial treatment alone.

There aren't sufficient data to evaluate the combination of psychosocial treatment with SSRIs, TCAs , and MAOIs.

Effective psychosocial treatment has been shown to reduce **relapse following discontinuation of benzodiazepines.**

Figure 1 (continued)

Draft PGC Panic Disorder Guideline.

Overall Clinical Management is Important

An essential component for either general form of effective treatment is **psychoeducation** for the patient and, when appropriate significant others, covering:

> An explanation of the **basis for panic** and anxiety.
> The **nature and course** of panic disorder.
> Rationale for the treatment, likelihood of a positive response, and expected time frame for response.
> **Likelihood of** experiencing some **residual anxiety** in the course of treatment.

If there is an **inadequate response** after an adequate trial of a first line treatment, **switch** to another evidence-based treatment. At this time it may be important to **obtain a consultation** and/or refer the patient to a specialist or subspecialist.

If panic disorder is more severe than other co-occurring conditions (as determined by impairment or interference with daily living, and distress from symptoms), **panic should be the initial focus** of treatment, regardless of chronological onset.

The presence of severe agoraphobia and certain personality disorders is a negative prognostic indicator, while co-morbid depression has no consistent effect.

Issues in Managing Psychosocial Treatment

A **positive response** typically occurs within **6 to 8 weeks**.

A **typical course** of treatment in research protocols is about **12 sessions**. However, in clinical practice, more or less time may be required.

> Some patients require only a few sessions to understand that panic is not dangerous, and improvement continues naturally from there.
> Others may require substantially longer than 12 sessions, especially if agoraphobia is severe.

Issues in Managing Pharmacological Treatment

> A **positive response** typically occurs within **6 weeks** (response to benzodiazepines occurs considerably

---

Figure 1 (continued)

Draft PGC Panic Disorder Guideline.

faster) but additional time may be required to stabilize the response

Because there is **comparable efficacy,** issues related to safety, tolerability, price, simplicity, and ease of discontinuation should guide **clinician choice** among effective medications

Medications, especially benzodiazepines, should be **discontinued gradually,** as it may be difficult and may provoke relapse or even rebound panic

If a patient has an inadequate response or is unable to tolerate the side effects of the medication, the potential difficulty in discontinuing the medication should be carefully considered

Switching medications, using augmentation therapy, or treating medication side effects **may be effective**

When used alone, **SSRIs, TCAs, and MAOIs should be continued for at least 6 months** following symptom remission, and longer if full remission does not occur.

Some clinicians advocate stopping medication only when the patient is in a stable life situation.

Longer use of medication may reduce the risk of relapse following discontinuation.

For patients with several episodes of panic, each responsive to medication, chronic medication use may be indicated.

Panic disorder patients may require **lower beginning dose and slower titration of SSRIs, TCAs, and MAOIs** compared to other patients receiving those medications.

How Do I Select Among Treatments?

We cannot predict which individual will respond best to which treatment. The following factors should be considered:

Suicide risk
Availability of provider expertise
Previous response
Concomitant medical conditions

Figure 1 (continued)

Draft PGC Panic Disorder Guideline.

and pharmacological treatments
Psychiatric co-morbidities,
    including substance use disorders
Patient preference
Chronic psychosocial problems
Risk/benefit ratio
Cost
Differential compliance to treatment modalities
Potential for pregnancy
Level of support from significant others

What About Prevention?

Early identification and treatment of the disorder is important in secondary prevention.

No known data exist on primary prevention of panic disorder.

Figure 1 (continued)

Draft PGC Panic Disorder Guideline.

guideline but with language designed for patients, and with a list of patient resources.

THE ROLE OF GUIDELINES IN ORGANIZED BEHAVIORAL HEALTHCARE

A self-amplifying loop between science and practice has never existed in behavioral health in the way that it has in some other areas of practical work. Behavioral health services are often delivered without significant regard for the nature and quality of the existing evidence. On the reimbursement and delivery systems side, sometimes cost containment has been more important in what services are paid for than clinical quality as defined by evidence of effectiveness and efficiency.

Practice guidelines, in combination with the industrialization of health service delivery across the spectrum of public and private agencies, hold out hope to change that picture. On the one hand, the combination of consolidation, accreditation, legislation, and regulation is increasingly linking the financial success of the health care industry to the production of quality outcomes. On the other, the behavioral sciences and professions seem finally ready to cooperate in non-proprietary efforts to create evidence-based practice guidelines. For the first time the elements for an evidence-based revolution in quality of care is in place.

Integrating science with practice in organized behavioral healthcare delivery has two components: drawing on the existing science to contribute to the effectiveness and efficiency of healthcare delivery, and developing new scientific knowledge in the context of managed care. In both areas, practice guidelines could form the warp and woof of such an integration. The first area is obvious (using practice guidelines as a means of drawing on the existing science) but the second could be even more important. Properly done, practice guidelines could create this exciting loop:

1) Implementation of practice guidelines leads to both clinical success and clinical failure.
2) Clinical work with treatment resistant population leads to
3) Clinical innovation leads to
4) Preliminary intensive testing with individuals leads to
5) Development of formalized treatment protocols leads to
6) Formal testing in defined populations leads to
7) Inclusion of these innovations into practice guidelines leads to
8) Implementation by managed care leads to
9) Training in guidelines with the practitioner base lead to
10) Assessment of penetration of guidelines in delivery systems leads to
11) Assessment of outcomes produced by guidelines leads to
12) Accreditation and quality care standards based on successful training and implementation, which hopefully leads to
13) Better quality healthcare care overall, at lower cost, and thus to economic success of the industry, but also leads to
14) Success with some clients and failure with others, which leads to
15) #2 above

This is a remarkable possibility and one that could fundamentally change behavioral health care in this country. Yet it is easy to overstate the relevance of practice guidelines. At present no one knows how to develop and implement them in a way that will produce changes in clinician behavior and, furthermore, it is not known if they will contribute to clinical outcome.

At present clinical practice guidelines in behavioral healthcare are more a focus of accreditation activity than of clinical excellence. But the possibility is there. Clinical practice guidelines, done well, could be a vital step toward a more empirical approach to behavioral healthcare delivery.

REFERENCES

Cummings, N. A. & Hayes, S. C. (1996). Now we are facing the consequences: A conversation with Nick Cummings. *The Scientist Practitioner, 6*(1), 9-13.

Drum, D. J. (1995). Changes in the mental health service delivery and finance systems and resulting implications for the national register. *Register Report, 20*(3) & *21*(1), 4-10.

Frank, R. G., McGuire, T. G., Notman, E. H., & Woodward, R. M. (1996). Developments in Medicaid managed behavioral health care. In R. W. Manderscheid & M. A. Sonnenschein (Eds.), *Mental health, United States, 1996.* Washington, DC: Substance Abuse and Mental Health Services Administration.

Gannett News Service (1996, November 11). *HMOs remain a mystery, poll says.* Reno Gazette Journal, 7a.

Hayes, S. C., Barlow, D. H., & Nelson-Grey, R. O. (1999). *The Scientist-Practitioner: Research and accountability in the age of managed care* (2nd ed.). New York: Allyn and Bacon.

Manderscheid, R. W. & Henderson, M. J. (1996). The growth and direction of managed care. In R. W. Manderscheid & M. A. Sonnenschein (Eds.), *Mental health, United States, 1996.* Washington, DC: Substance Abuse and Mental Health Services Administration.

Seligman, M. (1995). The effectiveness of psychotherapy: The Consumer Reports Study. *American Psychologist, 50,* 965-974.

Shoor, R. (1993, November). For mental health cost problems, see a specialist. *Business and Health,* 59-62.

Strosahl, K. (1994). Entering the new frontier of managed mental health care: Gold mines and land mines. *Cognitive and Behavioral Practice, 1,* 5-23.

Strosahl, K. D., Hayes, S. C., Bergan, J., & Romano, P. (1998). Assessing the field effectiveness of Acceptance and Commitment Therapy: An example of the manipulated training research method. *Behavior Therapy, 29,* 35-64.

Discussion of Hayes and Gregg:

Comment on Practice Guidelines

Duane L. Varble, Ph.D.
University of Nevada, Reno

Hayes and Gregg outline three major purposes in their chapter. Namely,...
"to convince the readers that practice guidelines are not an arbitrary development in the field"...to convince the readers that practice guidelines, done properly, hold out great hope for consumers, managers, payors and providers alike..."and "finally discuss where practice guidelines fit within an integrated system of evidence based care" (Hayes and Gregg page 1 of chapter 9).

This discussion will examine how well these three purposes are carried out. In addition specific issues of concern to behavioral healthcare providers will be highlighted.

THE NONARBITRARY NATURE OF PRACTICE GUIDELINES

Hayes and Gregg provide excellent examples of how industrialization works in manufacturing systems to produce cheaper costs and better quality. Their arguments that the industrialization of health care and especially behavioral healthcare, by means of managed care, will ultimately result in better quality for consumers is less convincing. Most of the empirical evidence to date indicates managed care has grown because of increased cost cutting measures not increased quality. In fact the perception that decreases in quality are occurring as a result of managed care has many consumers putting pressure on their congressional representatives to pass a patient's bill of rights.

Hayes and Gregg address this problem in their discussion of the industrialization process in terms of stages. Their contention is that managed health care delivery is not at a mature level yet but will reach maturity in the future. The fact that health care delivery is changing is certain but it is not so clear that practice guidelines or even managed care will be major components in the future.

Hayes and Gregg's argument that practice guidelines will help ward off threats to successful industrialization makes sense if their scenario that consensually based guidelines can be developed that will actually guide practices across professional disciplines is achievable. Not only are there substantial problems with developing meaningful diagnostic systems that have treatment implications but the history of mistrust and poor cooperation among the major behavioral healthcare professional disciplines makes such consensus unlikely at the practice level. What seems more probable is a top down approach where the behavioral healthcare turf is carved up by legislation based on the desires of special interest groups and/or a few very large managed care organizations reaching an agreement about who will treat what problems and what the reimbursement rates will be. EAP programs and preauthorization requirements already serve some of these functions and could easily be expanded. No consensus building is required under this scenario and those providers who are in the medical fields with prescription privileges, such as nurse practitioners and physician's assistants as well as physicians will be doing the lions share of treatment. This saves money and has already started to occur in some settings such as Veteran's Administration Medical Center Mental Health Clinics.

In concluding this section, Hayes and Gregg have made convincing arguments that practice guidelines are not an arbitrary development in the field *if* industrialization of behavioral healthcare occurs in the way they envision. Their assumptions that industrialization will occur in the relatively smooth straight forward fashion they would like are not convincing. Unfortunately, there are good reasons to predict that there will be precious little that will be behavioral in behavioral healthcare delivery. This point will be elaborated on in the next section.

If Done Properly, Practice Guidelines Hold Out Great Hope for Consumers, Managers, Payors, and Providers Alike

Hayes and Gregg let their idealism run wild in this regard. There is general agreement that the present behavioral healthcare delivery system is inefficient and only marginally effective. There is confusion among consumers, managers, payors and providers alike. Consumers do not know what benefits are available for what problems and have no rational idea who is best trained to deliver specific treatments. Managers are focused on keeping costs to a minimum by limiting the types and lengths of service. Payors have inadequate systems for handling changing benefits, variable benefits and multiple options for different companies. Providers magically appear and disappear on provider lists as managed care companies buy and sell each other. Almost any change would be an improvement if it produced stability and predictability.

Hayes and Gregg persuasively argue that practice guidelines could help provide needed predictability if they are done properly. The first question is: if done properly by whose definition? The key concern here is whether it is realistic to assume that meaningful practice guidelines that incorporate more than pharmacological treatments can be developed *and* put into practice. Hayes and Gregg describe the enormous difficulties of achieving the necessary cooperation among a diverse group of stakeholders to arrive at some generic guidelines for two sets of symptoms, anxiety and back pain, in their discussion of the Practice Guidelines Coalition process. To achieve consensus these guidelines are so broad that they are minimally helpful to providers in addressing individual cases.

Consumers are not likely to consult behavioral healthcare providers for such symptoms because what they see advertised tells them otherwise. Open any magazine, but especially any magazine targeted to women and you will find advertisements for Prozac, Paxil etc. "Having trouble sleeping? Just don't enjoy your job anymore? Feel tired? This medication may help you get back on track" One of the advertisers for the NBC Today morning news show, the television industry leader, is the company that makes Buspar..."feeling upset lately? maybe a little anxious? Ask your doctor about Buspar, research studies show that it is not addictive or habitforming..." They are not talking about seeing your psychiatrist. "Ask your doctor" means see your primary care physician or his/her nurse practitioner or physician's assistant and they will likely prescribe Buspar if that is what you as the consumer patient requests. If you, as a consumer, requested that you be referred to a psychologist or a social worker the referral might be made but where are the advertisements for systematic desensitization or exposure and response prevention? The pharmacological companies have the money, the public acceptance of the biological model-based on "scientific evidence" and a huge headstart over any kind of behavioral healthcare. Furthermore, it is in the managed care companies cost cutting best interest to utilize pharmacological treatments whenever possible because it is faster and cheaper, at least in the short run.

In conclusion, I agree with Hayes and Gregg's contention that practice guidelines, if done properly, could benefit everyone involved in the provision of behavioral healthcare eventually. However, it seems very unlikely that practice guidelines that have an important role for the behavioral in behavioral healthcare services will be developed and utilized in the foreseeable future.

The Fit of Practice Guidelines Within a System
of Evidence Based Care

Just as in the last section the paramount questions here are what evidence and whose is it? Hayes and Gregg do an excellent job of pointing out the difficulties of obtaining agreement between scientifically oriented researchers who want to limit uncontrolled variables and providers who are faced daily with fuzzy diagnostic categories, overlapping symptoms and multiple influences of cultural and environmental factors. Researchers tend to frame the issues in terms of treatments for disorders while providers typically frame the same issues in terms of treatment of clients or patients. This variant of the debate about nomothetic versus idiographic emphasis has a long history and there are good arguments that the disorder treatment focus and the patient treatment focus are not mutually exclusive philosophically. The implications in practical terms are important, however. Hayes and Gregg present the dilemma well, i.e., in order to obtain the necessary money do the research the experimental model, including strict adherence to treatment manuals, is required but providers who are responding to the life event changes in their clients or patients find the inflexible treatment manuals to be inadequate or inappropriate and do not use them.

Hayes and Gregg provide some interesting strategies for dealing with this dilemma, namely, implement the practice guidelines in specific settings and evaluate client outcomes. Their example of the "manipulated training method"(Strosahl, Hayes, Bergan and Romano, 1998) offered a glimpse of how this could be done. Positive client outcome data from general clinical population studies would be the most convincing to the clinicians who are providing services today. Future generations of providers may be less influenced by theoretical orientation loyalties and more by the practicalities of pocket book issues based on what treatments are reimbursed. This trend is already underway. Evidence of effectiveness would help providers, payers and the managed care companies reach agreement about which practice guidelines to apply. Evidence of effectiveness does not yet seem to be that important to consumers based on their willingness to pay large sums of money for alternative treatments such as herbs, vitamins, extracts etc.. Advertising and testimonials seem to drive these purchases not evidence of effectiveness.

The important point that Hayes and Gregg make, with regard to the evidence of effectiveness issue, is that practice guidelines that achieve sufficient penetration to be evaluated and modified in an ongoing improvement process could have much wider impact on evidenced based behavioral healthcare delivery than the more pure experimental models can ever achieve. I would argue that for such penetration to occur direct marketing including advertising to consumers has to be a part of the package. This means rethinking the ethical guidelines of the professional disciplines involved in behavioral healthcare delivery.

In conclusion, Hayes and Gregg make a good case for the role of practice guidelines in integrated evidence based behavioral healthcare. In fact, adoption of practice guidelines could make the evaluation of client outcomes in general clinical populations possible, which in turn, makes the acceptance of evidence based care by providers more likely.

Specific Issues of Concern to Behavioral Healthcare Providers

Behavioral healthcare providers did not receive much emphasis at this conference. They were not considered to be unimportant but the specific concerns of providers other than shrinking incomes as a result of managed care cost cutting did not get considered adequately in my opinion. Two managed care practices that are considered to be core issues for most of today's behavioral healthcare providers are non-clinicians making the decisions about the type and length of treatments through pre-authorization and re-authorization requirements and perceived interference in the relationship between the patient and the provider. Practice guidelines do not bear directly on these issues as long as they remain as guidelines and not standards of care. The fear of some providers is that practice guidelines will be portrayed as guidelines but acted upon as standards of care. In other words the provider who does not agree to follow the guidelines will be dropped from provider panels by the managed care companies. Most providers who deal with managed care companies on a regular basis have had some firsthand experience of disagreements between the company's case management plan and the clinician's. The pressure to comply with the company's plan is not subtle and if compliance is not perceived to occur the provider may not be dropped from the panel but does not receive any further referrals. The client or patient is often caught in the middle of such conflicts.

In summary, Hayes and Gregg do an excellent presentation on the benefits of developing and adopting practice guidelines for behavioral healthcare. The task is a difficult one. This discussion has attempted to point out some of the more germane issues and pitfalls.

If practice guidelines based on consensus are developed and implemented everyone in behavioral healthcare will be better off. If a top down approach is used pharmacological treatments and not behavioral treatments are likely to be the result. Prescription privileges for psychologists would almost be a certainty.

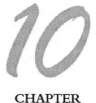

CHAPTER

Financial Risk and Structural Issues

Stephen P. Melek, FSA
Millman & Robertson, Inc.,
Denver, Colorado

Why Integrate?
Integration of Medical and Behavioral Healthcare
Behavioral Healthcare Service System Pricing
Potential for Medical Cost Offsets
Reimbursement and Risk-Sharing Models for Integration
    Example 1
    Example 2
    Example 3
Psychotropic Drug Risk Issues
    Challenges wtih Integration
Summary

Managed care has brought about substantial change in the cost of healthcare, in the ways healthcare providers practice medicine, and how healthcare providers are reimbursed for their services. The growth rate and consolidation in managed behavioral healthcare in the 1990s has been remarkable in the United States. Managed behavioral healthcare organizations are now involved in the management of mental health and substance abuse coverage for over 176 million Americans. In most settings, behavioral healthcare services are provided "off-site" from primary medical care and are considered specialty services. However, there is an increasing trend towards the integration of behavioral healthcare services in primary care settings. This paper will examine some of the supporting reasons behind this integration, and explore some of the financial, risk and structural issues related to such integration under managed care.

WHY INTEGRATE?

Why even consider integrating behavioral healthcare services in primary care settings? After all, aren't most behavioral healthcare services in managed care plans provided through managed behavioral healthcare companies on a "carve-out" basis? By design, doesn't this structure separate the delivery of primary medical and behavioral healthcare services and make such integration extremely challenging, if not practically impossible?

One driving force behind integration initiatives is the return of a challenging issue for many employers and payers - healthcare costs are back on the rise! After several years of low or no increase in the cost of employers' health benefit plans, costs rose by over 7% in 1999, by over 8% in 2000, and are expected to rise by even larger percentages in the year 2001 (average increase expected at 11%). Perhaps most significant is that the cost of managed care plans may grow as fast or even faster than the cost of traditional indemnity medical plans as insurers try to recover from under-priced plans in previous years.

Employers drive what happens in healthcare through their purchasing decisions. They are beginning to demand that healthcare providers focus on maintaining the health of their employees rather than on simply treating diseases. Interest is rising on how much health plans spend on disease treatment vs. early detection of disease and identification of people at risk for early symptoms. To be closely aligned with employers' desires and objectives is not only a business opportunity for healthcare providers, but an opportunity to influence benefit design and purchasing decisions for the good of consumers.

Consider the following statistics relating to medical and behavioral healthcare treatment in primary and specialty care settings:

> 60% to 70% of all medical visits have no medical or biological diagnosis which can be confirmed.
>
> An estimated 25% of patients seeking primary care treatment have anxiety and depressive disorders.
>
> HMO mental health specialty providers (in non-integrated settings) see only 3% to 6% of covered members in any given year, whereas at least 15% of all covered members are known to suffer from some type of psychological disorder during the year.
>
> More than 50% of patients with mental health problems are seen only in the general medical sector.
>
> Approximately 67% of all psychotropic medications are written by nonpsychiatric physicians.
>
> Primary care patients are non-compliant with behavioral healthcare referrals by anywhere from 50% to 90% of the time.
>
> Undiagnosed and untreated anxiety and depressive disorders result in significantly greater (up to 2 times) medical costs and greater social and vocational disability.
>
> Diagnosis and detection of behavioral disorders is missed in 33 to 50% of PCP outpatient cases.

Common symptoms of patients in primary care settings include:

Chest Pain	Fatigue	Dizziness
Headaches	Edema	Back Pain
Dyspnea	Insomnia	Numbness
Abdominal Pain		

The University of Wisconsin School of Medicine reports the following statistics related to the percent of certain symptoms that initially had no medical or biological explanation, but were subsequently found to be related to depressive or anxiety disorders (See Table 1).

These data clearly indicate that somatization (the translation of emotional problems into physical symptoms, or the exacerbation of a disease by emotional factors or stress) is prevalent in primary care settings. Such somatization inevitably results in overutilization of healthcare services, potentially even overloading the system.

	Unexplained	Depression	Anxiety
Headache	48%	53%	44%
Stomach Pain	46%	66%	50%
Dizziness	39%	66%	44%
Chest Pain	36%	66%	66%
Back Pain	30%	53%	40%
Joint Pain	26%	58%	48%
Dyspnea	25%	64%	44%

Chronic Condition	Age-Sex Adjusted Prevalence of Psychological Illness
Arthiritis	25%
Cancer	30%
Diabetes	23%
Heart Disease	35%
Hypertension	22%
Chronic Lung Disease	31%
Neurological Disorder	38%
Well (Baseline)	**18%**

Table 1

Findings from the University of Wisconsin School of Medicine.

Table 2

Prevalence of comorbidity in age-sex adjusted studies.

Besides the prevalence of psychological disorders among somatizing patients, there are observed levels of psychological illnesses among patients with chronic physical disease. Epidemiologic and other studies have reported the following age-sex adjusted (normalized) prevalence rates of comorbidity between psychological illness and chronic physical disease (See Table 2).

These data and observations provide supporting evidence that integration of behavioral healthcare services in primary care settings, where structurally possible, may have great potential for reaching and treating more patients with behavioral disorders, providing more appropriate healthcare services for the underlying illness or disorder, increasing awareness of behavioral disorders, increasing both medical and psychological wellness, and reducing medical, vocational and social costs.

What Could the Integration of Medical and Behavioral Healthcare Include?

The integration of behavioral healthcare services in primary medical settings could include or involve a fairly wide range of potential objectives and structures. The following list provides examples of what an organization could include in their integration of behavioral and primary medical care services:

> Mental health professionals are just "one of the docs", as on-site members of the medical care teams within the medical care plan.
> Use of behavioral professionals as on-site consultants to PCPs.

Smooth transition between the medical and behavioral health portions of care.

Coordination of separate but related behavioral health and medical agendas and care (inter-departmental and inter-clinic care planning, case management, and program development).

Behavioral health therapy groups run in primary care settings (e.g. adolescent psychotherapy groups run in pediatric as opposed to mental health settings; newly pregnant, substance abusing women treated and educated in OB clinics).

Creation of innovative care programs to increase patient self-management and awareness (e.g. hypertension management, asthma self-management, "skills not pills" and reconditioning exercise programs).

Multi-departmental treatment of chronic pain or ADHD, allowing providers to see a more global approach to care of patients, decreasing the possibility of certain treatment elements being overlooked.

Case-finding programs - the process by which certain cases or illnesses are sought out, with the idea that early intervention will prevent more costly care down the road (e.g. inpatient medical and surgical patients with evidence of alcohol or drug problems; ER patients seen for symptoms of panic disorder).

Joint staff meetings between medical and behavioral healthcare professionals.

Increased use of technology and online medical information.

Video conferencing teaching sessions related to behavioral healthcare for PCPs.

Integration need not involve the primary behavioral healthcare providers on a full time basis. However, there is a need for flexibility on their part in order to "capture the moment" when a medical PCP needs the behavioral provider. Many of the behavioral providers may spend only part of their day in the primary integrated care offices and the rest in their own personal behavioral healthcare practices. The behavioral healthcare provider would normally have a professional degree, state licensure, and be a member of important provider panels.

Behavioral Healthcare Service System Pricing: Traditional vs. Integration

The pricing of behavioral healthcare services in an integrated setting involves many new considerations beyond those typically found in pricing traditional carve-out services. The traditional way of providing segregated behavioral healthcare services primarily has an illness treatment focus. The development of expected costs related to these services include using historical utilization rates and referral patterns of PCPs and, at times, specialists to behavioral healthcare providers. Expected utilization rates of the various alternative modalities along the continuum of available behavioral healthcare services are also developed (i.e., inpatient acute, residential, day treatment, intensive outpatient, outpatient therapies, medication management, etc.). Demographic adjustments are considered, as well as considerations for the potential impact of Employee Assistance Programs.

Reimbursement rates for facilities are developed for the various inpatient and acute alternative services (per diems, case rates, program rates, or discounts to fee-for-service levels), and professional fee levels are also developed. Professional rates commonly vary by type of behavioral healthcare professional. Occasionally, professionals accept case rates for therapy or specialized treatment programs, but some type of fee-for-service reimbursement structure is the norm.

Risk-sharing arrangements are not common among behavioral healthcare providers, between behavioral healthcare providers and the managed care organization, or between the behavioral providers and the medical providers. The behavioral providers themselves have had little financial incentive (other than being removed from managed care provider panels) to manage utilization, develop wellness and prevention programs, and reduce medical or other costs through their healthcare and other activities. Risk-sharing considerations in traditional pricing are essentially nonexistent.

In an integrated behavioral and primary medical structure, there are many new considerations for the development of expected costs, including:

The existence of primary behavioral healthcare providers
An increased prevention and wellness focus
Treatment pattern and service shifts from historical levels
Potential medical cost offsets
Financial risk-sharing and other revenue sharing arrangements

Primary behavioral healthcare providers could be teamed with medical PCPs and be responsible for a selected predetermined profile of services, which could include diagnosis, brief testing, brief therapies, patient and PCP education, and referrals to other behavioral specialists. Behavioral healthcare PhDs and, in some cases, MSWs could serve in this capacity, with service profiles appropriate for their training and expertise. They would be actively involved with the early identification and treatment of behavioral healthcare disorders in the primary care setting alongside the medical PCPs. They could be considered as "partners" to the primary care providers in the treatment of all patients receiving care.

The integrated system has a greater focus on behavioral wellness and illness prevention. Education programs and materials are more proactively developed to inform covered members on various topics, including stress, depression, anxiety, alcoholism, chronic illness, and workplace and family relationships. Intervention and case-finding programs could be developed in emergency rooms, acute inpatient settings, schools, and OB/Gyn clinics.

Treatment pattern and service delivery shifts from historical levels must be considered in the pricing process. There will likely be changes in the following pricing factors:

> Diagnosis rates of behavioral disorders
> Average lengths-of-stay for inpatient and acute alternative services
> Average lengths-of-treatment for outpatient services
> Rx vs. therapy service shifts
> Case management
> Referral patterns and patient flow among providers
> Overhead costs
> Case-finding results
> Professional provider mix in service delivery
> Education and prevention costs

The contract period is also a very important consideration in pricing. There will likely be start-up costs, which could be considerable in size, resulting from the integration process. The contract period needs to be long enough for the potential savings in medical costs to materialize and offset the start-up costs.

Potential for Medical Cost Offsets

Various studies related to the potential for medical cost offsets of effective behavioral healthcare service delivery and interventions continue to emerge. These studies on the effects of mental health and substance abuse treatment on medical and surgical utilization date back to the 1960s and can readily be found in the behavioral and medical journals and literature.

One particular recent study by Ron Z. Goetzel and colleagues examined how health risks affect medical costs and whether behavioral modification can produce savings. The study found that the two risk measures that had the largest percentage differences in mean annual medical expenditures between high and low risk levels were depression and stress level. Employees determined to be at high risk for depression had mean medical expenditure that were 70% higher than those of the employees that were determined to be at low risk for depression. In 1996 dollars, this translated to an annual difference of about $1,200 per employee after adjustments for group differences. Employees confronting high levels of stress had mean medical expenditures that were 46% higher than those of the employees that had low levels of stress. This translated to an annual difference of more than $700 per employee.

The study also found that multiple risk factors were extremely significant for cost levels. Individuals at high risk for psychosocial problems (high stress and depression) had predicted annual medical expenditures that were 147% higher than individuals without these risk factors.

The data from this study suggest that potential exists for reducing healthcare costs by implementing programs which address these two psychosocial factors which accounted for the greatest difference in healthcare costs between the high and low risk individuals.

Medical cost offsets are emerging and being reported through integrated programs that have been recently developed. The achieved reductions in various medical costs and utilization rates for one particular aggressive program for a large employer are summarized in Table 3.

These offsets or reductions were developed from the differences in actual utilization rates of various medical and surgical

Treatment Category	Reduction
Total ambulatory care visits	17%
Office visits - minor illness	35%
Office visits - acute asthma	25%
Office visits - arthritic patients	49%
Pediatric acute illness visits	40%
Average inpatient surgical length of stay	1.5 days
Cesarean section delivery rates	56%
Epidural Anesthesia	85%

Table 3

Reductions seen in various medical costs and utilization rates.

services for a given group of covered lives after the integration of behavioral healthcare services as compared to rates prior to such integration. These medical/surgical utilization reductions translate to the following per member per month cost reductions for a typical managed care plan under relatively conservative actuarial assumptions (See Table 4).

Service Category	PMPM Cost Savings
Medical Office Visits	$1.10
Emergency Room Visits	$0.60
IP Surgical Days	$1.30
C-Section Deliveries	$0.40
Anesthesia - Labor/Deliveries	$0.05

Table 4

Various programs and their utilization reduction rates.

The total savings for these medical and surgical service reductions amount to $3.45 per member per month. This is larger than the *total* amount of expected behavioral healthcare costs of between $2.00 - $3.00 for the typical managed care carve-out plan.

However, medical cost offsets through increased or integrated behavioral healthcare interventions are by no means guaranteed. The HCFA Hawaii Medicaid Project reported remarkably different impacts of increased mental health treatments on medical care costs. When such increased mental health treatments were unmanaged, nontargeted and unstructured, medical costs increased by 17%. However, when these increased mental health treatments were targeted, focused and brief, and delivered in a managed care setting, the cost of creating the managed behavioral healthcare system was recovered by medical-surgical savings within 18 months, and the significant reduction in medical interjection continued thereafter with no additional behavioral care required to maintain the cost savings.

The keys to obtaining real medical cost offset savings have been proven to include:

> High specificity and focus in psychological interventions
> Proper training of behavioral healthcare professionals
> Organized settings for healthcare delivery
> Collaboration with primary care providers

Reimbursement and Risk-Sharing Models for Integration

These levels of potential medical and surgical cost savings for integrated programs suggest that new models for reimbursement and risk-sharing arrangements will be needed for successful integrated systems of care to better align the incentives between the behavioral and medical healthcare providers.

The reimbursement and risk-sharing arrangements for the behavioral and medical providers under an integrated scenario should be designed to motivate all providers to deliver cost-effective and efficient healthcare. They should also encourage early diagnosis and appropriate treatment of behavioral disorders in the primary care setting, provide for educational and prevention programs related to behavioral and medical wellness, and be fair to all participants. A few examples of potential integrated reimbursement and risk-sharing models for various provider risk arrangements are described below.

Example 1 - Integrating Full-Time Behavioral Healthcare Into a Heavily Capitated PCP Group that Participates in Risk Pools in a Mature Managed Care Marketplace

A medical PCP group receives a capitation for all covered members within their group and participates in risk-sharing of surpluses and deficits of external facility, nonbehavioral physician specialty, and prescription drug pools. There are 20 PCPs in the group. They receive capitation revenues of $5,000,000 per year covering 30,000 commercially-insured and Medicare members based on actuarially calculated rates from health plans. The medical PCPs are all salaried, receive payment adjustments for certain high member risk (via risk adjusters) as well as productivity-related adjustments, and participate in the risk-pool sharing.

Two full-time primary behavioral healthcare providers (PBCPs) join the primary care team, each with their own service profiles for behavioral healthcare services. The integrated group receives $300,000 per year in additional capitation payments from the health plans for these primary behavioral healthcare services for their existing capitated members. The primary behavioral providers are given a salary consistent with their service responsibilities and the new capitation revenues. They also participate in member risk adjustments, productivity adjustments, and risk-pool sharing in the same way as the medical PCPs. They will each have service responsibilities for the covered members of 10 medical PCPs in the group. Referrals to other behavioral providers outside of the primary care group are treated like any other professional specialty cost. Funding for new educational and prevention programs and materials may be taken from the joint revenues received by the integrated group, or may be negotiated with the managed care plan or payer under the premise of future medical and behavioral cost savings.

In this example, both the medical PCPs and the primary behavioral providers participate in all healthcare cost results through the risk pools and through their own capitation structure. Any medical cost offset savings would naturally flow through these pools. Additionally, "saved" medical PCP services would free up the PCPs to potentially take on more covered lives under the per member per month capitation arrangements, which would also increase the capitated revenue for the primary behavioral healthcare services. An actuarial analysis produces the following summarized business model for the integrated group (See Table 5).

The business model that was developed projected that the PCP group would receive nearly $665,000 in the first year and nearly $1.2 million in additional revenues in the second year after the primary behavioral healthcare integration. This amount, arising from additional covered capitated lives and risk-sharing revenues from medical cost offsets paid through the risk pools, would be available to fund the start-up costs of the integration, educational and prevention programs and materials, compensation to the primary behavioral healthcare providers, and additional profits for the entire integrated group.

The integration will likely result in more behavioral services being provided per member in the initial stages due to increased awareness, diagnosis, education, etc. Care should be exercised to properly reimburse the behavioral providers for this productivity, as well as any associated reduction in medical services per member provided by the medical PCPs.

Item Description	Before Integration	Year 1 After Integration	Year 2 After Integration
Number of PCPs	20	20	20
Number of Full Time PBCPs	0	2	2
Capitated Lives	30,000	31,500	33,000
PCP Capitated Revenue	$5,000,000	$5,250,000	$5,500,000
PBCP Capitated Revenue	$0	$315,000	$330,000
Risk Pool Sharing:			
Facility Pool	$250,000	$300,000	$500,000
Specialty Physician Pool	$250,000	$275,000	$300,000
Prescription Drug Pool	$0	$25,000	$50,000
Total Revenues	**$5,500,000**	**$6,165,000**	**$6,680,000**
Increase in Revenues	**$0**	**$665,000**	**$1,180,000**

Table 5

A summarized businees model for the integrated group.

Example 2 - Integrating Part-Time Behavioral Healthcare Into a Mixed Capitation and Fee-For-Service PCP Group Without Existing Risk-Sharing Arrangements in a Less Mature Managed Care Marketplace

In this example, the 20 medical PCP group receives a straight capitation per member per month for their managed care business, and does not participate in any other risksharing arrangements. They also have a substantial amount of fee-for-service (FFS) business. They are salaried and receive high member risk adjustments and productivity-related adjustments within their group.

Four part-time behavioral healthcare providers join the PCP group and the group's capitation payment for their managed care business is adjusted by the health plan (payer) for the service profile responsibilities of the behavioral providers. They are paid salaries by the PCP group for these services based on the new capitated revenues and their part-time nature. The integrated group negotiates with the managed care plan (payer) for a new risk-sharing arrangement related to specific medical and surgical utilization and cost targets. Instead of broad-based risk pools, specific targets are agreed to for selected services such as inpatient surgical days, C-section rates, ER visits or psychotropic prescription drugs. They will then share in any savings that result from these specific services, presumably partly, or even substantially, due to their efforts and interventions. They will also share in any losses that arise due to cost increases in these service areas.

The behavioral providers also negotiate an arrangement with the medical PCPs in the group related to reduced office visits for primary medical care services to the managed care members. If such reductions result and the medical PCPs can take on more covered members, the behavioral providers will share in the additional capitated income to the group from these new members. Additionally, if the behavioral providers bring in fee-for-service medical business for the PCPs arising from their own private behavioral practice patients, they will share in the additional medical fee-for-service income of the integrated group from these referrals. Expenses for educational and prevention programs would likely be shared within the new group. An actuarial analysis produces the following summarized business model for the integrated group (See Table 6).

The business model that was developed projected that the PCP group would receive nearly $240,000 in additional revenues in the first year and nearly $500,000 in the second year after the primary behavioral healthcare integration. This amount, arising from additional covered capitated lives, fee-for-service revenues and risk-sharing revenues from medical cost offsets

Item Description	Before Integration	Year 1 After Integration	Year 2 After Integration
Number of PCPs	20	20	20
Number of Part Time PBCPs	0	4	4
Capitated Lives	6,000	6,300	6,600
PCP Capitated Revenue	$1,000,000	$1,050,000	$1,100,000
PCP FFS Capitated Revenue	$5,000,000	$5,100,000	$5,250,000
PBCP Capitated Revenue	$0	$315,000	$330,000
Risk Pool Sharing:			
Inpatient Targets	$0	$20,000	$50,000
Specialty Physician Targets	$0	$5,000	$10,000
Prescription Drug Targets	$0	$2,000	$10,000
Total Revenues	**$6,000,000**	**$6,240,000**	**$6,486,000**
Increase in Revenues	**$0**	**$240,000**	**$486,000**

Table 6

A summarized businees model for the integrated group.

paid through the specific risk-sharing targets, would be available to fund the start-up costs of the integration, educational and preventive programs and materials, compensation to the primary behavioral healthcare providers, and additional profits for the entire integrated group.

Example 3 - Integrating Full-Time Behavioral Healthcare Into a Multi-Specialty Group With a Global Cap in a Moderately Mature Managed Care Market

Here, full-time primary behavioral healthcare providers join a multi-specialty group and work alongside the medical PCPs. The entire multi-specialty group receives a global capitation payment for all professional services as well as all Rx costs. They also participate in an external risk pool for facility costs. The medical PCPs and primary behavioral providers are salaried and have their own service profile responsibilities. Other specialists are salaried or paid on a discounted fee-for-service basis. Like in example 1, the PCPs and the primary behavioral providers participate in all of the risk pools, with the difference being that the specialty and Rx risk pools are internal within the group, rather than external. This provides more flexibility for the group to determine the specific details of the risk-sharing arrangements. Expenses for new educational and preventive behavioral programs may be funded out of the global capitation amounts.

Psychotropic Drug Risk Issues

The risks related to the assumption of risk responsibilities for psychotropic drugs among the medical PCPs and the primary behavioral providers in an integrated setting should be carefully considered. The integrated group may believe that they may in a good position to control appropriate utilization and costs related to these drugs with more hands-on input from the behavioral providers. They would be well-served to analyze the expected impact of several factors on historical cost and utilization levels:

> The high cost of new and improved drugs with reduced side effects (e.g. generic drugs for treating depression may cost as little as a few dollars per month ... to a few dollars per day for Prozac, Paxil, Zoloft or Wellbutrin ... to even more for new drugs like Luvox, Celexa, Effexor or Serzone).
>
> The impact on consumer education and self-selection of drugs from increased activities of direct-to-consumer advertising from pharmaceutical companies
>
> The impact of managed care plan activities to limit access to newer drugs
>
> The trade-off of medical (medication) vs. therapeutic treatment approaches to behavioral disorders
>
> Benefit plan specifications related to drug co pay differentials, and benefit limits on generic, brand and mail order scripts.

Trends have continued to increase regarding psychotropic drug use. Costs typically exceed $1.00 pmpm in a managed commercial population group, and in many loosely managed groups may approach or even exceed $2.00 pmpm. This may be related to the prescribing patterns of non-behavioral physicians, the desire among the user population for "feel good" enhancers, and the exclusion of psychotropic drug costs in most behavioral healthcare carve-outs (managed and reduced therapy services typically leads to higher medical/psychotropic treatment costs). Consideration should be given to such ongoing trends in any analysis of psychotropic drug risk responsibilities.

Challenges with Integration

While there is ample evidence that the integration of behavioral healthcare into primary medical settings may have significant potential, as described above, many challenges may exist which could make such integration very difficult to achieve. These challenges could include the following:

Start-up costs. Who will provide the funding for the implementation expenses associated with the integration? Even if the model does pay for itself "down the road", if the managed care plan or payer will not provide capital for implementation costs with the anticipation that it will lead to lower future healthcare costs, do the behavioral and/or medical providers have the resources to handle these expenses?

Aligning physician incentives. It is usually not easy to implement financial incentive structures which will be perceived to be win-win among all the participants.

Changing management thinking. Integration typically has to overcome a few, if not many, hurdles in the thought and management processes of managed care plan executives, payers, and providers.

Marginalization of behavioral healthcare. There is still a prevalent tendency among managed care plans, payers, and medical providers to want to marginalize and separate the cost and delivery of behavioral healthcare.

Mental health vs. substance abuse fragmentation. There is still disagreement and friction within the behavioral healthcare community between these two segments.

Need for integrated technologies. The current technological capabilities of the medical and behavioral providers will likely be quite different, yet the need for common, integrated technological systems exists.

Need for co-location. Will it be easy to move primary behavioral providers into the bricks and mortar environment of the medical PCP group (even if it is not on a full time basis)? Are high front-end overhead costs associated with the co-location, and who will handle any such costs?

Two different departments, two different organizations. Can you successfully bring together members of two entirely different organizations or departments for the sake of the common good?

Provider credentialing. Medical PCPs may have difficulty determining the skill levels needed by behavioral healthcare professionals. They may be uncertain on how to identify and select behavioral healthcare professionals who would have the capabilities to make the integration effort successful.

Outcomes tracking. This necessary capability is still not present in many behavioral healthcare practices.

SUMMARY

While the focus of this paper has been on managed care plans and capitated PCP structures, many of the issues also apply, with some variation, to fee-for-service systems. For example, psychoeducational programs and public stress screenings may be provided direct to consumers by the integrated providers at very low or no cost to the public in order to increase awareness and potentially lead to more fee-for-service business in the integrated setting. While many challenges may exist that may make the integration of behavioral healthcare services in primary medical settings a difficult and, perhaps, seemingly impossible task, such proactive activities may lead to much higher degrees of medical and behavioral healthcare wellness in our population than exists today. A more seamless system of meeting both primary medical and behavioral healthcare needs may be just what the some employers and patients are seeking. Motorola, for example, has been going straight to healthcare providers for these services, bypassing the health plans. Patients seem to like the "one-stop shopping" aspect of the integrated programs.

Behavioral health prevention programs that integrate medical and behavioral health are on the rise. Quaker Oats has launched their "Live Well Be Well" program, a risk appraisal program, and integrated behavioral and physical health prevention efforts. Group Health Cooperative is integrating behavioral and general health prevention by identifying high-risk populations and by merging depression and anxiety screening/treatment with general health maintenance. Digital Equipment has mandated that prevention and early intervention services be included in the behavioral health services it purchases. And Kaiser is implementing a major redesign project to integrate behavioral care in primary care settings. These are but a few examples of the trend towards increased attention to prevention, early treatment and integrated behavioral healthcare in primary care settings.

Discussion of Melek:

Integrated Care:
Potential Disaster or Golden Opportunity?

Jeanne Wendel
University of Nevada, Reno

Stephen Melek examines the implications of the trend toward increased integration of behavioral health care and primary care services and addresses the question, does this trend present potential disaster or a golden opportunity for behavioral health care providers?

Melek begins by noting that some innovative providers have produced good patient outcomes by integrating behavioral health care into a primary care setting. To the extent that behavioral health care providers can successfully reduce patient medical expenditures via improved mental health, improved compliance with medical care instructions, and improved management of chronic diseases, behavioral health care providers may offer the solution to the fundamental dilemma posed by managed care: how can medical costs be managed and reduced without reducing the quality of patient health outcomes?

WILL INTEGRATED CARE SUCCEED IN EFFICIENT DELIVERY OF HIGH QUALITY CARE?

The potential role for integrated care in the nation's health care system will be defined gradually as providers, managed care organizations and researchers begin to answer detailed questions about the impact of integrated care. Which types of patients benefit sufficiently from behavioral health care to experience sizeable medical cost offsets? What treatment programs impact patient behavior consistently and effectively? Whose costs will be reduced by behavioral interventions? Is the time between delivery of the behavioral health

Integrated Behavioral Healthcare: Positioning Mental Health Practice with Medical/Surgical Practice

care service and the medical cost reduction short enough to justify provision of these services by managed care companies or employers with high turnover rates? How should risk be shared among providers, insurers, employers, and households? How should incentives be structured to induce optimal actions by members of these groups?

Melek assumes that continued exploration of integrated care will yield positive results. He assumes that providers and insurers will develop treatment patterns, organizational structures, and risk-sharing arrangements to develop the potential for quality and efficiency offered by the concept of integrated care. These assumptions raise a broad range of questions. If the trend to integrated care continues, how should providers respond? What public policy issues must be addressed in response to this trend? How should educational institutions adjust their programs to prepare new providers and veteran providers for the emerging market?

How Should Providers Respond to this Trend?

Successful integration of behavioral health and primary care will require business acumen as well as innovative clinical approaches. Managed care companies and providers are increasingly utilizing contracts that shift risk to the provider. This presents a spectrum of opportunities to providers ranging from traditional fee-for-service to case reimbursement, in which the provider is paid a given amount per case treated, and further to capitation, in which the provider is paid a given amount per enrolled member. Providers may contract with managed care companies directly, or as members of integrated primary and behavioral health care groups. Providers facing this broad spectrum of contract options, or - in the short term – facing a decision of whether to sign a given contract, must assess whether the specified services can be delivered at the contract price. Thoughtful analysis of this question requires in-depth understanding of the contract population, the distribution of potential service utilization rates, and service delivery costs.

Since actuarial analysis of these issues typically relies on historical cost and utilization patterns, cost and pricing analysis is problematic during periods of rapid innovation. Providers currently face an environment of ongoing shifts in treatment patterns that may affect diagnoses rates, average length of inpatient stays, and tradeoffs between alternate treatment approaches. Assessing the potential impacts of new risk-sharing arrangements is also hindered by the sizeable gaps that exist in the body of scientific knowledge about the relationships between patient characteristics, provider interventions, and patient health outcomes. Analysis of price, risk, and contract terms in this environment requires particular care.

In addition, Melek advises providers to give careful consideration to the non-price contract specifications such as the length of the contract. A contract period of several years may be needed to recoup the program's setup costs, but a lengthy period of contractually-fixed price increases the risk posed by uncertainty about pricing and utilization.

To build the capability to assess new programs and understand cost, risk and price, providers (who traditionally treat one patient at a time and record the results of that treatment in individual patient files) must develop new methods for efficient analysis populations of patients. While such analysis has traditionally been conducted by researchers, innovative risk-bearing providers will find it useful as well.

Developing a computerized infrastructure for collecting and analyzing outcomes data is essential for such analyses. Without computerized medical records, collecting sufficient data on ongoing outcomes tracking is problematic: information about large groups of patients that is stored in individual patient charts is only accessible at high cost, while electronic information can be retrieved readily if an appropriate system has been set up. Designing such a system requires thoughtful consideration of the types of information that may be useful.

First, if the expected benefit of behavioral health care includes reduced utilization of physician office visits, medications, and hospital services, for example, the data tracking system must be sufficiently comprehensive to encompass care obtained at all of these sources.

Second, effective programs reduce utilization of medical services while improving patient health outcomes or, at minimum, without impacting patient health outcomes. The outcomes tracking system must therefore be sufficiently comprehensive to include data on relevant dimensions of patient health status, both medical and psychological, to assess the quality of innovative programs.

Third, meaningful outcomes assessment must include consideration of variations in initial health status among different patient groups. If patients participating in a weight-loss program, for example, make fewer appointments with primary care physicians, it is important to assess whether the program effectively improved their overall health status or whether we are simply observing fortuitous selection of relatively healthy patients. This raises the complex issue of risk-adjustment. Development of meaningful risk-adjustment systems is not inexpensive, and use of partial risk-adjustment mechanisms creates opportunities to earn profits via clever patient selection rather than delivery of quality health care.

Finally, if variations in patient characteristics exert significant impacts on program outcomes, large samples may be needed to understand the impacts of alternate treatment protocols on patient outcomes. In such cases, it may be difficult to assess program innovations undertaken by small organizations or innovations that target small patient groups. Program assessments in these cases may require analysis by an independent researcher who collects comparable data from several cooperating integrated care groups.

The Federal Trade Commission (FTC) has explicitly recognized the importance of computer information system infrastructure as a key strategy for increasing efficiency in physician networks. The FTC's fundamental antitrust question regarding physician networks is: will the network succeed as a profitable business venture because the network structure facilitates efficient delivery of quality health care or because it increases the physicians' bargaining power as they deal with employers, insurers, hospitals, and other health care entities? Networks whose profit-potential stems from increased bargaining power may be challenged as unlawful mergers, while networks whose profitability stems from increased efficiency will not be challenged. The FTC horizontal merger guidelines for physician networks identify investment in computer infrastructure as evidence that the network is working to improve coordination and efficiency among providers.

How Should Policy Makers Respond to the Trend Toward Integrated Care?

Policy makers will face at least two issues as managed care plays an increasing role in the provision of behavioral health care. How will cost-based competition among providers and managed care organizations affect the quality of patient care? Will providers have sufficient information and resources to negotiate reasonable contracts with managed care organizations?

How Will Cost-Based Competition Among Providers and Managed Care Organizations Affect the Quality of Patient Care?

Several conference participants expressed deep concern that cost-based competition in the health care industry is driving high-quality care from the market. If hourly reimbursement rates continue to decline for behavioral health care providers, traditional one-on-one care may be substantially replaced by group treatment programs. This concern raises two questions.

First, how can high quality products survive in markets dominated by price competition? Second, how are the reimbursement rates set? Do managed care companies enjoy sufficient market power to dictate reimbursement rates that are insufficient to cover providers' costs?

The potential trade-off between cost and quality is not unique to behavioral health care or to the broader health care industry. Consumers face this trade-off in a wide array of markets. More powerful computers cost more than less powerful models. Expensive new cars may be safer than cheaper used vehicles. Airline passengers can buy higher-price first-class tickets if they value the extra leg-room enough to pay the higher price. In competitive markets in which buyers can accurately assess product quality, firms frequently offer a variety of models, with higher quality models tagged with higher prices. Each buyer is free to decide whether the additional quality offered by the luxury model is worth the higher price. While some firms offer a full range of price/quality combinations, other firms fill specialized niches, offering only luxury products or serving only the bargain-hunter market. Competitors are free to test whether consumers would prefer new combinations of price and quality. For example, the Wall Street Journal reported recently on a new chain store that plans to target customers who prefer to buy products that are cheaper and lower quality than the products typically sold in existing discount stores. One potential customer of the new chain reportedly explained that she does not want to pay for long-wearing fabrics for children's clothes that will be outgrown in a few months.

Government policy dictates the level of quality for some goods. Prior to 1977, federal regulation of airline pricing and routes essentially required interstate airlines to provide high cost/high quality service. The success of Southwest Airlines in the interstate market in Texas during the 1970's offers an interesting example of consumers choosing, instead, to forego some convenience in order to obtain lower prices.

Concern about price/quality choices made by consumers generally focuses on markets in which buyers cannot readily assess the quality of the goods offered for sale. Economists use the term, search goods, to denote goods that can be inspected and assessed before purchase. Buyers can easily make informed decisions about price/quality trade-offs for these goods. Buyers cannot assess the quality of experience goods, in contrast, until they purchase the item and experience its use. Restaurant meals, used cars, and hair cuts are experience goods because the buyer cannot inspect the quality of these goods until they have been purchased and experienced. Some goods, such as vitamins, are even more difficult to assess. Buyers are still unsure about the quality and impact of these goods after they purchase and use them.

Despite the difficulty of assessing product quality, high quality products frequently compete successfully against cheaper/lower quality competitors. The key to success for the higher quality products is that the extra quality must be valued by consumers enough to induce some of them to pay the higher price. Consumers assess product quality with a variety of market-based and regulatory consumer information and consumer protection strategies. Buyers obtain additional information from second opinion experts, from quality reporting services such as Consumer Reports, and informal word-of-mouth sources. Buyers reduce their risk of purchasing a low quality item via product warranties, department store return policies, and repeat purchases from known suppliers. Government policies assist purchasers via legal liability, safety standards, and regulations requiring government approval for items such as prescription drugs.

Applying this combination of market and government strategies to health care is problematic for several reasons. First, the employers who purchase health insurance and the employees' households who utilize the health care may not agree on the optimal level of quality to be purchased. (In assessing this problem, we should not rush to conclude that employers have no interest in providing quality health insurance and quality health care. Since employers offer health insurance as one component of a total compensation package, they have a profit incentive to consider household satisfaction and employee willingness to forego wage increases in order to obtain more comprehensive health insurance coverage.) Second, provision of multiple levels of health care quality present complex ethical issues. On the one hand, consumer selection of a low price/low quality option raises concerns about equity, the degree to which the choice was informed and voluntary, and the impacts of this choice on the consumers' family members. On the other hand, insistence on provision of only one level of quality may price some consumers out of the market entirely. For employees with automatic employer-provided coverage, mandating a single (high)level of quality will reduce employee wages. Some low-wage workers might be better off if they could reallocate some of their total compensation to wages by accepting lower quality health care. Third, it is difficult for employers or households to assess the quality of alternate treatment programs.

We will focus here on the third concern: can employers or households assess the quality of care offered by competing managed care companies? If quality cannot be assessed, buyers will not be willing to pay higher prices for higher quality services, and high quality providers will disappear from the market. More costly/higher price services will only be offered in a competitive market if providers, provider organizations, researchers, or government agencies demonstrate and/or guarantee the value of these services. How can providers help consumers and employers assess the quality of care?

The computerized data needed by providers to assess program quality and assume and price risk may also provide the basis for demonstrating program quality to employers and households. Since it is difficult for buyers to compare idiosyncratic pieces of information produced by individual behavioral health care providers, standardized "report cards" that provide comparable audited data for all providers may help buyers compare alternate plans. The difficulty in developing useful report cards lies in determining exactly what pieces of information are both available and useful to buyers. For example, it is relatively easy to report the proportion of HMO patients who receive anti-smoking counseling, but it might be more meaningful and more difficult to report the proportion of smokers who actually quit smoking in response to the counseling.

Development of meaningful and useful report cards will require a two-pronged effort. Providers and managed care companies must strengthen the infrastructure to support better data collection and analysis. Providers, consumer groups, and employers must also give thoughtful consideration to the dimensions of quality that are valued by consumers and the measurement of health outcomes.

Psychologists may make a particularly valuable contribution in developing an understanding of consumer perception and valuation of health care. One example of the stumbling blocks inhibiting development of meaningful quality measures is that consumer attitude surveys seem to indicate that consumers value the warmth and friendliness of the providers' office staff. If a consumer selects a physician whose office staff seems caring and supportive, without considering the physician's performance in producing health outcomes, is this consumer necessarily making a "wrong" choice? If a smoker understands the health impacts of smoking, but does not want to give up the pleasure of smoking, is a "quality" provider one who respects this choice or one who continually works to induce the smoker to quit? It will be difficult to assess the impact of innovative healthcare delivery programs until we have a better understanding of the consumers' concept of "quality healthcare".

Will Providers Have Sufficient Information and Resources to Negotiate with Managed Care Organizations?

Some conference participants expressed two concerns about the relative bargaining power of providers v.-a-vie managed care companies. First, providers may negotiate with managed care companies from weak positions if managed care companies have greater resources for collecting and analyzing outcomes, risk, and financial data. Second, managed care companies may present contracts to providers on a "take it or leave it" basis, rather than negotiating a mutually-beneficial contract if providers must compete vigorously to obtain managed care contracts.

The first concern raises two issues: Do managed care companies have access to better information than providers? Can the larger managed care organizations analyze data at lower cost per enrollee than the smaller provider organizations? Large size may confer significant efficiency advantages for two reasons: developing computerized medical records systems will require significant capital investment and larger organizations are more likely to have large enough patient samples to obtain statistically significant conclusions. The viability of small provider groups in the managed care marketplace may depend on their ability to obtain data collection and data analysis services at competitive prices.

The second concern focuses on the impact of cost-based competition, which places providers under intense financial pressure. As in any industry with excess capacity, competitive bidding pushes price down near average variable cost, which implies reimbursement rates that are not sufficient to cover average total cost. This type of intense competition is often described with the terms, "destructive competition" or "cutthroat pricing".

Should providers expect reimbursement rates to continue to decline? This vigorous competition, with reimbursement rates below providers' traditional average cost, resulted from decreased demand for behavioral health care services. With prices below traditional average cost, fewer students will earn the degrees necessary to enter the field and some providers will exit via early retirement or career changes. For areas in which traditional treatments continue to be the norm, this decrease in the supply of behavioral health care services will permit reimbursement rates to stabilize at levels that cover average cost.

This process is expected to occur in any industry in which demand for the product decreases; it is the normal process by which supply adjusts to the new level of demand. Destructive competition and cutthroat competition pose particular problems, however, in industries characterized by high fixed costs, large infrequent contracts, and fluctuating demand. Behavioral health care does not appear to meet the first or third criterion of high fixed costs and fluctuating demand, but increasing penetration of managed care may introduce the second characteristic to this industry. If providers feel pressured to successfully bid for one of a few large contracts, they are likely to feel pressured to ensure that the bid is low enough to obtain the contract. In this situation, they may bid at prices that are sufficient to cover variable costs (i.e. direct costs of providing patient care), but not total costs.

For areas of behavioral health care in which group treatment or integrated behavioral and primary care are successful in reducing cost, the introduction of a newer lower-cost production technology will lead to prices that approximate the average cost of delivering care via these new methods. Traditional methods will only be marketable in these areas if the providers can demonstrate that the extra cost is justified by higher quality outcomes. The burden of proof, in this case, will lie on the shoulders of providers who wish to continue using traditional treatment patterns.

How Should Educational Institutions Respond?

As managed care plays a growing role in the behavioral health care industry and primary and behavioral health care develop new models of integrated delivery, provider organizations will need to assess the results of innovative programs, develop computer infrastructures to support data collection and analysis, decide how much risk to bear, and evaluate alternate pricing methods. New graduates and continuing practitioners may require increased financial, business, and computer literacy. They may need additional quantitative and research methods skills to develop systems for analyzing outcomes data and cost data for populations of patients.

Educational institutions therefore face the age-old dilemma: if new topics are added to the curriculum, the institution must either reduce the time devoted to traditional topics or lengthen the course of study. Graduate schools may explore the possibility that students might study business, computer information systems, and quantitative methods as undergraduates. Alternately, it may not be efficient or effective for every behavioral health care provider to undertake outcomes studies, risk assessment, and cost analysis. Some providers may opt for overview summaries of these fields, and contract with consultants or hire business managers to provide these services. Conference participants, however, repeatedly returned to the question of how providers can exert more control over industry pricing and patterns of care. Providers in leadership roles area may require in-depth understanding of these additional subjects. Educational institutions may respond to the variety of provider preferences by offering specialized study tracks.

CONCLUSION

Do the increasing roles of managed care and integrated primary and behavioral health care present health care providers with potential disaster or a golden opportunity? Answers to this question depend on many factors, including the future evolution of the health care industry and the extent to which behavioral healthcare providers step into leadership roles.

Conference participants focused largely on the potential to exercise leadership in developing integrated primary and behavioral health care. If integrated care can consistently generate sufficient medical cost offsets to fund the cost of providing the behavioral care, these programs will help managed care organizations solve the fundamental problem of delivering cost effective plans to employers without sacrificing health outcomes.

In addition, behavioral health care providers may offer the expertise needed by managed care companies to understand consumer perceptions of health care and consumer values. It is clear that automobile manufacturers understand consumer demand in great detail. One manufacturer recently announced that it believes its target consumers are now more concerned about safety than style. It is designing its new cars to specify deliver higher levels of safety. This firm is responding to its customers' definition of "automotive quality". Current discussions of health care report cards indicate that health care providers do not have this type of sophisticated understanding of their customers' values. Behavioral healthcare providers may be ideally positioned to help managed care companies develop this understanding.

11
CHAPTER

Program Restructuring and Curricular Enhancement for Accountable Training

Warwick G. Troy, Ph.D., M.P.H.
Center for Health Care Innovation,
California State University, Long Beach

Integrated Behavioral Healthcare: Positioning Mental Health Practice with Medical/Surgical Practice

THE CHANGING PROFESSIONAL WORLD ORDER

The last decade has been witness to a dramatic revolution in health services organization and financing in the U.S. (Broskowski, 1995; Cummings, 1996; Shueman, Troy, & Mayhugh, 1994). The signal manifestation of this is the current dominance of organized systems of care, known generically as managed systems, as the prevailing medium through which health services are delivered. These systems differ in essential ways from the traditional models, a vast majority of which operated under fee-for-service reimbursement approaches.

Traditional models have been characterized by acute care services in physician-dominated hospital settings with their attendant dependence on technology and associated high costs. The new systems involve decentralization of services embracing community models of care, acknowledgment of the critical nature of disease management approaches to deal with chronicity, and a clear recognition of the roles of prevention and health promotion. They also require new approaches to clinical management, including the application of new, more cost-effective technologies, and increased inter-professional collaboration.

Above all, however, these new systems are based on an essential tripartite set of concepts related to professional service provision. These concepts are **professional responsibility, competence,** and **accountability**. They are based on a core set of attitude/value, knowledge, and skill competencies, and they lie at the heart of training program redesign. Attention to all three is required if purchasers, consumers, and other stakeholders are to be assured by the professions that providers have been prepared to plan, deliver, and evaluate in a consistent manner the quality of care under a significantly changed set of professional imperatives (Troy, 1994).

The changes in health services create significant opportunities for psychologists and other behavioral health professionals interested in exploring new professional roles (Broskowski, 1995; Cummings, 1996). At the same time, these role demands present significant challenges for professionals wishing to contribute to these new models of service delivery. Few behavioral health professionals have had opportunities to obtain the knowledge, skills, and values necessary to adapt to these new work environments, let alone exposure to the essential health care policy issues framing them. For many if not most, training has reflected a normative stance essentially antithetical to the needs of multi-disciplinary, comprehensive, and integrated systems of care.

Four aspects of new service models account for most of the variance in the challenge facing psychologists. These are: (1) human diversity; (2) chronicity aspects of disease and disability; (3) preventive approaches; and (4) alternative delivery models. Roles – but, particularly, new and emerging roles – derive from these challenges.

Characteristics of Managed Systems

Because the managed care industry is still in a formative stage of developmental, the financing and delivery systems representing the industry reveal a great deal of heterogeneity. These systems do, however, ascribe to a great extent to a common normative approach. Consequently, they tend to share certain features of structure and process (American Psychological Association, 1996). These include:

> Large highly articulated, integrated systems of care which include mechanisms for quality management and improvement.
> A blurring of the distinction between purchaser/payer and service planning/delivery functions.
> Multi-disciplinary work force involving routine inter-disciplinary collaboration.
> Formal mechanisms for process and outcome evaluation.
> Large management information systems supporting financial, clinical, and personnel subsystems.
> Minimal use of hierarchical modes of organization with differentiation of function across separate organizational sub-units.

Focus on prevention and wellness.

Emphasis on consumer empowerment.

Population-based approach to services planning and
delivery.

Erosion of the barriers between public and private sector
patients and facilities.

Increasing use of lower (training) level services
personnel.

Emphasis on primary (non-specialist) services.

Functional linkages between behavioral health and
primary medical care.

The service requirements of these new models, with an emphasis on
providers' working effectively as interdependent elements of integrated
systems, have developed well beyond the current capability of academic
programs to prepare clinicians for the current, let alone emerging systems of
care (Shueman, Troy, & Mayhugh, 1994). The failure in preparation can not
be attributed to training programs alone, however. On the contrary, related
developments within the federal government and professional associations
have resulted in a reduction in the capacity of these groups to offer their
traditional support for the development and implementation of innovative
training programs (Troy & Shueman, 1996).

Diminished Role for Traditional Sanctioners of Behavioral Health

Three stakeholder groups – academic training programs, professional
associations, and the federal government – have long been the primary
advocates, agents, and resource bodies for the science and practice of behavioral health (Troy, 1997). Through policy development, advocacy, funding,
and training activities, they have traditionally assumed the responsibility for
ensuring that professionals in training are appropriately prepared to work
within existing health systems. For a number of reasons, however, the changes
in health care have far outstripped their capacity and, in some cases, willingness to respond to the current and emerging system needs. In particular, three
sociopolitical developments severely threaten the capacity of this larger
training community to achieve educational innovation and appropriate
training program redesign.

Reductions in government support for training. The federal government as
a funding agent has had a significant influence in the of training of the health
care work force, including behavioral health professionals. Federal budget

pressures of recent years have significantly and negatively affected the direct financial support the government can provide for training – even for medicine. More importantly, funding level reductions severely threaten the continuation of demonstration projects that serve to enhance innovation in the training models and mechanisms for service delivery.

Diminished impact of professional associations. To the uninformed observer, managed care appears to have caught professional associations and the practitioners they represent by surprise. The truth is, however, that internal conflict over participation in managed care has resulted in the various associations being unable to capitalize on the admittedly limited opportunities to shape the policy agenda. Furthermore, the associations have promulgated policies inconsistent with sound health care management and, through internal and external guild-focused lobbying efforts, have given professionals the message that it is better to fight these systems than to adapt to them. Because of the multi-disciplinary emphasis of organized care systems, single-profession associations, particularly non-medical professions, have also found themselves significantly restricted in their ability to influence developments in the field.

Disjunction within academic psychology. The education and training of professional psychologists has for decades been characterized by a disjunction between psychology's scientific foundations, on the one hand, and its emerging practical orientation, on the other. Academic psychologists, who are scientists as well as educators and trainers, reflect an ambivalence about training for practice. Professional psychology's most developed and prevalent training model, scientist-practitioner, has traditionally demonstrated more support for the scientist side of the training. Lacking medicine's and law's comfort with training for professional roles, psychology has had great difficulty developing and supporting an enduring model which acknowledges the practical while incorporating the scientific. This problem is intensified by the negative attitudes toward managed care held by many training faculty and to their lack of knowledge about these new models of service delivery (Troy, 1994; Troy, 1997; Troy & Shueman, 1996). Ironically, more recent education and training models generally associated with schools of professional psychology appear to have been no more effective in bridging this disjunction. Practitioner-scholar and practitioner have remained operationally distant from the world of health policy, public health concepts, and the vagaries and challenges of integrated systems of care.

A Serious Consequence: Degraded Infrastructure for Supervised Training

One of the most serious consequences of reduced government support combined with changes in methods of payment under managed systems is the increasing shortfall in the number of health service programs and sites that can be used for supervised practical training. This holds for internship level, post-doctoral, and post-licensure training sites. The problem is seriously exacerbated by the current American Psychological Association accreditation criteria that are based on an anachronistic model of practice. The inherent inflexibility of these criteria with regard to structure of and supervisory process within training sites, makes it difficult for trainees to acquire the competencies appropriate for the professional challenges facing them during their sanctioned training experiences (Troy, 1997).

Because the managed care industry is relatively immature, changes will continue and will affect professionals long after their training years have concluded. The roles and skills acquired by current license holders during graduate and post-graduate training will become increasingly irrelevant. Consequently, the professional who wishes to continue functioning effectively must make a true functional commitment to his or her lifelong professional development.

Post-licensure continuing education of professionals typically occurs independently of the training establishment described above. Such training has traditionally been ad hoc, directed toward the individual, and not organized to prepare providers for new professional roles. To meet current and future demands of health services, training needs to be conceptualized on a pre-doctoral/post-doctoral/post-licensure continuum that draws for its development upon work force studies (Biegel, 1994) identifying emerging professional roles and the knowledge and skills supporting those roles.

The New Imperatives

What are the demands associated with the new systems that so significantly challenge service providers in behavioral health? From the perspective of behavioral health professionals, the current workplace environment requires understanding (although not necessarily mastery) of a variety of competency areas outlined below. These competency areas subsume attitudes/values, knowledge, and skills. (Note that these are generic factors, affecting all disciplines equally.)

The elements of health care organization, financing, and
provision.
The associations among provider, payment, and service:
the elements of services management.
Principles of comprehensive services development,
coordination, and continuity.
Health policy issues.
Essentials of community welfare, organization, and
intervention.
Population-based services planning and organization.
Structural and role interdependence in integrated care
systems.
Technology for effective clinical management.
Technology for quality assessment and management.
Outcome evaluation and health services research.

One of the most difficult aspects of training for the new world order relates
to the fact that psychology training programs, with the possible exception of
community psychology, have tended not to deal with the more macro, system
issues in health care. This would include, for example, financing, services
organization, and population-based planning. Such issues tend to be seen as
the concern of managers rather than clinical professionals. The new demands,
then, will require that these professionals adopt a broader perspective on
health services (or at least understand the "big picture").

Observations on the Current Status of Professional Training

It is clear that psychology training programs have not demonstrated that
they can be appropriately responsive to the changing requirements for
professional competencies in the dynamic world of health care. The gap
between competencies required and competencies acquired is wide, raising
concerns that we are training professional psychologists for a world that has
largely ceased to exist. Programs certainly have the capacity to evolve,
however, but psychologists who are involved in training need to be increasingly sensitive to the educational requirements inherent in the new health care
delivery systems. Accountability to their consuming public, other stakeholders, and their own students demand it.
The essential challenge to training in professional psychology is to
develop providers who can work effectively as salient elements of service
systems characterized by accountability and interdependence of roles. This

requires a significant commitment to the induction and support of an appropriate values stance as well as to the acquisition of a new technology of generic practice. A reflection of such a values stance might, for example, include an emphasis on and understanding of the necessity for balancing quality of care issues with limited resources, quick response times, working within interdisciplinary teams, and utilizing family members as primary service providers. Dealing effectively with cognitive and attitudinal resistance to change on the part of providers (and faculty) will remain a challenge into the foreseeable future. In addition, the necessary retraining requires a commitment to a training sequence in order to master a new set of skills associated with a different kind of work life: a set of demands both strange and alienating to many solo practitioners. Investment in such retraining is often more than providers wish to give, and the change in daily work is not what they would chose.

Many providers have professional concerns (e.g., the quality "trade-off" made in the interest of cost-effectiveness) that are as yet unanswered. A major task, then, is to overcome this resistance to change. Not insignificant numbers of independent practitioners have already chosen, and will continue to choose, to work outside the world of health care. For those who see for themselves as true health service professionals, the appropriate training sequences referred to above need to be developed and they need to have the capability to flexibly acknowledge the professional role requirements of these personnel. The challenges to those charged with designing and implementing post licensure professional development are very real indeed.

New Roles for Professional Psychologists

In this section we take a closer look at the role demands that will be placed on psychologists now and in the future. These roles are best seen as a mix of the traditional, the new, and the emerging which, collectively, reflect the challenges and imperatives of the changing professional world. A reformulation for professional roles is outlined below, using the tripartite division of traditional, new, and emerging (see Table 1).

It is important to note that there is a generic (core) component to roles within each classification. This core component reflects the changing structure of health services and involves the capacity to understand and contribute to the realities of large integrated systems of care which emphasize intra-system linkages and interdisciplinary collaboration. The successful psychologist, therefore, must be equipped to engage in a combination of core and specialized roles through the acquisition of generic competencies. Indeed, the

Traditional Role Function	New Role Function	Emerging Role Function
- Testing and assessment	- Health systems design and monitoring	- Quality management
- Specialties and proficiencies	- Development and use of clinical protocols	- Disease management
- Alternate treatment modalities	- Development of profiling techniques	- Development of MIS
- Case formulation and clinical management	- Development of consumer-oriented treatment materials	- Strategic planning
- Special populations	- New program development	
- Consumer education and advocacy		
- Consultation and supervision		

Table 1

Traditional, New, and Emerging Roles for Psychologists in Managed Health Systems

modern psychologist's ability to exercise the specialist roles – many unique to psychologists – depends upon his or her full understanding and acceptance of the realities and imperatives of these role functions within highly articulated systems of care. This is the essence of the "generic" role component. It is the key to operational fluency and influence for psychologists in a changing professional world.

Traditional Role Functions

Some of the traditional role functions discussed below are typically viewed as unique to psychologists (e.g., traditional psychodiagnostic assessment), while some are responsibilities shared with other behavioral health professionals (case formulation and clinical management). As becomes clear in the discussion, managed models of health services organization, financing, and delivery will have a significant effect not only on the creation of new roles but also on opportunities for behavioral health professionals to continue to engage in these traditional activities.

Assessment. Traditional psychodiagnostic assessment as well as the routine administration of test batteries are much less likely to be supported under new and emerging delivery and financing systems. Skills in the functional assessment of disabilities as well as those involved in behavioral assessment will be critical, however. The utility of assessment in treatment planning will be the critical factor. Ad hoc testing which does not directly inform treatment planning will rarely be endorsed, while regular and ongoing targeted assessment necessary for treatment planning and outcomes monitoring will be. In addition, with the increasing recognition of the mind-body connection, the role of behavioral health in physical health, the focus on prevention, and the need for competent biopsychosocial assessment will be paramount in both primary health care and behavioral health care.

Specialties and proficiencies. Within the framework of organized health care services, open-ended psychotherapeutic services have only a marginal place. On the other hand, services planned, provided, and monitored by well-trained health psychologist sub-specialists and those with proficiencies in behavioral medicine will constitute an integral part of behavioral health, medical-surgical rehabilitation, and preventive care. It is likely that opportunities for doctoral-level clinical and counseling psychologists as direct service providers in the developing health system will be increasingly restricted to professionals with formal preparation in clinical health psychology or behavioral medicine.

Alternate treatment modalities. This function has been associated largely with organized care settings, particularly public sector and community-based programs. Operationally, the emphasis here is on the development of programs, rather than one-on-one interventions, which are organized in ways that maximize efficiency of service delivery (i.e., the ratio of service units to resources used to provide services). Maximizing service access while minimizing service costs through use of efficient modes of delivery is a goal as well as a constant challenge for organized delivery systems. Again, the skills involved are technical: the use of media or indirect targets which maximize service outreach or case finding; the development and utilization of psycho-educational programs; use of treatment groups, workshops, handbooks/manuals, and electronic products for self-management; use of mutual support groups, etc.

Case formulation and clinical management. This critical clinical service function is related to, but not identical to, traditional assessment and diagnostics. With the increasing accountability focus of service delivery, optimizing the incidence of desired outcomes is critical. The capacity to employ assessment findings in case formulation, to monitor with precision the course of treatment, and to fine-tune inputs in ways that maximize outcomes have always been central components of effective clinical work. Clinical health psychologists must avail themselves of the growing technology supporting clinical management.

The current move away from fee-for-service payment to "at risk" arrangements will place inordinate emphasis on the effective use of empirically-supported, replicable clinical protocols. Case formulation, treatment planning, and monitoring will increasingly take into account the use of such protocols as well as provider competence in the identification and use of collateral resources. This role function will become the arena in which the true clinical decision-making skills of the specialist psychological provider will be on display for other disciplines to see, and can only be validated by the achievement of specific outcomes associated with improved health status.

Special populations. This speaks to the capacity of professional psychologists to plan, provide, and monitor interventions which reflect sensitivity to the needs of a variety of special populations. Such populations include traditionally under served and at-risk groups. Persons with disabilities, including those with severe mental illness, are examples of vulnerable groups whose health benefit will increasingly move from the public to the private sector as public services become increasingly "privatized." And, as the large pharmaceutical companies and health plans continue to differentiate and increase their involvement in, for example "disease management," psychologists who have acquired knowledge-skill-value based professional competencies which focus on the concerns and resources of consumers with special needs will play significant roles in service planning and delivery, at both individual and program levels.

Consumer education and advocacy. The accountability imperative so central to emerging health systems embraces fiscal and professional responsibility as well as a commitment to the patient as an empowered consumer. The model holds that the delivery system is accountable to the purchaser of services who, in turn, represents and is influenced by the consumer. The model also holds that, as the consumer becomes increasingly discriminating through education and empowerment, health plans will increasingly incorporate consumer preferences in the benefit package. While a full implementation of such a model is most unlikely, an informed consumer empowered by a collaborative partnership with his or her provider, plays a critical role in the generation of desired treatment outcomes in the longer haul.

It is important to note the essential role of psycho-educational services in the behavioral health-physical health link. With the increasing awareness of the role of psychological processes in physical health and the focus on prevention, patient education will become increasingly important and psychological interventions which increase patient awareness and treatment compliance will be highly valued.

Professional consultation and supervision. This heterogeneous mix of role functions, long associated with professional psychologists working within and outside of organized systems of care, is likely to assume a much more structured and less opportunistic form in the years ahead. Increased opportunities for intra- and interdisciplinary activities provide, in turn, increased opportunities for consultation and supervision by psychologists. Again, the focus of intervention can be at both the individual and the system level. Finally, professional preparation for activities subsumed under this general role function will come to utilize a far more formalized and strategic approach to skills development than has generally been true for most training to date in this area.

New Role Functions

New roles exist on a continuum with the "traditional" role functions previously considered. The difference is that these "new" roles generally derive from, and are embedded in, the imperatives of the new, accountable health systems. At the same time, this set of professional role functions also invokes generic aspects of the established roles for psychologists as previously considered. A degree of speculation is involved in the identification of the set of roles, particularly with those considered emerging. Further, in some instances the inclusion of role functions in a particular category is arbitrary.

Health systems design and monitoring. Core aspects of the training curricula of community, clinical, counseling, and I/O psychology programs would seem to prepare certain psychologists well for this function. For the more immediate future, much of the content, as opposed to the conceptual formulation and understanding of system processes, will necessarily be acquired on the job.

Development of clinical protocols. This is becoming an increasingly important function as organized systems of care attempt to reduce uncontrolled variation in interventions across providers and thereby enhance the probability of obtaining desired outcomes for particular disorders. Scientist-practitioner trained psychologists have already contributed to the development of evidence-based clinical protocols for specific disorders. The critical thinking skills and analytic abilities developed through psychologists' research training is invaluable in this area.

Development of models of provider profiling. This function involves the development, and implementation of empirical models permitting the evaluation of the "success" of individual providers or practice groups in providing cost-effective care across a variety of behavioral health disorders. At its best, this involves the integration of clinical research into clinical practice, with documented outcomes associated with providers and their treatments. Increasingly, as the role of integrated practice groups develops, this function will be routinely incorporated within the practice group itself rather than remaining a "control mechanism" currently associated with managed care organizations.

Development of consumer-oriented treatment materials. As more efficient means of service delivery are used, and access to what might be called "nontraditional" service modalities increases, psychologists who can develop, for example, manuals for client self-assessment and self-management, or materials involved in psycho-educational program development will be valued.

New program development. Central to this function is the increasing need for preventive services, partially involving outreach and health promotion activities. Community-clinical psychologists have traditionally been involved in the development and implementation of primary and secondary prevention programs for at-risk persons. In this regard, inter-system linkages – involving, for example, schools, housing, and income support – constitute a core component of successful program planning and implementation, particularly in community settings. As the public-private sector linkages increase, with private sector providers involved in what previously have been public services, the need for new programs and for linkages between service sectors will increase dramatically. In addition, the use of community-based interventions is likely to increase, requiring new approaches to problem resolution.

Emerging Role Functions

The bulk of these role function opportunities involve specialist, technically-oriented competencies and their applications within changing health care systems. Since a number of these functions can be discharged by disciplines other than psychology, the challenge to our profession is to demonstrate our effectiveness by targeting such role functions and providing the competencies associated with their appropriate realization.

Quality management. There exists a great variety of mechanisms associated with these critical areas including quality assessment and improvement, utilization management, and outcomes monitoring. Since the behavioral health care industry will increasingly be called upon to compete on quality rather than price, the systems-oriented psychologist with applied science skills is in an advantageous position to contribute to the process rapidly becoming an industry rallying cry—continuous quality improvement.

Disease management. This function requires the application of behavioral science to problems of patient compliance with drug or treatment regimens, secondary prevention, and rehabilitation. It has multiple foci including applied research, human diversity, consumer empowerment, prevention and health promotion, and inter-professional collaboration. The wider issue involved in any consideration of this role function is health care's most significant challenge: the displacement of acute care services by services oriented toward the clinical management of **chronicity**. Disease management is an exciting and rapidly developing field which offers challenging professional opportunities for psychologists with specialist or proficiency preparation in community clinical, health/behavioral medicine, applied social, applied developmental, and counseling psychology.

Development of management information systems (MIS). An effective MIS is an indispensable precondition to a service system's capacity to accept financial risk, whether it be capitation, case rate reimbursement, or any other payment arrangement. The MIS serves clinical management needs as well as other functions including human resource management and accounting. The key to successful role involvement in this area is the capacity to work with computer systems personnel on the designation of criteria for clinical outcomes monitoring as well as on processes to maximize user friendliness and efficiency of data retrieval. Psychologists are also well qualified to assist organizations in evaluation and interpretation of data.

Strategic planning combining needs and resource analysis. These and related functions, such as organization development, are endemic to the operational effectiveness of complex systems such as large organized care settings. The challenge, particularly for organizational psychologists, is to increase the penetration of their specialty as systems managers and consultants.

Obstacles to Reform

Above, we identified a set of imperatives with which professional education and training needs to contend. Also discussed were some of the challenges facing training programs in professional psychology. Before progressing to an analysis of prerequisites for training program redesign, we revisit some of the obstacles that stand in the path of training reform and training program redesign.

It is surely more than the claimed indifference of those in academia to the "outside world" or the bureaucratic inertia common to large institutions that makes change difficult. Likewise, there is more to it than the prevailing conflicts academic training programs have had with the notion of applied or professional endeavors. Whatever the complex of explanations - including the general absence of formal academic contingencies supporting external outreach and other program development activities by program administrators and core faculty - the time is long past for the training community to begin a process of significant program redesign. Nonetheless, it seems incontestable that academics tend to view the marketplace, even the non-corporate world of organized care settings, with significant unease: they don't know much about it, nor care to learn much; and they know they feel out of place in or near it.

Costs of Professional Training "Non-Compliance"

There have been costs associated with the prevailing absence of formally accountable training in behavioral health other than the critical failure of the larger profession adequately to serve sanctioners. These costs have accrued to both the behavioral health workforce and the profession. Although the economic costs to practitioners arising from the vagaries of managed care arrangements have been high, another cost has been higher and far more serious. This is the cost of under preparedness – a significant threat to the collective efficacy of the profession.

It is little wonder that rank and file behavioral health practitioners have for the past decade exhibited confusion, helplessness, rage, and lack of strategic competence in the face of the cataclysmic changes within health care. Absent an understanding of the new world of health care, the bulk of the behavioral health care workforce had no capacity to control or adapt to, let alone influence, a game (they claimed) whose rules had changed after it had commenced. This state of powerlessness was exacerbated by the exceedingly ambiguous attitudes held by so many providers toward the world of health care. Drawn into and trained in traditional psychotherapy rather than as health care providers, per se, these practitioners utterly lacked an armamentarium permitting them some realistic chance of both negotiating the labyrinth of the (non) system of health care in the U.S. and of playing a constructive and enduring role in it.

Accountable Education and Training in Behavioral Health

It would seem axiomatic that professional education and training for the behavioral health workforce, to be deemed truly accountable, would take direct account of professional role imperatives derived from the current environment of health care organization, financing, and provision. It would also seem reasonable for such programs to explicitly acknowledge the substance and pattern of the changes confronting health care systems, payers, providers and consumers. Professional preparation across the behavioral health disciplines has acknowledged neither. While there has been episodic attention given to individual issues, professional education and training have seen no true systematic incorporation of either of the above within the broad scope of its programs.

Again, there are good reasons why this has been so, not the least of which is the pragmatic one of sheer difficulty. Dealing effectively and in an intellectually honest fashion with either of the above, requires both a knowledge base and an operational infrastructure significantly beyond the province of the vast majority of professional training programs. Also lacking is a policy-oriented vision of the scope and pattern of health care in its emerging state. Such vision can not reasonably be expected of program leadership in traditional academic settings sustained by traditional contingencies.

Nonetheless, these issues must be confronted if the behavioral health workforce is ever to acquire the appropriate professional armamentarium. This target involves the wherewithal, not only to effectively adapt to a changing world, but also to actively contribute to such a world - one as replete with professional challenges as perplexities. If, then, this is the general way to operational accountability in professional training, what might the road look like?

Recognizing Accountability in Training Programs

Achieving accountability requires the identification of professional roles appropriate to the demands, or imperatives, of a complex health care environment, as well as program redesign which anticipates and provides for the establishment of a framework for a changing professional world. These are our twin criteria earlier identified.

In this context, accountability also involves responsibility to multiple stakeholders. And these include not only consumers and their careers, but payers, health plans, provider organizations, state and federal governments, non governmental organizations, professional organizations, licensing and credentialing authorities, consumer advocacy organizations, and the community at large.

Accountable professional education and training is also characterized by a values stance that explicitly acknowledges the program's responsibility for its products, within both proximal and distal time frames. Indeed, this is one of the ways in which the autonomy traditionally accorded professions is repaid to their stakeholders and sanctioners. Finally, in the accountability criteria outlined above, there is no place for the narrow guild interests of the professions or of academia, and none for the economic welfare of the provider community. Professionals have obligations to their sanctioners and those they serve, and accountable education and training programs seek to reflect this routinely, and in multiple ways, both formally and informally.

In the next section we present the substantive elements of accountable training program redesign. A normative approach is proposed, one that provides a platform for incorporating the criteria for the design of accountable training programs discussed above. What follows may be regarded as a kind of template for education and training for the behavioral health workforce. Importantly, however, it is also designed to be directly responsive to the needs of a variety of stakeholders. We hope that this product might be useful as a road map of sorts for program redesign in clinical health and community psychology.

A Template for Training Program Redesign

In this section, we identify core instrumental approaches to training program redesign. These are essentially the prerequisites for a true strategic approach on which enduring accountable program redesign must be based.

Beyond Curriculum Development

Innovation in **program** design involves a great deal more than curriculum and instructional design work. Collaboration with sanctioners (including, for example, formal alliances with consumer advocacy groups), new models for faculty roles, recruitment, and performance assessment, service and training network development with community based organizations, faculty practice plan development, risk contracting, and alliance building with health plans, are only some of the activities associated with the strategic planning enterprise at the program level. In this latter guise the proposed platform is a structural, generic approach useful for linking present and emerging professional role imperatives. It also provides a framework for the essential continuity of pre-doctoral education and training and post licensure competency development. Nonetheless, curriculum development is at the very core of program redesign and a framework for it is suggested below.

Curriculum redesign: Four approaches. There would seem to be four essential approaches to curricular innovation in the interest of accountability. The first involves the identification of a foundational **normative stance**: a professional values base which overtly acknowledges certain core imperatives guiding accountable training. The second approach seeks to identify a **core set of formal competencies** sufficiently generic to serve professional roles - traditional, new, and emerging. Central to our third approach to program redesign is a formal treatment of the complex **context of health care** - its developmental path, characteristics, and policy content. The fourth approach involves a clear recognition of the centrality of **collaborative and**

enduring relationships with the multiform world of health care. The strategic incorporation of all four approaches would seem indispensable to the development of behavioral health education and training programs that can truly be said to be accountable.

Generic Foci for Education and Training

The foci that are the elements of the following classification scheme are extremely broad content areas incorporating a combination of professional knowledge, values, attitudes, and skills with implications for training program development. As identified below, the foci are those substantive areas which need to be designated as the content targets for professional education and training programs seeking to become accountable. Deriving from a normative base and reflecting the changed characteristics of U.S. health care, these imperative based foci collectively indicate the road along which professional preparation for the behavioral health workforce must now travel, and for the foreseeable future.

These foci can also serve as the source for professional roles, new and emerging. **Taken together, they constitute the general content mix to which trainees and professionals need to be formally exposed in order to interpret their professional world, to practice responsibly and effectively, and to exert a constructive influence upon the behavioral health field.** These foci are the very issues to which the vast majority of trainees and practitioners in behavioral health have been thus far so inadequately exposed through formal training and supervision.

In summary, these generic foci are intended to perform a conceptual service role that, over 40 years ago, the great cognitive theorist, David Ausubel, referred to as "advance organizers." Alternatively, the entire set of foci, organized by domains, may be seen as constituting a kind of professional world view – a glimpse from the mountaintop, as it were. It provides a "big picture" with an orienting function. Whatever the metaphor, the generic foci are designed to assist trainees, students, faculty and practitioners alike, to better interpret the world of health care in general and behavioral health in particular. Because the foci are so broad, the areas nested within them may be substituted for others to be in accord with changing times, imperatives, funding arrangements, service delivery structures, and new players.

Imperatives-Driven Training Foci: A Classification Scheme

Finally, the scheme is proposed as a pedagogic base for training program redesign in professional education and training. It should be noted, however, that these foci do not themselves constitute a curriculum. As we have earlier noted, the foci are designed to serve as a substantive template for subsequent curriculum development and instructional design. They are also intended as a guide for ongoing competency development for practitioners working with the imperative of lifelong learning.

The domains constituting this model are presented in Figure 1. The first four domains listed in this figure are best seen as forming a pyramidal hierarchy from Domain 1, the normative base of the structure, up through Domain 4. Domains 5 and 6 stand separately on the edifice made up of the first four.

The first four domains are presented in order of *increasing specificity* (alternatively, decreasing scope of focus) upward from Domain 1, the most general and pervasive, to Domain 4. Each successive domain is subsumed by the growing structure beneath it. For example, from a pervasive values base (Level 1), up through the wide contextual backdrop of health care (Domain 2), and community organization (Domain 3), we reach the more focused world of integrated delivery systems (Domain 4). Nonetheless, the main point of this scheme is that the content of the first four domains are, collectively, to be considered as the core, irreducible, values-and-knowledge base essential at the macro level to the understanding of the world of health care. The macro base of the first four domains is also the prerequisite for informed professional practice of behavioral health in a changing world as treated in the foci nested within Domains 5 and 6.

Domains 5 and 6 provide for the "technologies" essential to the planning, delivery, monitoring and evaluation of (behavioral) health care. This is what was signified above by "informed professional practice." The acquisition of these primarily skills-oriented technologies depends significantly, as has been noted, on trainees' having been already exposed to the more foundational domains.

It is important to note that the individual foci within the six domains are not themselves professional competencies. They are too broad for that. For competencies to have value as part of an instructional design model, they must be functional. Within the proposed scheme, individual foci are actually general content areas containing potentially many discrete competencies. For curriculum development purposes, however, operational competencies of a far more specific kind are necessary. Such competencies may be derived from each of the content areas (foci) listed, but not directly.

Domain 1. Foundation Values Base

- Consumerist orientation
- Commitment to accountability to multiple stakeholders (including consumers, payors,and the public at large) by providers and care systems
- Commitment to the care of undeserved populations
- Respect for and awareness of issues of human diversity
- Commitment to a programmatic public health approach to services development in addition to the traditional focus on personal health

Domain 2. The Contextual Framework of Health and Human Services

- Fundamentals of health care organization, financing, and provision
- Association between providers and payers as well as health care organization and outcomes issues in (behavioral) health policy

Domain 3. Adjunctive Community Approaches

- Essentials of the community health, welfare, and organization
- The role of intersectional linkages in behavioral health services planning and provision
- Population-based approaches to services planning and provision, including disease state management approaches to prevention and consumer education
- A model for primary care in behavioral health

Domain 4. The Locus of Care: Integral Delivery Systems

- Structures and function of health services delivery systems
- Parameters of services contracting: capitation and the assumption of risk
- Professional role interdependancies
- Consumer-focused, interdisciplinary copllaboration
- Interplay of provider, fiscal, and human resources sub systems in the service of quality

Domain 5. Technologies for Health Services Planning and Delivery

- Essentials of services development, coordination, and continuity
- Advanced technologies for clinical management
- Consideration of family, work, and community in individual service planning

Domain 6. Technologies for Assessing and Managing Outcomes of Care

- Use of evidence based protocols for clinical assessment and management
- Quality assessment and management
- Program evaluation
- Use of data management systems for clinical, fiscal, and resources decision-making

Figure 1

Imperatives-Driven Training for Accountable Program Redesign

Specific competencies to be derived from foci from the core macro base (Domains 1 through 4) would, with few exceptions, be values- and knowledge-based. Conversely, we would expect that competencies derived from foci clustered within higher levels of our scheme would see more skills-based representation, since such foci are more specific, more instrumental.

To reiterate, the competencies that may be developed from the foci within Domain 1 would be largely values-based, with a leavening of some knowledge-based competencies. For Domain 2, they would be largely knowledge-based. For Domains 3 and 4, they would be mainly knowledge-based but with some skill-based competencies. And, given their relative specificity (more focused nature) in comparison with areas in the macro base, we would expect that those professional competencies developed from foci within the "technology" domains - would be largely skills-based.

The Next Challenge

The challenge is now at the door of the curriculum developers. The foci as presented do not prescribe any particular curriculum. Rather, they're to be used as a foundational base for professional competency development, the next step in an epicyclic process of curricular enhancement. The foci, as clustered within their particular domains, indicate the essential scope of the redesign of training programs and the enhancement of existing curricula in the name of accountability.

Program Redesign and Infrastructure Development: Finding Partners

The capacity of psychology to begin to assume a degree of control over the complex policy agenda of health service systems (to become, in other words, a player) will depend upon its success in influencing the respective agendas of a very diverse group of stakeholders. The issue of managed care carries a level of emotional intensity within organized psychology and other behavioral health professions such that change and the change-agent function can easily subverted or otherwise imperiled. Accordingly, stakeholder groups must be encouraged to keep the "eye on the prize." A seat at the health care policy table can only be earned by a manifest commitment to designing approaches to professional competency development which embrace accountability to consumers, payers, and other stakeholders as a key plank in the platform.

Collaboration in the Public Interest

Professional psychology must explore ways to participate in government-supported and, possibly, private foundation-supported multi-disciplinary funding programs. The profession must also collaborate with managed care organizations to identify sources for extramural funding of training initiatives.

Given the significant reduction of the impact of the three large institutional players – the federal government (particularly in its role in funding demonstration grants for training innovation), the professional associations, and the academic training programs – the health care industry itself must step up to contribute. Doing so will clearly advance the interest of the industry, resulting as it will in the development of an appropriately trained professional work force for behavioral health services. The profession, however, must commit itself to the development of complementary role functions. Accordingly, academic training programs and managed behavioral health care organizations must seek to collaborate on ways that will enhance the professional psychological training curriculum, including the sharing of expertise, collaborative research, and the provision of "real world" training opportunities within the industry.

Let's Not Forget Post-Licensure Training

Currently, post licensure professional competency development, in the form of continuing education, suffers from a number of deficiencies.

> CE activities are characterized by an ad hoc and disjointed approach.
> CE programs lack a unifying theme and are oriented to enhancing skills which psychologists already have for roles which are quickly diminishing.
> The process is driven by market forces: programs are typically targeted at the individual provider according to a kind of smorgasbord approach.
> Work force requirements rarely derive development of CE activities.

Two major entities have little if any influence on the process: the managed behavioral health care industry and organized psychology (whose once central role has increasingly been assumed by state associations).

Post-licensure training activities do not systematically build on, complement, or extend doctoral level preparation.

Accordingly, there is a critical need for the development of arrangements between doctoral and post-licensure training activities such that the current approach is replaced by a mode of organization in which doctoral and post-licensure training content and formats lie on a continuum. Doctoral level education and training deals necessarily with broad generic approaches while post-licensure has a more focused approach to preparation for these roles.

There needs to be a generic professional values base which transcends training level peculiarities and provides a foundation for both levels. Absent this, we are forced to contend with current phenomenon in which those post-licensure trainees seeking to acquire knowledge and skills associated with new forms of health services are forced, in essence, to "unlearn" values and attitudes that do not apply to the changing professional world. This is extremely problematic: it is at once grossly inefficient and generates intense opposition in practitioners who feel patronized and, in many instances, betrayed and abandoned. **To reassert: both doctoral and post-licensure training redesign must be predicated upon a common professional values base. This values base reflects the new contextual imperatives and the development of competencies deriving from an acknowledgment of the professional roles associated with the massive changes in the health care industry.**

The Role of Regulatory Bodies

It is clear that changes of the scope recommended here require a system approach. Accordingly, the equation for change must include collaborative responses by regulatory and quasi-regulatory agencies that are currently at the periphery of professional education and training – namely licensing, credentialing, and accrediting authorities.

Historically, a number of formal accountability mechanisms have been associated with professional responsibility and competence - albeit indirectly. These mechanisms include: regional and specialty accreditation of institutions and training programs, respectively; accreditation of institutions and facilities providing professional services; ethical codes of professional disciplines; discipline-specific practice standards or guidelines; federal and state regulations; and professional licensing and credentialing criteria. The very number of such mechanisms and their essentially self-regulatory nature have, however, precluded their being responsive to the marketplace and to the many forces that drive the health care system. As a consequence, the effective impact of these mechanisms has been slight.

Changes brought about by the evolution in health services financing and delivery give cause for questioning the true value of many of these regulatory and quasi-regulatory structures and processes that have, for years, been taken for granted by many in the professional community. For example, one could question the effectiveness of state licensure, its relationship to quality control and consumer protection, and its role in large, highly organized and inte-grated entities with their own credentialing and quality assurance activities. One may similarly question the value of specialty credentialing. One might also ask how organized psychology can assist both providers and organized delivery systems in effective credential evaluation and management.

Recent analyses by the Association of State and Provincial Psychology Boards (ASPPB) as well as the American Psychological Association Presidential Task Force on Education and Training for Work in Organized Delivery Systems (APA, 1996) focused on professional activities and knowledge bases required for current practice. While the ASPPB recommendations were more broad-based, the professional activities and knowledge bases were quite consistent. This suggests that revisions in the licensing exam would support the changes necessary for effective participation in the changing world of health care.

The increasing emphasis on documentation of specialty capabilities requires that professional psychology adapt credentialing mechanisms to the current environment. The APA's College of Professional Psychology has a useful part to play in this regard. The College's success, however, will depend on the development of additional proficiency areas and on the extent to which the service delivery system accepts its certification products as evidence of relevant professional competencies.

It is through a process of review and negotiation between representatives of such entities, together with those from academic and internship training programs, consumers and the service delivery system, that an enduring template for the redesign for accountable education and training must be written. Training programs, health plans, practitioners, and consumers all will be forced to contend — albeit, in very different ways — disturbing deficiencies in professional competencies among behavioral health practitioners absent a confrontation of this shortfall by the relevant agencies and organizations. At the same time, it will be the community of empowered consumers and purchasers in their demands for outcomes management who will ultimately drive system accountability in behavioral health care. There is a corresponding need for the training and regulatory bodies within the behavioral health disciplines to be more effectively integrated with service delivery systems and their accountability requirements. At the same time, practitioners who increasingly participate in organized care settings must demonstrate the values and behaviors that drive both professional service and marketplace accountability.

Infrastructure Development: A Final Note

The only effective means for dealing with the current challenges to members of the psychological profession and threats to quality in behavioral health services would seem to be through the establishment of collaborative relationships among behavioral health training programs, the behavioral health care services industry, relevant governmental and regulatory agencies, and consumer advocacy groups. This would help ensure accountability for program redesign. Organized psychology could usefully seek the input of individuals familiar with the industry and engaged in interdisciplinary study of training and service delivery (Troy, 1997) in order to create additional opportunities for such collaboration.

Professional associations would also do well to consider underwriting with the assistance of the federal government and private foundations, the establishment of training resource entities to assist training programs in the difficult and protracted process of program redesign, and curricular enhancement. Absent such a venture, current resources and contingencies likely do not permit wholesale departures from the traditional nature and scope of education and training in behavioral health.

The successful development of such operational linkages, combined with a refocusing of professional education and training in the interest of the consumer and treatment outcomes, will pose significant challenges to all parties, unused as they are to interdependent roles. It is a process that will be entered into cautiously, will be characterized by diversity of arrangements, and will take time. It is, however, a process that must, ultimately, be confronted. The challenge of developing innovative professional training models that are responsive to the new imperatives, and of integrating necessary changes within existing models, requires the diffusion of multiple innovations within a very large, multifaceted community involving institutions as well as organizations. Such a process is fraught with obstacles - structural and operational – and, if achieved at all, requires strategic approaches for the very long haul.

REFERENCES

American Psychological Association (1996, December). *Presidential Task Force on Education and Training for Work in Organized Delivery Systems.* Unpublished report presented to the Board of Professional Affairs.

Beigel, A. (1994, June). *The challenges facing psychiatric education in the changing health care and medical education environment.* Center for Mental Health Services (Substance Abuse and Mental Health Services Administration). Unpublished report.

Broskowski, A. T. (1995). The evolution of health care: Implications for the training and careers of psychology. *Professional Psychology: Research and Practice*, 26(2), 156-162.

Cummings, N. A. (1996). The resocialization of behavioral healthcare practice. In N. A. Cummings, M. S. Pallak, & J. L. Cummings (Eds.), *Surviving the demise of solo practice: Mental health practitioners prospering in the era of managed care.* Madison, CT: Psychosocial Press.

Shueman, S. A., Troy, W. G., & Mayhugh, S. L. (Eds.) (1994). *Managed behavioral health care: An industry perspective.* Springfield, IL: Charles C. Thomas.

Troy, W. G. (1994). Developing and improving professional competencies. In S. A. Shueman, W. G. Troy, & S. L. Mayhugh (Eds.), *Managed behavioral health care: An industry perspective*, 168-188.

Troy, W. G. (1997). Training the trainees: The new imperatives. *Administration and Policy in Mental Health*, 25(1), 27-35.

Troy, W. G., & Shueman, S. A. (1996). Program redesign for graduate training in professional psychology: The road to accountability in a changing profession world. In N. A. Cummings, M. S. Pallak, & J. L. Cummings (Eds.) *Surviving the demise of solo practice: Mental health practitioners prospering in the era of managed care.* Madison, CT: Psychosocial Press.

Discussion of Troy:

Continuing Education: Opportunities for Enhanced Family Relations

Victoria Follette
University of Nevada, Reno

A model for the training of the next wave of psychologists to work in the managed care setting is essential. At the same time, education regarding behavioral managed healthcare is also needed for existing practitioners. Troy (2000) addresses some of the post licensure education needs in his chapter on curriculum restructuring. However, more should be said on the relationship factors that might impede the collaboration of academics and practitioners on these matters. Much has been written about the relation of science to practice and the continued need for the strengthening of the essential bond between these two domains. Less has been said regarding how this relates to the role of the academy in the continuing education of existing practitioners. In this rapidly changing era, it is increasingly important for those in the academy to forge an alliance with practitioners that enhances the potential of both groups to thrive in the years ahead.

The disruption in the relationship between the two groups is an interesting one to consider. An examination of the interactions between members of the academy and practitioners in the "real world" suggests that some therapy is in order. A contextual or systemic therapy model is useful in understanding the issues and potential solutions. Using the analogy of family relationships provides some interesting comparisons. Remembering that most current practitioners were in fact educated in fairly traditional academic settings, the often-contentious relations that have emerged are particularly troubling. To

Integrated Behavioral Healthcare: Positioning Mental Health Practice with Medical/Surgical Practice

continue the analogy, it is not unlike children who have left the family business to pursue other dreams. Both sides seem to feel disillusioned with the lack of understanding shown by the other for their current plights. An examination of the problem may suggest some possible remedies.

A thorough contextual analysis requires an assessment of the individual participants, the relationships between them, and the contexts in which they exist. At an individual level, both private practitioners and academicians have a number of strengths. Both have demonstrated cognitive and emotional capabilities. Certainly, surviving the rigors of graduate school is a testament not only to intellectual capacity but also the ability to endure periods of prolonged stress. Additionally, both groups are comprised of individuals who have dedicated themselves to alleviating human suffering. While the form this work takes can vary significantly, the function remains essentially the same.

While there is some interaction between the two groups, both have a number of interactions with other groups on a more regular basis. Client involvement is central to both groups. Even those academics involved in work that is more basic than applied are generally working on problems related to clinical issues. Both groups are involved in work directed toward advancing our ability to provide efficacious treatment. Given the complexity of the majority of clinical problems, collaboration is essential.

Historically private practitioners have been more likely to interact with third party payers, frequently managed care companies, and academics have worked with government funding agencies. However, increasingly these two external systems have similar goals and interests. The recent support of federal agencies for the development of practice guidelines is an excellent example of the intersecting goals of the two groups. Another area of shared interest, is the emphasis on accountability that is common to both groups of funding sources. Thus, there is more than ever an opportunity for the development of a mutuality that would benefit both members of the academy and the practice community. Given this basic premise, how can these two groups that have often found themselves in conflict work to enhance their relationship.

As any well-educated family therapist knows, communication is the sine qua non of good relationships. However, practitioners and academics seem to rarely have a forum for interaction about these issues. Private practitioners have a wealth of experience in dealing with the daily exigencies of providing care to a diverse client population. These practitioners are not able to use complicated and specific exclusion and inclusion criteria for participation in their treatment programs. Rather, they must deal with clients as they present, often with multiple and complex problems. Thus, it behooves the academic community to learn more from the practice community about typical patterns of presenting complaints and the specific needs that practitioners face in regard to intervention with those clients. Academics also have something to bring to the table in this regard. The nature of our daily work necessitates that we remain current about the newest innovations in assessment and treatment. Academics also have a central role in the development and implementation of strategies for program evaluation. We need more forums, such as the Nevada conference, in which these two groups can interact about issues related to the assessment and delivery of treatment. Increasingly, we have a shared agenda of survival in a more demanding environment and developing a collaborative stance will enhance the functioning both groups.

There are a number of areas of training that the academy can address. Providing education about physical health care and its interactions with psychological processes will assist those working in these new arenas. Information on program evaluation as well as single subject design will also augment the ability of all to be active participants in this new context. More research is needed on effective supervision of providers without doctoral training. Treatment acceptability and assessment of outcomes will be key issues and there is a significant increase in the data on these topics that has been published in recent years. Also providers need education about some of the newer technologies, such as Dialectical Behavior Therapy (Linehan, 1993). DBT is an excellent example of a treatment that may appear expensive on the face of it. However, research has demonstrated decreased costs associated with fewer numbers of hospitalizations. Additionally, while the treatment is quite intensive it is also effective in the long run, leading to decreases in demand for services over time.

A contextual analysis should also consider an awareness of the larger societal framework in which these systems are imbedded. As Troy indicates, there is a danger that specialized populations will be neglected as health care becomes increasingly privatized. Practitioners and academics need to work together to influence managed care policy in relation to developing inclusive programs. They can play an essential role in serving as a conscience in developing guidelines that address the needs of the poor and minorities. Other groups whose requirements have not always been adequately addressed are the elderly and women. The needs of the chronically mentally ill must also be remembered in evolving principles for comprehensive treatment. Lessons from the community mental health care systems of the 1960's can provide some direction. Moreover, those with CMI can also be significant users of physical health care resources. Demonstrating that attention to psychological problems can result in cost savings in the medical arena can provide the impetus for directing funds toward comprehensive treatment plans. Integrated delivery of services is an advantage for individuals and the culture. We have the opportunity and the ability to demonstrate the economic advantage of these comprehensive programs.

In summary, it is not only important to train psychologists for the future but also to address post licensure training. No group can simply demand a seat at the table as issues related to integrated health care are addressed. Rather we must earn it by demonstrating our unique talents and abilities to contribute to the overall system. Some have discussed the developing crisis that integrated managed care brings. While there is danger inherent in these changes there is also opportunity. There is an opportunity to forge a new alliance that moves beyond old rivalries with a resulting rapprochement between the practice and academic communities. More importantly, we have the opportunity to work within the system to ensure that the highest level of care is provided. We can do this not only because it is right but also because we can demonstrate the efficacy of such care in leading to decreased costs and enhanced physical and psychological outcomes. The opportunities are many and varied. Rather than viewing the changes as dangerous and limiting our opportunities, we can serve as leaders in taking both doctoral and post licensure training to the next phase in the evolution of psychology.

REFERENCES

Linehan, M. M. (1993). *Cognitive-Behavioral Treatment of Borderline Personality Disorder.* New York: Guilford Press.

CHAPTER

Managed Care:
Implications for Clinical Training

Michael S. Pallak, Ph,.D.
Foundation for Behavioral Health

Integrated Behavioral Healthcare: Positioning Mental Health Practice with Medical/Surgical Practice

The relatively rapid evolution and re-organization of services under managed health and mental health care has left traditional clinical and service provider training well behind the needs of the current mental health service delivery system. Graduate curricula have never been known for rapid response to changing external environments for several understandable reasons (below). Yet the gap in orientation between organized mental health services systems nationally and traditional training systems seems greater now than in the past and continues to widen. Mental health providers are faced with dramatically different orientations, roles, requirements and service demands in managed systems of care for which there has been little consideration in most graduate training systems. In addition, the organization of health and mental health care toward greater efficiency and cost-effectiveness underscores the perception that there is an oversupply of available providers. Such a picture makes salient the need for shifts in training that enable providers, and especially new providers, to fit more effectively into roles in a system of care for which they have had little hands-on preparation.

Discussions of change needed in graduate training curricula are necessarily general. It is difficult to characterize the graduate training system in any great scholarly detail given the great variety in graduate programs, as even a cursory look at various compendiums of programs underscores. Similarly, it is difficult to characterize the mental health (and health) service system even in terms of "managed care" in part because "managed care" means a variety of care systems and approaches. Thus any specific training program, service system or service provider may point to any number of exceptions to the necessarily general summary here. It is useful to underscore this point because many colleagues, reluctant to address these issues, have often pointed out that "their" training program doesn't fit these generalizations and that managed care is only the latest aberration ("forced by cost-cutting efforts") from the traditional clinical training believed to be fundamental to clinical work.

ASPECTS OF TRAINING PROGRAMS

In psychology, as in other provider training programs, the array of clinical programs represents differing emphases and foci. Training programs in traditional academic settings emphasize a research orientation along with pre-doctoral practice, traineeship and a pre- or post-doctoral internship experience. Academic based programs have an emphasis upon mastery of a body of knowledge with the goal of preparing the Ph.D. student to make independent scholarly contributions. Academic preparation takes place in formal coursework, formal seminars, research groups, and so forth. Depending on geographic locale, graduate students may be exposed to academic based clinics, typically serving academic populations, to more public populations in the form of clinics or CMHCs or, depending on locale, to hospital or VA patient populations, etc. Training and supervision takes place in the facility conducted by providers on-site. Overall responsibility for clinical development of students may remain with an academic based training director and with faculty in the home department.

Relative to traditional academically based programs, professional schools of psychology tend to focus on service provision with clients or patients much earlier and to a greater extent as part of the training experience. Often the process begins with a placement in a service or agency setting with the first year student providing volunteer services as a process of familiarization with issues outside the more formal academic course track. Coursework is often provided by an array of "core" and adjunct faculty (with varying contractually specified teaching loads) who may also supervise a student. In addition, as the student progresses to more hands-on clinical work and receives supervision at the placement site, designated faculty serve as liaison to the placement, monitor student progress, coordinate evaluations of progress and provide additional mentoring. The overall clinical training process is coordinated by a designated training director assisted by clinical faculty committees. In urban areas, students receive a substantial amount of experience in the public mental health system such as CMHCs and other components within the public system as well as with hospitals, clinics, etc..

Both types of training systems, of course, are structured, reinforced, and held accountable not only by the consensus of the faculty, but also by various accreditation standards enacted and evaluated by various groups as well by the implications of various state licensing requirements. While traditional training models may differ in emphasis between more academic and research goals on the one hand or more patient oriented experience and service provision on the other, both continue a focus upon long term treatment with a single patient. Clinical training and development are influenced by the implicit and explicit clinical model or orientation embedded in the training system by faculty, by the orientations of on-site supervisors, case conference directors, training supervisors, training directors, etc.

In short, the graduate training process is, in part, a socialization process with certain elements of "received wisdom" as the groundwork for the future provider's orientation, as is true in any training system in any profession. Although programs may vary, training remains oriented to direct clinical service that provides service to one patient at a time (often, implicitly looking toward futures in solo private practice) with long term treatment as the treatment orientation.

Our collective problem is that the body of traditional received clinical wisdom summarized here may not enable new providers to make the transition into a very different professional and services environment produced in part by the rapid advent of managed care. In addition, the majority of faculty, training supervisors, etc. by and large, have little experience with managed care systems and thereby have difficulty playing a leadership role in meeting the implications of managed care systems for the training of future providers. Training programs in psychology rarely incorporate the perspective of providing treatment within a service system where a number of aspects of service provision need coordination and follow-up. Similarly, psychologists rarely see their service provision either as a part of an overall service system or as part of a system that was derived from primary medical services models. Lacking a system perspective in general, the field has not moved to develop more effective approaches to care or to mental health policy or to public policy more generally. As a result, few of our colleagues understand the constraints imposed by the acute care hospital model that substantially biased medical and mental health service provision at least until the advent of managed care. Although the field has developed robust programs in health psychology, the perspectives of health care policy and health care systems are rarely reflected within the formal curriculum in psychology. Thus as a field, and as a training system, psychology has been passive in incorporating a curriculum revision process that would intellectually invigorate clinical training and align training systems with the implications of managed care more effectively.

Aspects of Managed Care Service Systems

The past fee-for-service (ffs) system was geared to an individual provider with a single patient, often for very long episodes of care. Lengthy, long-term episodes of care were considered the customary "gold" standard of care. On the one hand, insurance carriers were willing to carve out mental health services to ffs providers but usually with great limitations upon reimbursable benefits that could apply. Carriers were willing to "carve-out" services to specialty mental health providers because mental conditions were described as too ill-defined to be treated in the medical or primary care system. The solo provider was largely unaccountable, for a time, for the services rendered as long as the service provided fit benefit criteria (the attempts to manage costs by benefit design failed however). Within the several mental health provider communities this was the predominant service orientation and reimbursement model and this model was largely reflected within the clinical training system.

In parallel, many health care systems evolved toward an HMO staff model in which patients received services at a specific site or within a network of sites as expansion took place. Mental health services were often provided by mental health specialists attached to the HMO, or working in staff positions within the HMO, often upon referral by or in coordination with primary care providers.

Relatively more recently, the high cost of inpatient psychiatric care (especially for adolescents) and to a lesser and more complex extent, the advent of medication strategies for non-institutional maintenance led to a major shift away from inpatient care. Mounting evidence suggested that appropriate outpatient support could forestall lengthy inpatient stays and reinforced managed care efforts to implement effective non-inpatient treatment alternatives. At this point the business of managing care shifted the orientation in the private sector away from reliance upon a service delivery model composed only of inpatient and solo practitioner care options toward a staff model for mental health service (similar to HMOs) and then to networks of providers and group practices. In light of these alternatives, managed care companies could provide contracts that often assumed the cost-risk for both inpatient and outpatient care for a fixed or capitated fee per covered person per year.

Capitation financing provided some incentive for early strategies of demand management or prevention with regard to risky behaviors such as smoking, drug abuse, workplace and marital stress, etc. As evolution continued in managed care, many companies shifted to an amalgam of service and financing strategies by forming in-house provider networks and/or subcontracting for services with group practice organizations or preferred provider network organizations for defined services to a defined population at capitated rates. Within the preferred provider network as with other subcontractors, the overhead costs of maintaining an office or facility are assumed by the office based preferred providers who contracted to provide services under capitated reimbursement rates in return for preference in patient referrals.

Managed care also continued to evolve toward an integrated service delivery system, in which a patient might present to an inpatient facility or to an emergency room but remain only until stabilized and then be referred to a less intensive service program within the system. In this example, the patient may remain for a day or two (depending on severity) for assessment, diagnosis, stabilization and then be "stepped down" to a less intensive day treatment program, partial hospitalization, or appropriate outpatient care.

In general, given the availability of these additional organized and clinically effective treatment options, the need for very expensive inpatient stays dropped as a matter of routine. The evolution from a mental health treatment system that relied on inpatient treatment and office based outpatient treatment as the only treatment options represented large cost savings by providing effective treatment options that were less expensive than long stay inpatient treatment. These savings were more than large enough to finance these new treatment options including a robust managed outpatient treatment system with an overall financial picture that also included predictable profit margins.

Implicit and Explicit Assumptions in Managed Mental Health Care

Allowing for this general description, several aspects of managed care are worth pointing out. The first is that the provider is accountable for the treatment provided, i.e., a third entity is involved in authorizing treatment, setting goals and in helping establish limits regarding intensity and duration of treatment. Thus providers are required prospectively to demonstrate that a particular patient meets clinically derived criteria for intensity or duration of care. Providers are required to specify a treatment plan with specific goals and a discharge plan when those treatment goals are met.

More importantly, when the patient's clinical condition varies from the treatment guides or norms, the provider is required to describe the manner of the variation and to justify why more intense or longer treatment may be required to return the patient to some previous level of functioning. Within integrated systems of care, treatment decisions to "step up" treatment (moving the patient to a more intense level of treatment) or to "step down" treatment, or to discharge the patient from treatment, require appropriate documentation. Discharge planning as well as treatment planning are an integrated part of service provision.

As part of the treatment authorization and treatment goals process, the steps involved in assessment, treatment and discharge planning, and to a more, or less, intense level of treatment, each require wording in very specific symptom or behavioral terms rather than in more global terms such as "reduce anxiety or tension". The advantage is that a much more quantifiable clinical record is available to justify treatment, as well as treatment change, and thereby a record potentially is available for aggregation and evaluation of more quantifiable data as a result.

A second explicit concept that varies from traditional service orientations is that of "restoration of function" as opposed to "cure", as others have eloquently elaborated (cf. Cummings, Pallak, Dorken & Henke, 1992; Cummings & Sayama, 1995). This conceptual system represents a fundamentally different view of presentation of symptoms, clinical processes and treatment goals when contrasted to the generic long-term treatment training in the typical graduate curriculum. Thus patients present when coping mechanisms are no longer adequate to handle the patient's issues. The focus of treatment is then on restoration of function by enhancing coping skills to meet those problems rather than on long-term strategies for personality change. Psychodynamics, in this view, provide a "roadmap" and an orientation by which to help gauge the patient's status and progress clinically without automatically or necessarily involving long term episodes of care that either may not be needed or may be counter-productive clinically.

Thus a third perspective is that patients' may not need or want (or be ready for the work of) traditional long-term oriented treatment, but rather may seek help to solve a particular problem or to resolve a particular crisis. Thus patients who opt out of treatment after one, two or three sessions may represent an effective treatment episode for that patient's problem or crisis rather than a treatment "failure" (as might be assumed, often, in a long-term orientation). Similarly, when the patient returns to treatment or services when the next crisis occurs, one would not assume a failure of previous treatment since the smart thing for the patient is a return to treatment when necessary. As a result, the first treatment session is critical in terms of rapid assessment and maximum help to the patient in contrast to more traditional long-term or generic approaches.

A fourth perspective is that rapid effective initial assessment, triage, and patient-provider matching is critical in making treatment and service provision both clinically effective and cost effective. Successful and effective treatment in managed mental health is represented by those models of service provision that are clinically driven by patient needs rather than by preconceived notions of what appropriate treatment ought to be or by a particular theoretical or clinical orientation. Similarly, treatment is determined by the patient's clinical need rather than determined by benefit design or benefit limits. Treatment tailored to the patient's clinical needs has been amenable also to the establishment of empirical guides, norms, or benchmarks that enable effective matching of treatment resources (intensity, duration, etc.) to patient need, on the average. These empirically derived guides help to make treatment more efficient and represent a basis by which to identify patients who fall outside the average or usual pattern, thereby enabling more efficient and earlier intervention than might otherwise occur. As a result, providers can identify in advance the types of presenting problems that can be addressed more rapidly and effectively by alternative behavioral, cognitive, psychodynamic, family systems, and/or medication strategies. In short, rather than unfolding a pre-conceived (usually long term) treatment approach, an eclectic approach assumes that one type of treatment strategy does not fit all types of patients and clinical issues.

A fifth perspective is that as the clinical underpinnings for managed care continue to develop an evidence base, it has also become clear that not all service provision must be rendered by a doctoral level provider for all patients. Rather, doctoral providers may be part of treatment teams in which non-doctoral providers render services under protocols supervised by doctoral level providers. The analogy, as presented elsewhere in this volume, is developing in primary care where the primary care treatment team may include a physician, a psychologist, a social worker, family counselor, etc. involved in developing appropriate care for the patient much of which may not require the physician's direct efforts other than as an overall supervisor for the treatment team for that patient. Managed care systems are also more likely to make clinically effective use of group therapy approaches especially for substance abuse. These may often be conducted by non-doctoral providers under overall supervision and coordination of doctoral staff. This flexibility in approaches to treatment strategies ensures greater access to more appropriate care for patients across a range of clinical issues.

A sixth perspective involves the implications of working in an organized system of care. In general, mental health service provider training provides little exposure to issues of operating successfully in an organization, or about the social psychological aspects of human functioning in organizations. Very often providers who deal with managed care report feeling enmeshed in a bureaucracy and feeling that they have little ability or experience to make sense out of organizational priorities, procedures, vulnerabilities or to role-play where representatives of the organization have their priorities. A large part of the frustration involves the transition from solo practice orientations that do not fit readily into systems that rely on treatment planning and case management in general (ideally the case manager follows the course of treatment and ensures coordination with other treatment resources). As a consequence, the frustration, sense of powerlessness, and psychological gap between provider, the case manager and the organization may widen, especially for providers with a solo practice and long term treatment orientation. Equally importantly, providers with little orientation to issues of systems of care are unlikely to assume positions of leadership within those systems of care. For example, provider experience within managed care enables new avenues for applying the wisdom of one's background in these new managed care situations. With appropriate experience, providers may also play roles as directors of various operations such as intake processing, clinical case management, clinical supervision, quality assurance, or quality improvement operations where a substantive clinical perspective is valuable. Similarly, providers have the opportunity to move into senior management roles regarding clinical operations, as well as senior roles in other managerial aspects of the organized system of care. In general, clinically informed management makes more effective managerial decisions. As yet the training system provides little orientation that would be helpful in taking advantage of these opportunities to make further use of clinical experience.

TRAINING CURRICULUM EVOLUTION: NEXT STEPS

Since there are as yet only a few graduate programs at best grappling with these issues, the foregoing represents themes regarding a substantially changed service provision world that can be addressed by an evolutionary process in clinical training. Of course, these issues are often bound up with the inertia and resistance to change common to any social system faced with greatly changed external circumstances, and graduate programs are no different. The challenge for training programs is to initiate a process that develops more effective training for providers by delineating and shaping core clinical content that translates to new, more effective, orientations and practice approaches that maximize clinical benefit for patients. Of necessity, some traditional content will have to receive either less attention or be translated into less time consuming formats.

A proposed series of course modules and training experiences is summarized here. In general, these are designed to meet the gaps or holes in graduate clinical training experience identified by a substantial number of providers who have made an effective transition into managed care. In addition, these experiences and approaches are also derived from the extensive two year ongoing post-doctoral training, re-training and supervision program that was developed by Nick Cummings as part of the Hawaii Project (Cummings, Pallak, Dorken & Henke, 1992) and continued to be developed at American Biodyne, Inc.

The goal of the staff training program was to facilitate a shift in clinical orientation to brief treatment when clinically appropriate, and to understand the conditions under which brief treatment was clinically appropriate and effective. Training also included experience in each of the components necessary for effective managed mental health care. That training program continued to develop as we found that it was far more difficult for more senior traditionally trained clinicians to make the transition to the managed care approaches discussed here. We found that relatively new clinicians made the transition more easily, thereby underscoring the need for exposure to these approaches as part of the pre-doctoral graduate training experience.

In light of the often heavily structured traditional academic course sequence that is typical of training programs, the proposed experiences may be unfolded in a much more flexible format in terms of "modules" and in terms of ongoing pro-seminars, weekend classes, case conferences and case supervision. The more flexible format is useful as an experience more closely akin to the treatment team and multi-professional experiences typical of the managed service provision world and may contrast to the more traditional, scholarly oriented semester long graduate course. Hopefully this perspective forestalls some of the expected groans on the part of graduate students and faculty about adding more courses to an already substantial course load.

Foundation: History and Systems of Health and Mental Health Care

This course module traces the development of health and mental health policy and services in this century in both public and private sectors. The perspectives developed include the shift in policy assumptions and the consequences for mental health services and for provider orientation. These include societal assumptions and perspectives for organization and financing of services which led to reliance on the acute care model evolved from acute care hospitals as the paradigm for mental health service. In contrast, the more public health orientation developed population based perspectives regarding longer term health issues. The shift from long term inpatient mental hospitalization in the latter half of the century and the development of the CMHC movement are developed as a major precursor of current managed mental health care. Contrasts, using a small number of case examples, between traditional generic treatment approaches and managed care approaches are developed with examples drawn from both private and public sectors.

Comment: The goals of this module include an understanding of mental health services in the context of overall health policy and in the context of an overall system with multiple components involving varying degrees of coordination and fragmentation. A second goal is familiarization with managed care as a clinically viable approach to service provision and patient care. A third goal is an understanding of accountability on the part of the service system, and on the service provider balanced by an evidence-based analysis of traditional and managed care approaches. Participants are encouraged to develop an orientation that both contrasts, compares and integrates these approaches as an orientation to their own clinical orientation. While the course is geared for first year students, students at any level should benefit since this material is rarely part of the perspective in graduate training.

Managed Mental Health and Behavioral Health Care

This module builds upon the former by presenting a systematic analysis of the evolution of managed care approaches, systems, service delivery processes and focus on patient outcomes. Specific emphases include organizational and clinical issues faced by clinical administrators, financing and managerial staff, and treatment providers (and treatment teams) in ensuring effective services. In particular, case examples that illustrate issues and processes in rapid assessment, treatment planning, discharge planning, follow-up and outcome assessment in managed care are incorporated and contrasted with traditional long term care approaches. Examples in both the public and private sector are included in order to illustrate differing issues in both systems including provider orientation, the role of rehab services and coordination with families and social services. Finally, public sector issues in transitioning to managed care systems are developed with an eye toward the difficulty of translating approaches derived from a private care system to the public system responsible for services to a more clinically complex and often more culturally diverse population.

Comment: The goals for participants include a thorough familiarization with the nomenclature and perspectives within managed care. A second goal is an appreciation of the markedly different clinical perspective regarding patient problems, the treatment process and treatment goals represented by managed care The third goal is an understanding of the processes relating to accountability for patient treatment. The fourth goal is an understanding of the dilemmas facing the public mental health system as that system begins to grapple slowly with implementation of managed care procedures. The fifth goal is an understanding of the current systems regarding mental health as a response to meet societal and patient needs rather than as an evidence based logically derived entity. Finally, case examples reinforce the value of brief treatment and coordinated care as tools in meeting patient needs.

Brief Treatment: Maximizing Patient Progress

This module is probably the most critical in the evolving training curriculum. Ideally it should be available to participants throughout the graduate experience after the first year and the foundational course above. The format should be that of an ongoing case conference seminar and may be sectioned for more and less advance students. The module is developed to review the literature regarding rapid assessment and brief treatment in terms of combinations of patient variables (presenting problems, clinical needs, implicit resistance), provider variables (rapid establishment of therapeutic bond) with an eclectic view of alternative treatment approaches. Dependent upon assessment of patient needs, behavioral, cognitive, family systems, psychodynamic, problem-solving, etc. approaches may be most effective in the shortest time, consistent with the goal of maximizing treatment impact. In addition, illustrations of group treatment approaches and the conditions under which group therapy is appropriate in managed care is incorporated. Most importantly, traditional treatment approaches are contrasted with brief treatment approaches in terms of treatment goals based upon patient need, motivation and patient restoration of function.

A significant component of this module is an ongoing case conference and treatment supervision format that illustrates brief treatment strategies. Participants regardless of their practice, traineeship or internship placement setting should be expected to make periodic case presentations and to formulate alternative brief treatment and traditional treatment approaches. Presentations and case examples may be drawn from treatment and supervisory settings that may be long-term in orientation and may not be amenable to brief treatment interventions in practice. Participants should be expected to provide periodic case follow-up and update presentations and to discuss patient progress from both perspectives.

Comment: The goal for participants is to develop the clinical acumen necessary to see a specific case (other case presentations) and an array of cases from multiple perspectives regarding clinical assumptions and case formulation. A critical goal is that of developing the perspectives that permit rapid assessment in terms of an eclectic outlook about treatment alternatives and to make use of clinical information in order to gauge patient progress and outcome. Finally, participants should develop alternative perspectives regarding "termination" issues and issues of re-presentation for further treatment. Ideally participants begin implementing brief treatment techniques in their own clinical efforts.

Professional Issues Seminar (a revised "pro-sem")

The seminar is designed to provide a flexible ongoing forum for discussion of managed care and professional issues throughout the training experience. The pro-seminar format is familiar to most training programs and usually meets twice per month in a 2 hour block of time. The format includes presentations by, and discussions with, managed care providers, staff, managers, directors of various managed care operations, public mental health officials, and other relevant senior officials. These ongoing discussions are designed to provide participants with an orientation to problems, perspectives, and issues faced in the external service provision organization on an everyday basis. In addition, presentations and examples that illustrate coordination between primary care, mental health and behavioral health care should be included.

Comment: The goal of the pro-sem is to foster an appreciation of the problems faced in a managed care and public mental health system on an operational basis. Similarly, participants are exposed to issues and operating functions in an organization that are central to managed care but are rarely brought into focus in the more traditional clinical graduate sequence. As a result, the pro-sem format should foster the development of an organizational perspective and the coordination of information within an organization necessary for a comprehensive treatment and service delivery system.

Ideally the format also fosters discussions about the manner in which participants and the academic program may assist managed care in terms of services evaluation, re-training, etc. and develop a sense of common ground in areas of mutual interest.

From Managed Care to Integrated Delivery Systems

This module develops general clinical, behavioral health and service delivery issues involved in the effective integration of services from crisis, emergency room, inpatient, partial hospitalization, day treatment, residential treatment, intensive outpatient, outpatient, rehabilitation services, follow-up, community-based and social services. Examples are drawn from primary medical settings as well as from public and private mental health settings. Problems faced in secondary service settings such as skilled nursing facilities (recovery, nursing home, etc.) are included. Additional perspectives include (a) the delivery of services in multi-cultural and ethnically diverse settings; (b) effective case management and coordination of information within service delivery systems; (c) the integration of multi-disciplinary treatment teams and treatment approaches; (d) integration of mental health, behavioral health with primary care and medication strategies; and of course (e) "medical cost offset" — the effect of psychologically based interventions on medical services utilization especially for patients with chronic medical conditions.

Comment: The goal is a more hands-on development of a system and organizational perspective regarding the coordination of services for patient progress. A second goal is a greater familiarization with components of service delivery and their integration than traditional provider training may provide. The third goal is a much fuller understanding of the value of integrated primary and mental health care in providing more effective treatment and in managing overall health and mental health costs in a defined population.

Managed Care: Program Evaluation, Information Systems and Information Integration, Research Strategies and Outcomes Evaluation

This module is designed to foster both a program focus and a more traditional patient focus by contrasting and then integrating three often disparate perspectives:

1. Program evaluation in terms of evaluating program effectiveness in providing services to a population defined by regulation, legislation or contract negotiations. This component includes issues of quality improvement as well as program improvement and the development of estimates of incidence and prevalence in the population served. The focus is upon evidence-based strategies to meet program goals in terms of access, utilization and program evolution to enhance service provision.

2. Information utilization in terms of a common set of indices useful for clinical assessment, triage, treatment planning, treatment process evaluation, treatment discharge and follow-up by which to inform clinical decision-making. The module emphasizes strategies of data collection, utilization of software systems (from charts to on-line aggregation), data summary and interpretation for multiple purposes including clinical, program, outcome, service utili-

zation, financial and organizational functioning. The module develops strategies for development of clinical norms, guidelines, and clinical pathways in the service of clinical and managerial decision-making.

3. Outcomes measurement and evaluation in terms of strategies and data by which to assess (and document) patient progress in response to treatment and services. Available evidence-based tools for outcomes assessment are reviewed and presented in the context of closing the loop from previous quality assurance and quality improvement approaches to evaluating whether the services provided resulted in improved patient status. Research strategies in the ongoing world of treatment provision are discussed in the context of overall research design issues. Retrospective and prospective case study techniques are examined as a tool by which to assess program functioning, information needs and changes in patient-family functioning.

Implications for Departments and Training Programs

The proposed modules above are designed to provide a minimum content and experience core that balances traditional training and to provide a basis for thinking about provider roles in a broader context. There are clearly additional modules that one might wish to include especially a module dealing with social psychology in terms of attitude change, communication processes, group and organizational dynamics and resistance to change. Since one tendency in some departments will be to react by pointing out the fact that since the current "course A" may have features about "topic B" in "module X" there may be little need for curriculum evolution. As a result, it is important to emphasize the overall thematic perspective represented here: successful clinically driven managed care (and unless clinically driven, managed care will be ultimately unsuccessful) necessitates a fundamentally different orientation, one that contrasts sharply to traditional views of the clinical process represented in training programs.

Tempering this resistance to this set of issues is the realization that these issues are similar to basic social science approaches in this arena that would ask "under which conditions, assumptions and processes, for which patients, may patient benefit be maximized in terms of restoration of function?" Casting these issues in this framework structures the discussion of these issues into an evidence-based perspective with regard to the underpinnings for clinical services and clinical management.

An additional theme is that of the national transition from public mental health care as generic treatment (increasingly narrowed to the severely and persistently mentally ill) to some form of managed care strategy. The transition represents a profound re-orientation for public mental health at all levels with major opportunities for providers who understand managed care to assist that transition process.

A shift to incorporate managed care perspectives into clinical training offers several problems and opportunities for departments and clinical training programs. One problem is that the need for a substantial amount of clinical training in managed care implies that the training program has training faculty and training supervisors experienced in managed care. The second is that successful training implies training in managed care systems and sites, both public and private, along with on-site experience in multi-disciplinary treatment team settings (cf. Dorken & Pallak, 1994). Not only will programs need to consider comprehensive integration of managed care perspectives in the training sequence, but also programs will need to consider their role as a training institution in relation to managed health and mental health care.

There are several roles that would be helpful, constructive and would facilitate closer substantive roles in relation to managed care organizations. For example, the business of managed care is unlikely to play a role in supporting training due to expense and the impact on the bottom line of business operations. As a field, however, our strong suit has always been our collective capacity to integrate research and evidence-based literature and to draw implications for patient treatment. At present, the business of managed care views the process of upgrading substantive knowledge as the responsibility of the provider and not that of the business. Thus training departments and programs have a role in providing research and literature integration in the service of improving the managed mental health "product" marketed by the business entity.

A second major role, of course, is represented by the innate capacity of departments and training programs to provide research and evaluation services in the service of developing "best practices," evidence-based clinical norms, guidelines, clinical pathways and evidence-based treatment interventions. Finally departments and training programs are in a position to develop comprehensive patient and family outcome assessment strategies and services in an ongoing process of improving clinical services and clinical decision-making. Of course much of that research as yet will be conducted as retrospective case studies since the managed care business entity will not or can not undertake the legal and ethical exposure attendant upon unfolding more traditional randomized experiments or controlled trials with patient populations. However, departments can be in an excellent position to offer enhanced training in new treatment protocols, e.g., in prevention, and then provide evaluation of the impact of that training enhancement on patient/ family services and outcomes.

The advantage of the proposed modules lies in adding to the quality of the training experience by providing managed care perspectives and experience. The format is flexible and is closely modeled on both an evidentiary base and on the kinds of intervention techniques that seem most effective in bridging from traditional training to a managed care perspective. The format represented, relying on scholarship, critical discussion, case examples, and interactions with hands-on experts, represents the process by which we have all developed our professional careers beyond that represented in our own graduate training.

REFERENCES

Cummings, N. A., Pallak, M. S., Dorken, H., & Henke, C. J. (1992). *The Impact of Psychological Services on Medical Utilization.* (HCFA Contract No. 11-C-98344/9 report). Baltimore, MD: Health Care Financing Administration.

Cummings, N.A. & Sayama, M. (1995). *Focused Psychotherapy: A casebook of brief, intermittent psychotherapy throughout the life cycle.* New York: Brunner/Mazel.

Dorken, II. & Pallak, M. S. (1994). Using law, research, professional training and multidisciplinary collaboration to optimize managed care. In Cummings, N. A. & Pallak, M. S. (Eds.), *Managed care quarterly: Behavioral health care.* Frederick, MD: Aspen Publications.

Discussion of Pallak:

Clinical Psychology Curriculum and the Industrialization of Behavioral Healthcare

Jane E. Fisher
Jeffrey Buchanan
Jacob E. Hadden
University of Nevada, Reno

As Pallak cogently argues, change is clearly in order within current clinical psychology training programs if the next generations of clinical psychologists are to be adequately prepared to function within an industrialized health care system. Current curricula tend to focus on the individual as the unit of analysis. Programs essentially train students to be craftspeople in an outdated, cottage industry model of behavioral healthcare delivery. Through coursework and practica students are taught to assess, diagnose, and treat individual clients. Historically, this focus made sense. With the rise of managed care, however, psychologists are confronted with a much larger unit of analysis, namely an organized care system.

The question that emerges for educators is how to expand the focus to larger systems without losing sight of values regarding scientific rigor, ethics, and clinical competence. While the prospect of expanding from an individual to a systems level may at first appear daunting, the task is largely one of applying methods of the methods of clinical science to larger units of analyses. In the section that follows we provide an outline of some of the issues that emerge when one's unit of analysis is a system as opposed to an individual. Clearly our list is not comprehensive. Other skill sets that warrant consideration in this new age of service delivery will include personnel management skills and financial literacy. For the purpose this volume we focus our attention to the modification of clinical science curricula.

An issue that immediately emerges when one moves from an individual to a system of care is *identification of the constituency.* In other words, one must

Fisher, Buchanan, and Hadden

determine whom one is serving, i.e., who is/are the consumer(s). Currently, training programs emphasize an individual, couple, or family as the primary constituent. Accountability is based on the satisfaction of the person or persons who directly receive services. The concern is with achieving certain outcomes for our clients (e.g., symptom reduction), with less concern for the possible cost and/or benefits for other potentially affected parties.

Other parties may be considered consumers, although they are not themselves directly receiving services. For instance, the quality and cost of services delivered may have a large impact on several other agents including family members, employers, and the community at large. In addition to impacting the quality of life of the client directly receiving services, ineffective assessment and treatment programs can greatly impact these agents in terms of money spent on services, lost work days, and fewer resources being available to other individuals in need. A clinical psychologist practicing within an organized behavioral healthcare system must be prepared to first specify all interested parties.

Once the psychologist has identified potential constituents, he/she must next *identify the values of* each of these constituents and the outcomes associated with these values. Because current training emphasizes the individual client as the primary constituent, values tend to center around symptom reduction or behavior change. Therefore, targeted outcomes are consistent with the particular goals of the client (e.g., reduction in depression and anxiety, improved marital relationship, reduced back pain).

Of course, monetary costs to the client and possibly their insurance company are important, but, under the current model of training, clinicians may be better equipped to identify outcomes associated with the value of alleviating psychological distress.

However, as was mention above, in an organized behavioral care system there are a greater number of constituents, each potentially having a different set of values. In response, a different set of outcomes will need to be specified to reflect the values of individual constituents. In the early history of managed care cost containment was the primary goal. More recent trends indicate a shift toward striking a balance between quality care and cost containment. In other words, the focus is now on the value of services. Identifying outcomes in accord with this value is a complex task given our understanding of what are "quality services" along with the wide variety of outcomes associated with cost containment. For instance, possible relevant outcomes could include the cost of assessment/therapy services, cost of training therapists, days missed from work, client satisfaction, symptom reduction for presenting problems, number of return visits following termination, or number of emergency room or hospital visits.

Of course once relevant outcomes have been identified, it will be the responsibility of the Ph.D. level psychologist to operationally define these outcomes so that they can be measured. Current training emphasizes measuring certain indices related to the client's presenting problems, often through the use of empirically validated questionnaires or perhaps psychological tests. Outcomes may also be measured in terms of frequencies, such as increases in more functional behaviors (e.g., increases in job attendance) or decreases in certain symptoms (e.g., reduction in the number of panic attacks).

In the larger system of organized care, with its emphasis on cost containment and quality care, other outcomes warrant consideration. First, measures of relevant symptoms will need to be administered periodically in order to evaluate the effectiveness of a particular treatment program. Current training in scientifically oriented clinical psychology programs provide training in this aspect of measurement. These programs tend to emphasize the use of outcome measures with adequate psychometric properties (i.e., reliability and validity). Service delivery that is data generating as well as date based is emphasized.

An even more important characteristic of assessment instruments is treatment utility, which refers to the degree to which an assessment device or process is shown to contribute to beneficial treatment outcome (Hayes, Nelson, & Jarrett, 1987). If a particular instrument does not have treatment utility, there is no reason to use it because it costs money to administer while providing no useful information concerning treatment planning. It may be particularly important for psychologists in an organized behavioral health-care setting to investigate the treatment utility of certain assessment batteries that may be standard protocol. It may be that these batteries provide little or no useful information beyond that collected during intake interviews. This could potentially save a great deal of money and time by creating a more efficient assessment/triage process. The reader is referred to Hayes et al., (1987) for a more detailed discussion concerning how one may conduct a study to assess treatment utility.

In addition to having well-developed measures of symptoms to detect changes during treatment, measures of client satisfaction and life functioning should be employed. Client satisfaction may include satisfaction of the client, family, employer, or any other concerned party.

A challenge for the psychologist will be to design an assessment process that is psychometrically sound, practical, and user friendly. Although collecting a great deal of information may be desirable, it may not always be practical. Clients may be unwilling to complete lengthy assessment forms on a regular basis, practitioners may be unwilling to spend time administering them, and the administration may be opposed to the cost of such a process. Therefore, psychologists must be sensitive to issues of utility when developing outcome measures that will be administered frequently and with large numbers of individuals within a managed care system. An elegant, psychometrically sound assessment instrument has no utility if it gathers dust in the clinician's desk drawer.

Another challenge faced by clinical psychology training programs is teaching *research methods that are applicable at the systems level.* Currently, many programs provide extensive training in research methodology. However, the typical methods taught in these courses emphasize group design comparison studies (i.e., randomized control trials or efficacy studies). These studies, however, are impractical for an organized behavioral healthcare setting because they require random assignment to groups and often require a control group that either receives no treatment or is put on a waiting list. These studies also usually require a large number of individuals that meet very specific inclusion criteria. Therefore, randomized control trials can be very expensive and it can be difficult to find an adequate number of appropriate subjects.

Due to the limitations of this method, it would seem necessary to train psychologists in alternative research methodologies that may be more suitable for the managed care environment. Two such examples will be discussed. The first is single-case methodology (i.e., interrupted time-series designs). With these designs, only one or a few subjects are needed in order to evaluate the effectiveness of an intervention. These designs have two potential uses in the organized care context. First, because therapists within managed care are being held accountable for therapy outcomes, single case methods provide a means for tracking the progress of individual clients or several clients that suffer from similar conditions. The reader is referred to Hayes, Barlow, and NelsonGray (1998) for a more in-depth discussion of specific methods and how they can applied within in a managed care system.

A second use for single case methods is evaluating the effectiveness of a program at a systems level. In other words, the "subjects" in single case designs do not have to be individual clients, but can be an entire group receiving a particular treatment program or even an entire organized healthcare company. For instance, if a new program for substance abusers has been developed, one way to test its efficacy is to conduct a multiple baseline design across groups or companies. In this type of design, the intervention is first implemented in one group and not the others. Then, once treatment gains seem to be occurring in this first group, the treatment program is implemented in the next group. This process continues until treatment has been implemented in all groups. The advantage of this kind of design is that although treatment is withheld from one or more groups for a period of time, treatment is implemented after a period of time in which the treatment appears to be having the desired effect. In other words, there are no "no-treatment" control groups or "waiting list" control groups in which treatment is withheld for long periods of time. The reader is referred to the work of Anthony Biglan and his associates (Biglan, 1995) who have utilized such designs to evaluate the effectiveness of community-wide smoking prevention programs, using entire communities as subjects.

An alternative type of research methodology that may be more adaptable to the managed care system is field effectiveness research. Effectiveness studies are designed to determine if a particular treatment works in the field, for instance, in a managed care company (Seligman, 1995). Put another way, efficacy studies determine if a treatment works under highly controlled conditions, effectiveness studies determine if a treatment works in actual mental health settings (Strosahl, Hayes, Bergan, & Romano, 1998).

Surveys are one method utilized in effectiveness studies. Seligman (1995) describes a survey study conducted by *Consumer Reports* that assessed client's self reported improvement (or lack thereof) and satisfaction with psychotherapy services. Advantages of this method are that one can collect a large amount of data about client's reactions to psychotherapy as it is conducted in the field with relatively little effort. However, some drawbacks include possible sampling bias and lack of control groups (Seligman, 1995).

Another excellent example of an effectiveness study was conducted by Strosahl and associates (Strosahl, et al., 1998). They performed an effectiveness study within a managed care company in Washington state to evaluate the effectiveness of Acceptance and Commitment Therapy (ACT) utilizing a method called the manipulated training method. Briefly, this method involves dividing a group of clinicians into two groups, those who receive a particular form of training (in this case training in ACT) and those who do not. Prior to training, the two groups are compared on some outcome measure(s), with training then being provided. Finally, the two groups are compared after training using the same outcome measure(s).

Although a certain degree of experimental control is compromised in this type of research, there are advantages such as the use of heterogeneous patient samples, treatment length is not pre-determined, therapists do not have to adhere strictly to treatment manuals, and "usual care" is the comparison condition. Another advantage is that very simple and broad dependent variables can be used (e.g., brief Likert-type scales designed to measure severity of distress), which reduces cost and burden on clients and therapists.

As can be seen, single-case methods and effectiveness studies seem to provide attractive alternatives to the more typical training in randomized clinical trials one receives in most doctoral training programs. Therefore, it appears as if many training programs may need to modify training in research methods to include these other methodologies that are more applicable to a systems level unit of analysis.

References

Biglan, A. (1995). *Changing cultural practices: A contextualist framework for intervention research.* Reno, NV: Context Press.

Hayes, S. C., Barlow, D. H., & Nelson-Grey, R. O. (1998). *The scientistpractitioner: Research and accountability in the age of managed care* (2nd ed.). New York: Allyn and Bacon.

Hayes, S. C., Nelson, R. O., & Jarrett, R. (1987). Treatment utility of assessment: A functional approach to evaluating the quality of assessment. *American Psychologist, 42,* 963-974.

Seligman, M. (1995). The effectiveness of psychotherapy: The Consumer Reports study. *American Psychologist, 50,* 965-974.

Strosahl, K. D., Hayes, S. C., Bergan, J., & Romano, P. (1998). Assessing the field effectiveness of Acceptance and Commitment Therapy: An example of the manipulated training research method. *Behavior Therapy, 29,* 35-64.

Index